OXFORD PROFESSIONAL PRACTICE HANDBOOK OF

Quality Improvement in Healthcare

T0202145

OXFORD PROFESSIONAL PRACTICE HANDBOOK OF

Quality Improvement in Healthcare

EDITED BY

Peter Lachman

Lead Faculty of Quality Improvement, Royal College of
Physicians of Ireland, RCPI, Dublin, Ireland

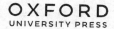

OXFORD
UNIVERSITY PRESS

OXFORD
UNIVERSITY PRESS

Great Clarendon Street, Oxford, OX2 6DP,
United Kingdom

Oxford University Press is a department of the University of Oxford.
It furthers the University's objective of excellence in research, scholarship,
and education by publishing worldwide. Oxford is a registered trade mark of
Oxford University Press in the UK and in certain other countries

Published in the United States of America by Oxford University Press
198 Madison Avenue, New York, NY 10016, United States of America

British Library Cataloguing in Publication Data
Data available

Library of Congress Control Number: 2023946381

ISBN 978–0–19–286638–7

DOI: 10.1093/med/9780192866387.001.0001

Printed in the UK by
Ashford Colour Press Ltd, Gosport, Hampshire

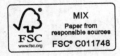

Foreword

This book invites improving the contribution that healthcare service can make to better the health of people. The authors explore the multiple knowledge systems and diverse practices to make desired changes happen. It enables inquiry into quality improvement as an *'object'* that stands alone and as a *'subject'* related to the persons holding the question or needing an answer.

Over the last century, those working to improve quality have been driven by different questions. In the early 1920s, the question that the American College of Surgeons addressed was *'What is a "good" hospital?'*. They defined its characteristics in one page (Roberts, 1987). Fifty years later, the quality gains from enterprise-wide efforts in other economic sectors, such as the automotive industry, led health leaders to ask, *'What enterprise-wide systems might offer optimal service for diseases/conditions?'* (Batalden and Stoltz, 1993; Berwick, 1989). More recently, as this book opens, the driving question seems to have changed again. Now, the question of *'How might we improve the value of the contribution that healthcare service makes to health?'* re-invites curiosity about the nature of co-produced 'service' itself (Batalden et al., 2015).

When *'service-making'* was a new emerging economic force, Victor Fuchs observed that it took two parties, leading others to recognize the phenomenon of co-production (Fuchs, 1968; Gersuny and Rosengren, 1973; Ostrom and Ostrom, 1977). The *science* of healthcare service-making includes the empirical study of how the biology of the underlying condition works, how the experience of having an illness unfolds, and how an intervention might be designed for access, reliability, and 'fit' with the need it addresses (Batalden et al., 2021). The *logic* of healthcare *'service-making'* considers its differences and similarities to *'product-making'* and the ecosystems that enable each. The *architecture* or design of healthcare service-making includes clarity about whose health is being served and of the roles that various actors, contexts, and arrangements make to their health.

The integration of the central themes—thresholds, enterprise-wideness, and co-production—invites curiosity, reflection, and learning. New ways to define, assess, and accredit emerge. New approaches to professional development and pedagogy are invited. New systems of work emerge. New ways to measure are developed. The further development and local application of these will benefit from the shared, collaborative work of people working together.

The book offers practical access to the work of improving the quality of healthcare service. It can be read from beginning to end or by starting anywhere. Read the material, use the references, discuss with a colleague. Historically, collaborative circles helped innovators learn, develop, and apply their thinking (Farrell, 2003). As you make a bridge between ideas in this book and your local application setting, consider a collaborative circle of people with whom you can explore, discuss, and apply what this book opens. Enjoy!

Paul Batalden, MD
Professor Emeritus
The Dartmouth Institute for Health Policy
and Clinical Practice, Hanover, NH, USA

The Jönköping Academy for the Improvement
of Health and Welfare, Jönköping, Sweden

References

Berwick, D.M. (1989). Continuous improvement as an ideal in health care. *New England Journal of Medicine*, 320(1), pp. 53–6. doi: https://doi.org/10.1056/nejm198901053200110.

Batalden, M., Batalden, P., Margolis, P., et al. (2015). Coproduction of healthcare service. *BMJ Quality and Safety*, 25(7), pp. 509–17. doi: https://doi.org/10.1136/bmjqs-2015-004315.

Batalden, P., Ovalle, A., Foster, T., and Elwyn, G. (2021). Science-informed practice: an essential epistemologic contributor to healthcare coproduction. *International Journal for Quality in Health Care*, 33, Supplement_2, pp ii4–ii5. doi: https://doi.org/10.1093/intqhc/mzab054.

Batalden, P.B. and Stoltz, P.K. (1993). A framework for the continual improvement of health care: building and applying professional and improvement knowledge to test changes in daily work. *The Joint Commission Journal on Quality Improvement*, 19(10), pp. 424–47. doi: https://doi.org/10.1016/s1070-3241(16)30025-6.

Farrell, M.P. (2003). *Collaborative Circles: Friendship Dynamics and Creative Work.* Chicago, IL: University Of Chicago Press.

Fuchs, V.R. (1968). *The Service Economy.* New York, NY: National Bureau of Economic Research (distributed By Columbia University Press).

Gersuny, C. and Rosengren, W.R. (1973). *The Service Society.* Cambridge, MA: Schenkman Publishing.

Ostrom, V. and Ostrom, E. (1979). Public goods and public choices. In Savas, E.S. *Alternatives for Delivering Public Services: Toward Improved Performance* (1st ed.), pp 7–50. Routledge, New York. Ebook (2019) https://doi.org/10.4324/9780429047978.

Roberts, J.S. (1987). A history of the Joint Commission on Accreditation of Hospitals. *JAMA*, 258(7), pp. 936–40. doi: https://doi.org/10.1001/jama.258.7.936.

Contents

Contributors

Ahmeda Ali

General Practitioner & Assistant
Scheme Director, Irish College
of General Practitioners. Dublin,
Ireland
Chapter 10: The Lens of Psychology
Chapter 11: How to make change
happen

John Brennan

General Practitioner, Gowran
Medical Centre, Co. Kilkenny,
Ireland
Chapter 4: Implementation Science
and quality improvement
Chapter 14: The Lens of Knowledge:
Methods used in quality improvement

Isabella Castro

Patient Advocate, Rio de Janeiro
Brazil
Chapter 8: Co-producing health and
person-centred care

Edward Corry

Gynaecological Oncology
Consultant UCD Gynaecological
Oncology Group, Mater
Misericordiae University Hospital &
Saint Vincent's University Hospital,
Dublin, Ireland
Chapter 1: Introduction to quality in
healthcare
Chapter 2: Challenges for quality
improvement

David Crosby

Consultant Obstetrician and
Gynaecologist, Subspecialist in
Reproductive Medicine & Surgery
and Reproductive Genetics,
Assistant Clinical Professor, National
Maternity Hospital, Dublin &
University College Dublin, Ireland
Chapter 3: Improvement Science
Chapter 9: Standards in healthcare:
(Quality 1.0)

Eoin Fitzgerald

Paediatric Fellow, Children's Health
Ireland and Temple Street Hospital,
Dublin Ireland.
Chapter 13: The Lens of
Understanding Variation
Chapter 15: Strategies for
measurement

John Fitzsimons

Consultant Paediatrician and
National Clinical Director for
Quality Improvement HSE, Children
Hospital Ireland Temple Street,
Dublin, Ireland
Chapter 12: The Lens of Appreciation
of Systems
Chapter 19: Quality improvement,
research, ethics, and publishing

Eimear Gilhooley

Consultant Dermatologist, The
Mater Misericordiae University
Hospital, Dublin, Ireland
Chapter 6: Sustainable quality
improvement

Bradley Hillier

Consultant Forensic Psychiatrist,
States of Jersey, Channel Islands;
Hon. Consultant Forensic
Psychiatrist, West London NHS
Trust United Kingdom
Chapter 16: Measurement of person-
centred care

Samira Barbara Jabakhanji

Postdoctoral Researcher, Healthcare
Outcomes Research Centre, School
of Population Health, Royal College
of Surgeons of Ireland, RCSI Dublin,
Ireland
Chapter 7: Economics of quality
improvement

Peter Lachman

Lead Faculty of Quality Improvement, Royal College of Physicians of Ireland, RCPI, Dublin, Ireland

Catherine Lynch

Paediatric Registrar, Emergency Department, Children's Health Ireland at Crumlin, Dublin, Ireland

Anne Mahony

Consultant Respiratory Physician, Cork University Hospital, Cork, Ireland

Siobhan McCarthey

Lecturer, Graduate School of Healthcare Management (GSM), Royal College of Surgeons of Ireland, RCSI, Dublin, Ireland

Sinead McGlacken-Byrne

Paediatric Endocrinology and Diabetes SpR, Great Ormond Street Hospital for Children NHS Foundation Trust, London, United Kingdom

Frances Mortimer

Medical Director, Centre for Sustainable Healthcare, Oxford, United Kingdom.

Paula Murphy

Consultant Forensic Psychiatrist, East London NHS Foundation Trust, London United Kingdom

Patricia O'Connor

Honorary Professor, Professor at University of Stirling, Scotland, United Kingdom

Sinead O'Donnell

Consultant/Senior Lecturer in Clinical Microbiology, RCSI and Beaumont Hospital, Dublin, Ireland
Chapter 12: The Lens of Appreciation of Systems

Liam O'Driscoll

Senior Clinical Fellow in Trauma Anaesthesia Addenbrooke's Hospital Cambridge, United Kingdom
Chapter 12: The Lens of Appreciation of Systems

James F. O'Mahony

Assistant Professor at the School of Economics at University College Dublin, Ireland
Chapter 7: Economics of quality improvement

Jane Runnacles

Consultant Paediatrician, St Georges University Hospital NHS Trust, London, United Kingdom
Chapter 17: Application of QI methods: Preparing your QI project
Chapter 18: Application of QI methods: Next steps

Laurentina Schäler

SpR Obstetrics and Gynaecology at Royal College of Physicians of Ireland, RCPI, Dublin Ireland
Chapter 9: Standards in healthcare: (Quality 1.0)

Ulfat Shaikh

Professor of Pediatrics and Medical Director for Healthcare Quality, University of California Davis Health, Sacramento, CA, USA
Chapter 5: Equity and quality improvement

Jan Sorensen

Director of the Healthcare Outcomes Research Centre, Healthcare Outcomes Research Centre, School of Population Health, Royal College of Surgeons of Ireland, RCSI, Dublin, Ireland
Chapter 7: Economics of quality improvement

Victoria Stanford

Quality Improvement Educational Fellow, Centre for Sustainable Healthcare, Oxford, United Kingdom
Chapter 6: Sustainable quality improvement

Lisa Zubkoff

Associate Professor Division of Preventive Medicine, Department of Medicine, University of Alabama at Birmingham, Birmingham, AL, USA
Chapter 4: Implementation Science and quality improvement

Abbreviations

AQLQ	Asthma Quality of Life Questionnaire	IBS	irritable bowel syndrome
ASCO	American Society of Clinical Oncology	ICER	incremental cost-effectiveness ratio
CAMHS	Child and Adolescent Mental Health Services	ICU	intensive care unit
		IHI	Institute for Healthcare Improvement
CBA	cost–benefit analysis	IOM	Institute of Medicine
CE	cost-effectiveness	ISO	International Organization for Standardization
CEA	cost-effectiveness analysis		
CFIR	Consolidated Framework for Implementation Research	IV	intravenous
		LGBTQ+	lesbian, gay, bisexual, and trans+
ChASE	Child and adolescent service experience		
		LHS	learning healthcare system
COPD	chronic obstructive pulmonary disease	LMWH	low-molecular weight heparin
		MFI	Model for Improvement
COVID-19	coronavirus disease 2019	MLHFQ	Minnesota Living with Heart Failure Questionnaire
CQC	Care Quality Commission		
CT	computed tomography	MSQLI	Multiple Sclerosis Quality of Life Inventory
CUA	cost utility analysis		
CVC	central venous catheter	NCI	National Cancer Institute
DMAIC	Define, Measure, Analyse, Improve, and Control	NHS	National Health Service
		NICE	National Institute for Health and Care Excellence
DoH	Department of Health		
EBCD	experience-based co-design	NICU	neonatal intensive care unit
ED	emergency department	PARIHS	Promoting Action on Research Implementation in Health Services Framework
EHR	electronic health record		
ENABLE	Educate, Nurture, Advise, Before Life Ends		
		PCC	person-centred care
ERIC	Expert Recommendations for Implementing Change	PDSA	Plan–Do–Study–Act
		PEQ-ITSD	Patient Experience Questionnaire for Interdisciplinary Treatment for Substance Dependence
ESO	European Stroke Organisation		
EU	European Union		
GDPR	General Data Protection Regulation		
		PFA	patient and family association
GHG	greenhouse gas	PICC	peripherally inserted central catheter
GIRFT	Getting it Right First Time		
HADS	Hospital Anxiety and Depression Scale	PIPEQ-OS	Psychiatric Inpatient Patient Experience Questionnaire—On Site
HCAHPS	Hospital Consumer Assessment of Healthcare Providers and Systems		
		PMDI	pressurized metered-dose inhaler
		PMOS	patient-reported measure of safety
HCRW	healthcare risk waste		
HFE	human factors and ergonomics	PPE	personal protective equipment
HIW	Healthcare Inspectorate Wales	PREM	patient-reported experience measure
HRQL	health-related quality of life		
HSE	Health Service Executive		

PRO	patient-reported (health) outcome	SHO	senior house officer
PROM	patient-reported outcome measure	SMART	Specific, Measurable, Achievable, Relevant, Time-bound
PROQUOLID	Patient-Reported Outcome and Quality of Life Database	SOPK	System of Profound Knowledge
PTSD	post-traumatic stress disorder	SPC	statistical process control
QALY	quality-adjusted life year	SPO	structure–process–outcome (model)
QI	quality improvement		
QoL	quality of life	SQUIRE	Standards for QUality Improvement Reporting Excellence 2.0
RCPI	Royal College of Physicians of Ireland		
RE	resilience engineering	SusQI	Sustainability in Quality Improvement
RE-AIM	Reach, Efficacy, Adoption, Implementation, and Maintenance	TA	technical assistance
		TOC	Theory of Constraints
RQIA	Regulation and Quality Improvement Authority	TQM	total quality management
		VLC	virtual learning collaborative
SD	standard deviation	VRE	video-reflexive ethnography
SDH	social determinant of health	VTE	venous thromboembolism
SDM	shared decision-making	WHO	World Health Organization
SEIPS	Systems Engineering Initiative for Patient Safety		

Introduction to quality in healthcare

Key points
- Healthcare has variable and inconsistent quality outcomes.
- The quality improvement movement aims to improve quality in seven cross-cutting domains.
- The approach to achieving quality has three phases:
  - Setting standards for care delivery;
  - Introduction of improvement science and systems thinking;
  - Co-production of health.
- Quality improvement must develop a sound evidence base to demonstrate its efficacy.
- Policies can facilitate and promote quality improvement.
- Leadership for quality at every level is essential to achieve quality.

The rationale for quality improvement

'Heal thyself or heal thy system.'

Donald M. Berwick, 1992

This book aims to provide the improver with the *nuts and bolts* about how to improve the quality of care where one works. The reason we need a book on quality in healthcare is the significant variation in the quality of care delivered to patients.

Over the past 100 years, the life expectancy of people has increased in every country in the world, as shown in Figure 1.1.

- Most of the improvement is related to improved housing, nutrition, sanitation, clean water, etc..
- Advances in medical science have provided cures for infectious diseases, cancer, and many genetic disorders.
- As a result of this success, there are new challenges in managing people with long-term conditions, as well as an elderly population with many comorbidities.
- To address this challenge, healthcare has been 'industrialized', broken down into component parts, and often delivered in silos.
- Modern healthcare is hospital-focused, as most people with chronic conditions can be treated in the community.
- The experience of care received by people has been variable.

The quality improvement (QI) movement in healthcare has become significant over the past 20 years, following the landmark reports on the quality and safety of care delivered, as well as the experience of people receiving care (Table 1.1).

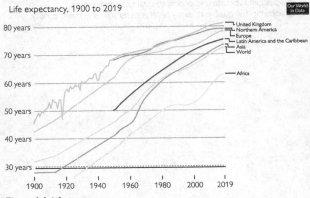

Figure 1.1 Life expectancy.

Max Roser, Esteban Ortiz-Ospina and Hannah Ritchie (2013)—'Li fe Expectancy'. Published online at OurWorldInData.org. Retrieved from: 🔗 'https://ourworldindata.org/life-expectancy' [Online Resource] Updated 2022.

Table 1.1 Key reports on quality and safety of care

Report	Main findings and recommendations
United Kingdom *An organization with a memory* (Department of Health, 2000)	Quality and safety are variable in the NHS. Four steps are recommended: • Improved reporting • An open culture • Mechanisms to learn and improve • A systems approach for solutions
United States *To Err is Human: Building a Safer Health System* (Kohn et al., 2000)	Safety is a major challenge in healthcare; for example, over 100.000 lives lost yearly in the United States due to adverse events. • Standards for safe care to be developed • A move from studying errors to improvement and safety • Improved reporting and a culture of safety • Design for safety with standardized processes • Not to rely on memory or vigilance • Developing safe teams and involving patients and families (see ⊃ Chapter 2)
United States *Crossing the Quality Chasm: A New Health System for the 21st Century* (Institute of Medicine, 2001)	Assessed the quality of healthcare and recommended action across six domains (see ⊃ p. 16) Provided a roadmap for improvement Patients need to be in control of their health
Global *Crossing the Global Quality Chasm: Improving Health Care Worldwide* (National Academies of Sciences, Engineering, and Medicine, 2018)	The quality of healthcare in lower- and middle-income countries is variable. Up to eight million lives are lost each year due to poor quality of selected conditions. Recommendations included taking a systems approach to solutions, developing universal health coverage, empowering patients as partners in their care, using digital solutions, and ensuring that quality improvement is embedded in daily work
Global *High-quality health systems in the sustainable development goals era: time for a revolution* (Kruk et al., 2018)	The care that people receive is inadequate and of poor quality. The most vulnerable receive the worst-quality care Recommendations to build highly effective systems based on the foundation of governance, good platforms of care, skilled workforce accountability, and tools and resources for improvement to develop competent learning systems
Global *Handbook for National Quality Policy and Strategy* (World Health Organization, 2018)	Provides a template for policy development for high-quality health systems (see ⊃ p. 24)

NHS, National Health Service.

- People receiving care are now more focused on the quality of care they receive, concurrent with the spread of access to medical knowledge on the internet.
- During the coronavirus disease 2019 (COVID-19) pandemic, the inequity of delivery of care has been made apparent, with quality and safety of care being compromised.

What is the quality problem?

Many would contend that a lack of resources is the underlying reason for poor quality of care. Although this can be the case, there are many other reasons for care to be of poor quality. These can be related to:

- The way care is organized;
- The culture of the team or organization regarding quality and safety;
- How resources are used to deliver quality in care;
- Unwarranted variation in processes of care delivery;
- Knowledge about processes and outcomes;
- Lack of data to assess how well one is performing;
- Lack of expertise in quality and patient safety theories and methods.

How can we improve care?

The delivery of high-quality care is an aim of clinicians, nurses, and all healthcare workers. To achieve high-quality care, we must acknowledge that:

- Healthcare is dynamic within a complex environment;
- Healthcare is in constant evolution, which presents a challenge to all who deliver care;
- Healthcare systems are made up of people who have differing beliefs and attitudes;
- Knowledge and skills on how to improve are not universally known by providers of care;
- Learning how to improve is often difficult to achieve within the complexity of healthcare;
- We can learn from each other and from experience in other industries such as aviation and manufacturing.

Closing the knowledge gap

To close the knowledge gap, we will:

- Explain the theories of QI;
- Provide methods for clinicians on the front line to assess the quality of care provided;
- Discuss ways to improve care when indicated;
- Ignite curiosity and desire to continually explore how to improve and develop the services;
- Demonstrate how people who receive care can have great outcomes and experience in which they feel valued at every point of care.

Further reading

Kiney, M.-P., Evans, T.G., Scarpetta, S., et al. (2018). Delivering quality health services: a global imperative for universal health coverage. Washington, DC: World Bank Group.

References

Department of Health (2000). *An organisation with a memory. Report of an expert group on learning from adverse events in the NHS*. London: The Stationery Office.

Institute of Medicine; Committee on Quality of Health Care in America; Kohn LT, Corrigan JM, Donaldson MS, eds. (2000). *To Err is Human: Building a Safer Health System*. Washington, DC: The National Academies Press.

Institute of Medicine; Committee on Quality of Health Care in America (2001). *Crossing the Quality Chasm: A New Health System for the 21st Century*. Washington, DC: The National Academies Press.

Kruk, M.E., Gage, A.D., Arsenault, C., et al. (2018). High-quality health systems in the sustainable development goals era: time for a revolution. *The Lancet Global Health*, 6(11), pp. e1196–252.

National Academies of Sciences, Engineering, and Medicine (2018). *Crossing the Global Quality Chasm: Improving Health Care Worldwide*. Washington, DC: The National Academies Press.

World Health Organization (2018). *Handbook for national quality policy and strategy: a practical approach for developing policy and strategy to improve quality of care*. Geneva: World Health Organization. Available at: ℘ https://www.who.int/publications/i/item/9789241565561 (accessed 10 September 2023).

Development of quality in healthcare

How do we define quality?

The Institute of Medicine (IOM) defined six domains of quality, which identified the challenges faced by people receiving care.

- The domains of healthcare provide a framework to evaluate, assess, and deliver optimal healthcare.
- Patient-centred care has evolved into person-centred care (PCC).
- With the growing challenge of climate change, a domain to address this has been added (i.e. eco-friendly care).
- The interdependent domains are listed in Table 1.2.

Table 1.2 Domains of quality

Safety	Care where people are not harmed
Effectiveness	Evidence-based care
Timeliness	Care where people are not kept waiting
Efficiency	Care process which eliminates waste
Person-centredness	Care which focuses on what matters to people
Equity	Care which ensures everyone has an equal chance of quality care
Eco-friendliness	Care which focuses on climate change and is carbon-neutral

With the development of the quality movement, it has become clear that, to ensure improvement, one needs more than technical skills. The multidimensional QI model includes core values that underpin improvement in care (Figure 1.2). These values are:

- Being kind with compassion to develop a culture of psychological well-being;
- Respect for all in the system, both in receiving or delivering care;
- Integrating care to provide a holistic experience;
- Co-producing solutions with both healthcare personnel and patients and their families.

A quality system is supported by transparency, leadership, and resilience. In recognition that all care must be person-centred, the person-centred domain surrounds all the other domains and includes the wider community or kin that is part of the patient as a person (Lachman et al., 2021).

All improvement projects will have elements of each domain, though one domain may be dominant for that project. For example, a project to decrease waiting times will be mainly about efficiency, but also will include person-centredness, safety, and eco-friendliness.

In subsequent chapters, the domains of quality will be discussed in greater detail.

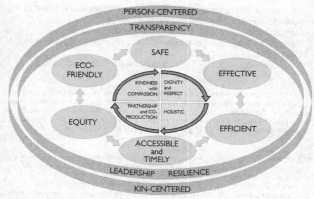

Figure 1.2 Multidimensional model of quality.

Lachman, P., Batalden, P., & Vanhaecht, K. (2020). A multidimensional quality model: an opportunity for patients, their kin, healthcare providers and professionals to coproduce health. *F1000Research*, 9, 1140. https://doi.org/10.12688/f1000research.26368.3.

The quality journey

Over the past century, the quality movement in healthcare passed through two main approaches to improvement and is now entering the third. These approaches are interdependent and are all required to deliver good care through three types of quality (Table 1.3).

Table 1.3 The quality journey

Approach	Description
Quality 1.0 (see ⟳ Chapter 9)	• Standardization and measuring performance against set standards • Involves regulation, certification, and accreditation
Quality 2.0 (see ⟳ Chapters 3, 10, 12, 13, and 14)	• Takes a systems approach and aims to improve defects in processes, so as to improve outcomes • Has been the dominant approach over the past 30 years, with lessons taken from other industries • The theories of Shewhart, Deming, and Juran inspired clinicians like Paul Batalden and Donald Berwick to introduce methods from the science of improvement to healthcare
Quality 3.0 (see Chapter 8)	• Co-production of health, as opposed to management of disease, is the latest phase of quality improvement • Aims to improve the value of healthcare service to deliver health • People as patients or providers of healthcare co-produce the desired outcomes based on their lived experiences • Involves sharing of power or agency

Adapted from Lachman *et al.*, 2021; Batalden, and Foster, 2021.

It is important to recognize that each approach adds value and that all are required to develop a high-quality system.
- Standards in Quality 1.0 are an essential foundation to QI.
- Many of the subsequent chapters will focus on improving systems as in Quality 2.0.
- Co-production in Quality 3.0 is an essential part of the solution.

Further reading

Institute of Medicine; Committee on Quality of Health Care in America (2001). *Crossing the Quality Chasm: A New Health System for the 21st Century*. Washington, DC: The National Academies Press.

Vanhaecht, K., De Ridder, D., Seys, D., *et al.* (2021). The history of quality: from an eye for an eye, through love, and towards a multidimensional concept for patients, kin, and professionals. *European Urology Focus*, 7(5), pp. 937–9. doi: 10.1016/j.euf.2021.09.001.

References

Batalden, P. and Foster, T. (2021). From assurance to coproduction: a century of improving the quality of health-care service. *International Journal for Quality in Health Care*, 33(Supplement 2), pp. ii10–ii14. doi: 10.1093/intqhc/mzab059.

Lachman, P., Batalden, P., and Vanhaecht, K. (2021). A multidimensional quality model: an opportunity for patients, their kin, healthcare providers and professionals to coproduce health. *F1000Research*, 9, p. 1140. doi: 10.12688/f1000research.26368.2.

The Quintuple Aim

The focus in healthcare improvement has often been on efficiency (e.g. decreasing waiting times, increasing throughput of patients). The concept of the Triple Aim addresses this approach by aligning three distinct goals of healthcare delivery (Berwick et al., 2008):

- Improving the experience of care for those who receive it, placing PCC at the core of all we do;
- Improving the health of populations;
- Reducing per capita costs of healthcare.

Two further aims have been added to transform the Triple Aim into the Quintuple Aim (Figure 1.3):

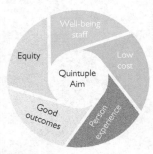

Figure 1.3 The Quintuple Aim.

- Care for healthcare workers, including psychological safety, to ensure that person-centred, safe, and effective care can be provided (Bodenheimer and Sinsky, 2014);
- Delivery of equitable care and programmes to deal with inequity in care design and delivery (Nundy et al., 2022).

The purpose of the five aims is to keep the focus of improvement on the person rather than on the process.

- It is essential that healthcare focuses also on population health, and not only on management of disease.
- Person experience is fundamental to the quality of care.
- Quality needs to be achieved within a defined budget. The aim of reducing per capita cost of care is probably the most controversial, given the often-held view that healthcare is underfunded (see ➲ Chapter 7). This aim focuses on decreasing waste within the system, so that more value is obtained.
- The aim of well-being of clinicians and healthcare workers has been added in recognition of the importance of protecting the well-being of all who work in healthcare (see ➲ Chapter 10)
- The aim of equity is in response to the inequity in care delivery and worse outcomes for disadvantaged groups in society (see ➲ Chapter 5).

The Quintuple Aim calls for good data, clear outcomes, and an understanding of how systems work from primary to secondary to tertiary care. In the following chapters, we will address each of these aims. In addition, addressing climate change (i.e. sustainable healthcare) will be a sixth aim.

Further reading

Bachynsky, N. (2020). Implications for policy: the Triple Aim, Quadruple Aim, and interprofessional collaboration. *Nursing Forum*, 55(1), pp. 54–64. doi: 10.1111/nuf.12382.

Itchhaporia, D. (2021). The evolution of the Quintuple Aim. *Journal of the American College of Cardiology*, 78(22), pp. 2262–4. doi: 10.1016/j.jacc.2021.10.018.

Sikka, R., Morath, J.M., and Leape, L. (2015). The Quadruple Aim: care, health, cost and meaning in work. *BMJ Quality and Safety*, 24(10), pp. 608–10. doi: 10.1136/bmjqs-2015-004160.

References

Berwick, D.M., Nolan, T.W., and Whittington, J. (2008). The triple aim: care, health, and cost. *Health Affairs (Millwood)*, 27(3), pp. 759–69. doi: 10.1377/hlthaff.27.3.759.

Bodenheimer, T. and Sinsky, C. (2014). From Triple to Quadruple Aim: care of the patient requires care of the provider. *Annals of Family Medicine*, 12(6), pp. 573–6. doi: 10.1370/afm.1713.

Nundy, S., Cooper, L.A., and Mate, K.S. (2022). The Quintuple Aim for health care improvement. *JAMA*, 327(6), pp. 521–2. doi: 10.1001/jama.2021.25181.

Efficacy of quality improvement

What is the quality improvement credibility challenge?

As one starts the QI journey, a word of caution—the evolution of QI also recognizes that, like any science within healthcare, it is not immune to criticism.

- Some of the criticisms have highlighted the need for scientific rigour to be applied to QI, as in other domains of healthcare.
- These criticisms highlight the potential of ill-advised and poorly thought-through QI projects consuming scarce resources without delivering for patients or healthcare workers (Dixon-Woods, 2019).
- Reviews of the rigour in application of QI methodologies in published QI reports have shown that there is a wide variation in the quality and rigour of application of the methods (McNicholas et al., 2019; Reed and Card, 2016).
- A systematic review of QI projects utilizing the Plan–Do–Study–Act cycle found that, while all studies claimed success in delivering improvement, only approximately 25% used defined quantitative measures (Knudsen et al., 2019).
- This failure of many studies to apply methodological rigour to QI projects impinges on the credibility of the science of QI and emphasizes the obligation of those involved in QI to understand the science behind QI.

What is the QI credibility solution?

- In healthcare, evidence-based medicine is the foundation of the care we deliver.
- Quality must demonstrate its effectiveness by using improvement and implementation science methodology in a rigorous way to build the evidence base for QI.
- QI methods should be applied in a detailed, measurable, and replicable manner, while taking into account the impact of the context.
- This can ensure there is fidelity between intervention and outcome.

Further reading

Chassin, M.R. and Loeb, J.M. (2011). The ongoing quality improvement journey: next stop, high reliability. Health Affairs, 30(4), pp. 559–68. doi: 10.1377/hlthaff.2011.0076.

Dixon-Woods, M. and Martin, G.P. (2016). Does quality improvement improve quality? Future Hospital Journal, 3(3). pp. 191–4. doi: 10.7861/futurehosp.3-3-191.

References

Dixon-Woods, M. (2019). How to improve healthcare improvement—an essay by Mary Dixon-Woods. BMJ, p. l5514. doi: 10.1136/bmj.l5514.

Knudsen, S.V., Laursen, H.V.B., Johnsen, S.P., Bartels, P.D., Ehlers, L.H., and Mainz, J. (2019). Can quality improvement improve the quality of care? A systematic review of reported effects and methodological rigor in plan–do–study–act projects. BMC Health Services Research, 19(1), p. 683. doi: 10.1186/s12913-019-4482-6.

McNicholas, C., Lennox, L., Woodcock, T., Bell, D., and Reed, J.E. (2019). Evolving quality improvement support strategies to improve Plan–Do–Study–Act cycle fidelity: a retrospective mixed-methods study. BMJ Quality and Safety, 28(5), pp. 356–65. doi: 10.1136/bmjqs-2017-007605.

Reed, J.E. and Card, A.J. (2016). The problem with Plan–Do–Study–Act cycles. BMJ Quality and Safety, 25(3), pp.147–52. doi: 10.1136/bmjqs-2015-005076.

Policies to support quality in healthcare

Policies to support quality in healthcare

What is required for policies to improve quality?

The development of policies to facilitate quality in healthcare is an important step in a quality management system, be it at national, organization, or team level. The tools of QI cannot deliver improvements in patient care in a vacuum. Leaders and policymakers need to facilitate QI.

To have a successful transition from policy to implementation, the World Health Organization (WHO) has recommended eight key steps in developing a strategy for QI. This can be adapted to every level in the system, from national to the frontline team (Figure 1.4).

National health priorities

Local definition of quality

Stakeholder mapping and engagement

Situational analysis

Governance and organizational structure

Improvement methods and interventions

Health management information systems and data systems

Quality indicators and core measures

Figure 1.4 Eight interdependent elements of the National Quality Policy and Strategy approach.
Published with permission of World Health Organisation.

The steps to take in developing a policy include the following principles:
- To develop a strategy for quality with set standards;
- Systems thinking is required to drive the redesign of healthcare;
- This will require an understanding and application of the principles of human factors and systems design;
- The skills of QI need to be combined with an understanding of the importance of culture and leadership in the workplace;
- To allow local contextualization of quality with definitions that are in keeping with national policy and standards. This will encourage local ownership of the policy;
- To develop strategies to engage with stakeholders in the community and the workforce and with patients;
- To accept there will be variations in quality and to undertake situation analyses so that these can be determined;
- To ensure there are strong governance and accountability processes in the quality programme;
- To use improvement and implementation science as the foundation for methods to improve quality of care;
- Implementation needs to be built on strong data systems, so that all change is data-driven.

The challenge in translating policy to action

For the frontline doctor or nurse or other health professional, day-to-day activities can seem divorced from the policies set at national and governmental levels.

To have a successful policy, this disconnect can be overcome with effective leadership for quality. Policies need to empower health workers and patients to co-design and continually evolve their own work environment.

Further reading

World Health Organization (2018). *Handbook for national quality policy and strategy: a practical approach for developing policy and strategy to improve quality of care.* Geneva: World Health Organization. Available at: ℘ https://www.who.int/publications/i/item/9789241565561 (accessed 10 September 2023).

World Health Organization (2020). *Quality of care in fragile, conflict-affected and vulnerable settings: taking action.* Geneva: World Health Organization. Available at: ℘ https://www.who.int/publications/i/item/9789240015203 (accessed 10 September 2023).

World Health Organization (2020). *Quality health services: a planning guide.* Geneva: World Health Organization. Available at: ℘ https://www.who.int/publications/i/item/9789240011632 (accessed 10 September 2023).

Leadership for quality improvement

The leadership challenge for quality

The ability of frontline clinicians and other healthcare workers to undertake QI initiatives requires support from the leadership of the team or organization.

- A learning health system allows the flow of ideas and solutions throughout an organization.
- Leaders have a critical role in developing a culture that empowers all members of the organization to continually improve care.
- The positive impact of QI in organizations in the delivery of care can only become secure when it is embedded in the culture of the organization.
- Leaders need to show hope, courage, respect, and humility, as they create the time and space for improvement (Lachman and Nicklin, 2017).

Bevan and Henriks (2021a, b, c, d, e) have proposed seven leadership activities and rules to foster a learning system:

- Creating a *common purpose* for the organization or clinical team (see the microsystem theory in ⊃ Chapters 12 and 17). This implies that there is a vision to which all subscribe (e.g. Zero Harm is one set by the WHO as an aspiration for safety programmes);
- Enhancing a *sense of belonging*—this provides team members the support and psychological safety to challenge and develop;
- Using data to allow *prediction and anticipation* of future performance, so as to encourage improvement;
- Developing *agency*, which empowers people to make decisions and be in control (see ⊃ Chapter 10);
- Promoting a culture of *continual improvement*, so that all place improvement at the core of their work;
- Accepting the inherent *contradictions* and tensions as part of improvement work and encouraging ways to address these issues;
- Creating a *culture of learning* in the team and wider organization, so that curiosity is central to all work undertaken.

QI has the potential to empower staff. It provides a platform for healthcare staff to contribute their ideas, insights, and critical eye through QI projects. Leadership for quality needs to place QI at the forefront of all activities.

Further reading

Drew, J.R. and Pandit, M. (2020). Why healthcare leadership should embrace quality improvement. *BMJ*, 368, p. m872. doi: 10.1136/bmj.m872.

References

Bevan, H. and Henriks, G. (2021a). Creating tomorrow today: seven simple rules for leaders Blog one. *BMJ Leader*, 1 February 2021. Available at: ℘ https://blogs.bmj.com/bmjleader/2021/02/01/creating-tomorrow-today-seven-simple-rules-for-leaders-by-helen-bevan-and-goran-henriks/ (accessed 10 September 2023).

Bevan, H. and Henriks, G. (2021b). Creating tomorrow today: seven simple rules for leaders. Blog two: Define our shared purpose. *BMJ Leader*, 16 February 2021. Available at: ℘ https://blogs.bmj.com/bmjleader/2021/02/16/creating-tomorrow-today-seven-simple-rules-for-leaders-blog-two-define-our-shared-purpose-by-helen-bevan-and-goran-henriks/ (accessed 10 September 2023).

Bevan, H. and Henriks, G. (2021c). Creating tomorrow today: seven simple rules for leaders. Blog 3: Root our transformation efforts in a sense of belonging. *BMJ Leader*, 24 March 2021. Available at: ℰ https://blogs.bmj.com/bmjleader/2021/03/24/creating-tomorrow-today-seven-simple-rules-for-leaders-blog-three-root-our-transformation-efforts-in-a-sense-of-belonging-by-helen-bevan-and-goran-henriks/ (accessed 10 September 2023).

Bevan, H. and Henriks, G. (2021d). Creating tomorrow today: seven simple rules for leaders. Blog 4: Predict and prevent: start at an earlier stage ('upstream') in the intervention or care processes. *BMJ Leader*, 24 December 2021. Available at: ℰ https://blogs.bmj.com/bmjleader/2021/12/24/creating-tomorrow-today-seven-simple-rules-for-leaders-blog-four-predict-and-prevent-start-at-an-earlier-stage-upstream-in-the-intervention-or-care-processes-by-helen-bevan/ (accessed 10 September 2023).

Bevan, H. and Henriks G. (2021e). Creating tomorrow today: seven simple rules for leaders. Blog five: Support people to build their agency at every level of the system. *BMJ Leader*, 16 June 2022. Available at: ℰ https://blogs.bmj.com/bmjleader/2022/06/16/creating-tomorrow-today-seven-simple-rules-for-leaders-blog-four-support-people-to-build-their-agency-at-every-level-of-the-system-by-helen-bevan-and-goran-henriks/ (accessed 10 September 2023).

Lachman, P. and Nicklin, W. (2017). Effectively leading for quality. *Healthcare Management Forum*, 30(5), pp. 233–6. doi: 10.1177/0840470417706705.

Top tips

- QI is defined in terms of seven domains.
- Person- or kin-centred care is within every domain of quality.
- Core values are respect, kindness, integrated care, and co-production.
- The response to the challenge of quality has been in three stages: setting standards; taking a systems approach to improvement; and co-production of solutions.
- Policies and leadership are required to support change.
- The Quintuple Aim brings together the key elements of improvement.
- The evidence base for QI is being developed.
- QI theory and methodology need to be integrated into the training of all clinicians.
- Leadership is an essential enabler for improvement.

Summary

Quality in healthcare is an essential part of what we do every day. However, we cannot assume that quality will happen without interventions that will ensure we have safe and effective processes of care.

In subsequent chapters, you will learn about:
- Theories underpinning improvement and implementation science;
- The challenges for healthcare:
  - Managing unwarranted variation
  - The importance of equity and sustainable healthcare
  - Co-production of health with people who receive care
  - The need to train for QI
- The economic cost and benefits of improvement programmes;
- The need for standards as the first step on the improvement journey;
- Engagement of people to improve and sustain improvement;
- The value of a systems approach to improvement;
- Ways to measure and decrease variation and how to develop a measurement strategy;
- Methods used in improvement, with examples of projects;
- Ethical issues to consider when undertaking an improvement project.

Challenges
for quality improvement

> **Key points**
>
> Quality improvement has concentrated on addressing the defects in systems and processes. The key focus in the future will be on the following challenges:
> - *Equity*: using quality improvement methodology to address inequity in healthcare delivery and outcomes;
> - *Safety*: addressing the complexity of safe care;
> - *Climate change*: making sustainable healthcare a priority, as healthcare is a major consumer of energy and producer of waste, with a negative impact on the environment;
> - *Variation*: addressing the problem of unwarranted variation;
> - *Person-centred care*: enhancing shared planning, decision-making, and co-production;
> - *Integration*: decreasing care delivered in silos and integrating needs around people receiving care;
> - *Training*: ensuring the healthcare workforce is skilled in the theories and methods of improvement.

Introduction

The past 20 years have seen rapid changes in the way we think about healthcare. In this chapter, we highlight the challenges on which quality improvement (QI) will need to focus in the coming years, moving from solving defects in the system to co-designing healthcare systems that meet all the domains of quality (Figure 2.1).

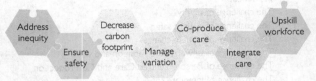

Figure 2.1 Challenges for modern quality improvement.

Each of these challenges will be discussed in subsequent chapters. The intention is to provide a brief overview of the challenges and provide a focus on what needs to be done.

In any QI project, we need to ask the following questions:

- Will the QI project close the equity gap?
- Will the project enhance patient and healthcare worker safety?
- Is the project decreasing unwarranted variation?
- What will the impact be on sustainable healthcare?
- Is the project co-produced with people delivering and receiving care?
- Will person-centred care be enhanced?
- Will the processes of care delivery be integrated as a result of the project?
- What will be the economic benefit of the project—is it cost effective?
- Do we have the skills to undertake the project?
- Do we have the leadership for QI?

An improvement project can therefore have multiple aims, which need to be managed. Innovation and change programmes and projects should define and deliver the parallel aims, as well as manage potential conflicts between them (Amalberti et al., 2022).

The solutions to the questions are all discussed in greater detail in subsequent chapters or in the *Oxford Professional Practice: Handbook of Patient Safety* and *Handbook of Medical Leadership and Management* companion books.

Reference

Amalberti, R., Staines, A., and Vincent, C. (2022). Embracing multiple aims in healthcare improvement and innovation. *International Journal for Quality in Health Care*, 34(1), p. mzac006. doi: 10.1093/intqhc/mzac006.

The challenge of equity

(See → Chapter 5.)

Why is equity important?

The social determinants of health (SDHs) have been studied in depth and play a major part in the outcomes that result from any intervention in healthcare. Most countries have an inequity challenge. For example, in England, despite equal access to care, the way the National Health Service (NHS) has been organized has resulted in structural issues leading to in-equitable care and outcomes (Box 2.1).

Box 2.1 Inequity in the NHS

A report by the UK NHS Race and Health Observatory concluded that:

'Ethnic inequalities in access to, experiences of, and outcomes of healthcare are longstanding problems in the NHS, and are rooted in experiences of structural, institutional and interpersonal racism.

For too many years, the health of ethnic minority people has been negatively impacted by:

- *lack of appropriate treatment for health problems by the NHS;*
- *poor quality or discriminatory treatment from healthcare staff;*
- *a lack of high quality ethnic monitoring data recorded in NHS systems;*
- *lack of appropriate interpreting services for people who do not speak English confidently;*
- *and delays in, or avoidance of, seeking help for health problems due to fear of racist treatment from NHS healthcare professionals.'*

Kapadia, D., Zhang, J., Salway, S., Nazroo, J., Booth, A., Villarroel-Williams, N., Bécares, L., and Esmail, A. (2022). *Ethnic Inequalities in Healthcare: A Rapid Evidence Review*. [online]. Available at: ℘ https://www.nhsrho.org/wp-content/uploads/2022/02/RHO-Rapid-Review-Final-Report_v.7.pdf. (Accessed 10 September 2023)

This analysis is not unique to one country, and wherever one is, one should question whether the care delivered and the outcomes achieved are equitable. Inequity not only impacts people from different ethnic backgrounds, but it can also be the result of age, poverty, where one lives, sexuality, learning difficulty, and other disabilities. In essence, inequity affects anyone who is not from the mainstream of society.

Therefore, QI programmes should consider how the projects may impact equity of service delivery and outcomes achieved. In addition, QI can be used specifically to decrease or eliminate the equity gap.

How can QI improve equity?

QI is not the panacea to the economic and structural inequalities that act as key determinants of health outcomes. Nonetheless, the delivery of high-quality healthcare consistently to all, with a focus on decreasing inequity, can make a difference. As shown in the case study in Box 2.2, QI and its implementation at a clinical organizational level can standardize care for all and can make a difference by ensuring that the inequities in care delivery are addressed as part of the QI programme.

Box 2.2 Case study on equity

Sarah has just started her registrar job at a gynaecological oncology service. The team have just readmitted a patient with a venous thromboembolism (VTE) 2 weeks following the latter's major pelvic surgery. Sarah learnt in her previous, more junior role in an oncology service that patients post-major pelvic cancer surgery are discharged on 4–6 weeks of prophylactic low-molecular weight heparin (LMWH).

However, when she asks the patient, she finds out that the latter had not received any instructions on discharge about taking LMWH. In addition, she did not understand what she needed to do on discharge. She had no support at home.

Sarah discovers that the service used to have an advanced nurse practitioner who discussed the risk of VTE with patients and educated them on injecting LMWH. Unfortunately, due to recent cuts to funding, the role had been terminated.

Being curious, Sarah wondered whether this complication affected disadvantaged people more and decided to look at the data. She discovered that people from different backgrounds had different outcomes, and she decided to start a QI project to close the gap.

In → Chapter 5, the challenge of equity is discussed in detail.

Signposting

Institute of Health Equity. Available at: ⅏ https://www.instituteofhealthequity.org (accessed 10 September 2023).

NHS England. *The equality and health inequalities hub.* Available at: ⅏ https://www.england.nhs.uk/about/equality/equality-hub/ (accessed 10 September 2023)

Public Health Scotland. *What are health inequalities?* Available at: ⅏ https://www.healthscotland.scot/health-inequalities/what-are-health-inequalities (accessed 10 September 2023)

World Health Organization. *Social determinants of health.* Available at: ⅏ https://www.who.int/health-topics/social-determinants-of-health#tab=tab_1 (accessed 10 September 2023).

Further reading

World Health Organization (2021). *COVID-19 and the social determinants of health and health equity: evidence brief.* Geneva: World Health Organization.

The challenge of patient safety

Patient safety is a cross-cutting domain of quality, as all services provided must be safe; for example, if a service aims to be highly efficient, safety cannot be compromised. The World Health Organization (WHO) has prioritized patient safety and provided an action plan to be implemented (World Health Organization, 2021). QI methodology is essential for testing new ideas and implementing solutions for patient safety.

Why is patient safety important?

Safe clinical care is the foundation of healthcare. Safe care is a fundamental right of people receiving healthcare. There is a moral and ethical responsibility to develop a system of care delivery that minimizes risk and protects people from harm.

- Healthcare is delivered in a complex system, and the risk of harm and adverse events will always be present.
- It is estimated that up to 15% of people receiving care will experience unsafe care and may be harmed (Panagioti et al., 2019).
- Many of the challenges healthcare systems face concern the safety of people receiving care and the safety of healthcare staff as they deliver care.
- The report by a team led by Don Berwick following the Mid Staffordshire inquiry highlighted the importance of applying improvement methods to develop safe care (Berwick, 2013).
- Implementation of patient safety theories and methods can make a difference to health outcomes.

How can QI improve safety?

The theories of patient safety and the methods used to ensure safe care align with the theories and methodologies of Improvement Science. In this book, many of the examples will show how one can use Improvement Science to improve the safety of the people receiving care and those providing care.

- Safety requires standards which set the process that is required to be safe (see ⊃ Chapter 9).
- Safety requires a culture that engenders teamworking and ensures people feel safe. This is essential in improvement of care (see ⊃ Chapter 10).
- Safety requires an understanding of how systems work and how the people within those systems interact with one another, the environment, and the tools and technologies they need to achieve their outcome (see ⊃ Chapter 12).
- The development of safe systems will require an understanding of variation, with methods to demonstrate, measure, and improve variation in safety (see ⊃ Chapters 13, 17, and 18).

In the *Oxford Professional Practice: Handbook of Patient Safety*, the theories and practical methods of patient safety are presented in detail.

Further reading

Canadian Patient Safety Institute (2020). *A guide to patient safety improvement: integrating knowledge translation and quality improvement approaches.* Edmonton, AB: Canadian Patient Safety Institute.

Available at: ⌖ https://www.patientsafetyinstitute.ca/en/toolsResources/A-Guide-to-Patient-Safety-Improvement (accessed 10 September 2023).

Leape, L.L. (2021). *Making Healthcare Safe: The Story of the Patient Safety Movement*. Cham: Springer. Available at: ⌖ https://library.oapen.org/handle/20.500.12657/49509 (accessed 10 September 2023).

References

Berwick, D.M. (2013). *A Promise to Learn: A Commitment to Act*. London: Department of Health and Social Care. Available at: ⌖ https://assets.publishing.service.gov.uk/government/uploads/system/uploads/attachment_data/file/226703/Berwick_Report.pdf (accessed 10 September 2023).

Lachman, P., Brennan, J., Fitzsimons, J., Jayadev, A., and Runnacles, J., eds. (2022). *Oxford Professional Practice: Handbook of Patient Safety*. Oxford: Oxford University Press.

Panagioti, M., Khan, K., Keers, R.N., *et al*. (2019). Prevalence, severity, and nature of preventable patient harm across medical care settings: systematic review and meta-analysis. *BMJ*, 366(366), p. l4185. doi: 10.1136/bmj.l4185.

World Health Organization (2021). *Global Patient Safety Action Plan 2021–2030*. Geneva: World Health Organization. Available at: ⌖ https://www.who.int/publications/i/item/9789240032705 (accessed 10 September 2023).

The challenge of climate change

(See ➲ Chapter 6.)

The WHO has declared that climate change is the greatest threat to human health of the twenty-first century, with healthcare as a major contributor to greenhouse gas emissions. Significant population benefits could be incurred by reducing the carbon footprint and limiting wasteful use of resources. In Box 2.3 a case study on how to start an improvement project aimed at decreasing the carbon footprint is provided.

Box 2.3 Case study on sustainable care

James is a registrar working on a busy respiratory ward. He notices that out of six patients with chronic obstructive pulmonary disease (COPD) admitted acutely, five are placed on intravenous (IV) hydrocortisone 100mg four times daily. All patients therefore require IV access (cannula, Y-connector, Clinell swab, Tegaderm, sterile swab) for administration of hydrocortisone (5mL sole-use syringe, filter needle, 10mL of normal saline flush).

The entire process seems wasteful (single-use plastic), time-consuming, and potentially harmful to patients. Most importantly, James notes there is no evidence for IV steroids in most cases of COPD exacerbation and current guidance advocates oral steroids.

With his curiosity aroused, James decides to calculate the carbon footprint for this intervention and to design a QI project to decrease the footprint, as well as the use of plastics in general.

Why is climate change important when implementing QI in healthcare?

- Healthcare has progressed rapidly over the last 50 years.
- Novel investigations, treatments, and technologies have led to a rapid increase in waste, carbon emissions, and prolonged healthcare usage, which further fuels the harmful effects of healthcare systems on the wider society and environment.
- The coronavirus disease 2019 (COVID-19) pandemic increased toxic waste and use of plastics (e.g. with extensive use of single-use plastics, personal protective equipment, and masks) (Graulich et al., 2021).
- There is difficulty with balancing urgent needs of the patient with the wider social responsibility of society to decrease the carbon footprint.

How can focus on climate change be achieved?

- Sustainable healthcare refers to the capacity of a health service to deliver healthcare over time, with considerations for future generations (Mortimer et al., 2018).
- Sustainable healthcare is a domain of quality in healthcare.
- Healthcare should consider current patients, as well as patients of the future.
- Frameworks for developing sustainable healthcare exist and are available to incorporate into QI programmes.

- Redesigning healthcare delivery can make a difference to the carbon footprint (e.g. with the introduction of telemedicine).

Role of the progressive healthcare professional

- The current generation of healthcare professionals needs to be progressive and mindful of the environment and its integral link to our current and future health.
- Healthcare professionals can be facilitators of change and champion a more sustainable approach to healthcare.
- Understanding the goals of QI and using this knowledge can bring about sustainable and real change. Simple projects can lead to waste reduction, improved patient care, and streamlined services.

In ⮕ Chapter 6, the challenge of sustainable healthcare is discussed in detail.

Signposting

World Health Organization. *Climate change*. Available at: ⌖ https://www.who.int/health-topics/climate-change#tab=tab_1 (accessed 10 September 2023).

Further reading

Purohit, A., Smith, J., and Hibble, A. (2021). Does telemedicine reduce the carbon footprint of healthcare? A systematic review. *Future Healthcare Journal*, 8(1), pp. e85–91.

Romanello, M., McGushin, A., Di Napoli, C., *et al.* (2021). The 2021 report of the Lancet Countdown on health and climate change: code red for a healthy future. *The Lancet*, 398(10311), pp. 1619–62.

References

Graulich, K., Köhler, A., Löw, J.C., *et al.* (2021). *Impact of COVID-19 on single-use plastics and the environment in Europe*. ETC/WMGE Report 4/2021. Boeretang: ETC/WMGE. Available at: ⌖ ttps://www.eionet.europa.eu/etcs/etc-wmge/products/etc-wmge-reports/impact-of-covid-19-on-single-use-plastics-and-the-environment-in-europe/@@download/file/ETC_4.1.7._Covid19-SUP_forwebsite.pdf (accessed 10 September 2023).

Mortimer, F., Isherwood, J., Pearce, M., Kenward, C., and Vaux, E. (2018). Sustainability in quality improvement: measuring impact. *Future Healthcare Journal*, 5(2), pp. 94–7.

The challenge of unwarranted variation and value

(See ⊃ Chapter 7 and 13.)

What is the problem?

- The persistence of unwarranted variation is one of the great challenges to be addressed in healthcare.
- Unwarranted clinical variation is variation that cannot be justified by the condition of the person receiving care.
- It concerns the appropriateness of the care delivered and this may have a value judgement.
- Unwarranted clinical variation decreases the value of the care provided and increases cost.
- QI programmes can play an important role in increasing the value of healthcare and in decreasing cost.
- Atlases of unwarranted variation in many countries have shown wide variation within hospitals, between hospitals, and between regions.
- Decreasing variation between both services and geographical locations is required.
- Variation may be based on the resources or skill sets in a particular area resulting in variations in effective care and patient safety, or due to individual choice of clinicians.
- In Table 2.1, a conceptual framework for unwarranted and warranted variation is presented, which shows the complexity of variation and how a deeper understanding of the reasons for variation is required.

Table 2.1 Warranted and unwarranted variation

	Warranted variation	Unwarranted variation
Capacity to deliver care	• Resource constraints • Proficiency-based service delivery (i.e. skill mix in local context)	• System design • Lack of technical ability
Agency and motivation	• Patient informed expectations • Patient needs dictating variation	• Provider needs and preference • Lack of judgement
Evidence base for intervention	• Equivocal evidence • Local context requirements are justified	• Unjustified deviation from evidence base • Lack of adoption of guidelines

Based on Sutherland and Levesque (2020).

Why is addressing variation important?

- Variation can be viewed at a global level across systems (Box 2.4) or within processes within a system.

Box 2.4 Decreasing unwarranted variation

In the United Kingdom, there have been several approaches to decreasing unwarranted variation.

- *NHS England*: the Getting it Right First Time (GIRFT) is a programme that aims to decrease unwarranted variation in medical and surgical care. The programme collects data, so that organizations can see where they sit in the spectrum of outcomes. The aim is to close the gap between the best-performing and the worst-performing hospitals or clinics. The data allow engagement with clinicians, so that they can join in solving the variation gap. Resources and training are provided, but the key is the data that show clinicians where there is opportunity to improve. Available at: ✍ https://gettingitrightfirsttime.co.uk (accessed 10 September 2023).
- *NHS Scotland*: the Scottish Atlas of Healthcare Variation highlights the geographical variation in the provision of health services and associated health outcomes. Like the GIRFT programme, the aim is to use data to start the conversation as to why there are differences in diagnosis, treatment, and resultant outcomes. Available at: ✍ https://www.isdscotland.org/products-and-services/scottish-atlas-of-variation/ (accessed 10 September 2023).
- *NHS Wales*: the NHS Wales Cardiovascular Atlas of Variation provides data on process and outcome variation for three cardiac conditions. Available at: ✍ https://www.isdscotland.org/products-and-services/scottish-atlas-of-variation/ (accessed 10 September 2023).

Similar programmes to decrease unwarranted variation exist in other countries, for example:

- *Australia*: Australian Atlas of Healthcare Variation Series, available at: ✍ https://www.safetyandquality.gov.au/our-work/healthcare-variation/australian-atlas-healthcare-variation-series (accessed 10 September 2023);
- *United States*: The Dartmouth Atlas of Health Care, available at: ✍ https://www.dartmouthatlas.org (accessed 10 September 2023).

- People receiving care experience variation at every stage of their health journey, be it in waiting times, investigations, or treatment. Some of the variation may be warranted and some is not.
- Healthcare professionals experience variation all the time, be it in the decisions made in investigation or in treatment of common conditions.
- Trainees move constantly between posts and much time is spent unproductively on learning how to order bloods and radiology and finding key pieces of equipment, and in different treatment approaches for the same conditions.
- Processes for simple tasks (e.g. taking bloods, inserting a cannula, ward rounds, prescribing) vary considerably and result in delays, safety concerns, and a poorly functioning, unproductive, ineffective team.
- Variation increases waste and this, in turn, decreases the value of the process and increases cost.
- This results in unsafe and poorly functioning health systems.

In ⟳ Chapter 13, the challenge of variation is discussed in detail.

Further reading

Cupit, C., Tarrant, C., and Armstrong, N. (2023). *Reducing Overuse* (series: Elements of Improving Quality and Safety in Healthcare). Cambridge: Cambridge University Press. doi: 10.1017/9781009310642

Wennberg, J.E. (2002). Unwarranted variations in healthcare delivery: implications for academic medical centres. *BMJ*, 325(7370), pp. 961–4. doi: 10.1136/bmj.325.7370.961.

Reference

Sutherland, K. and Levesque, J. (2020). Unwarranted clinical variation in health care: definitions and proposal of an analytic framework. *Journal of Evaluation in Clinical Practice*, 26(3), pp. 687–96. doi: 10.1111/jep.13181.

The Challenge of Person-Centred Care and Co-Production

(See ➔ Chapter 8.)

> 'must not only be prepared to do what is right [himself,] but also make the patient ... cooperate.'
>
> Hippocrates

Why is co-production important?

The evolution of person-centred care has been critical in the reassessment of the significant role patients as people can and must play in their own health.

- The concept of a passive patient receiving care without question or active participation is outdated and obstructive to optimizing the health of the patient.
- We need to understand the lived experience of the people receiving care, that is, the care "as is" rather than "as it should be as planned." The disconnect between "as is" and "as should be as planned" provides an opportunity for co-producing solutions together.
- Co-production recognizes that optimizing available therapies and techniques with the patient's own goals for their treatment can provide measurable improvement in their care. In Box 2.5 a practical example is given.

Box 2.5 Case study on person-centred care

Matt is a house officer (ST3) working on a busy oncology ward. Sean K is a person due to start chemotherapy but has declined treatment. The plan for chemotherapy was made 2 weeks previously when Sean K was informed that he had stage IV lung cancer.

Being curious, Matt asks Sean *what matters* to him. Sean K explains that as a child, he often had injections when he had juvenile idiopathic arthritis. Even though the methotrexate cured the condition, he now has a fear of needles and of chemotherapy in general. What mattered to him was that he would not experience what had happened to him as a child, that is, needles and the side effects of chemotherapy.

After discussing options, it is agreed that Sean K will return later that week for a peripherally inserted central catheter (PICC) line to be inserted to avoid the need for repeated venepuncture, and a plan to counteract the side effects of the chemotherapy was made. Sean K agreed to start the chemotherapy that day.

How to co-produce 'what matters' to people?

- The transition of co-production from a concept to the active participation of people in the design and delivery of healthcare systems requires a change in how healthcare is perceived by healthcare providers and people receiving care.
- People as service users need to be involved in every part of healthcare delivery and design.

- The goals should be designed together in a reciprocal relationship, taking into account the lived experience of professionals and patients.
- This requires the patient to be treated as a person, with expertise and knowledge that can assist in deciding the best course of action.
- Healthcare professionals have the responsibility to consider patient concerns on a continual basis.
- Empowered patients need to take ownership of the management of their own health, to ensure their voice is heard on their healthcare journey (Elwyn et al., 2020).

Benefit of co-production in healthcare QI

- Healthcare is 'service'-driven and in providing a service, we must partner with patients as people in order to provide high-quality, high-value care.
- The goal is to co-create value and facilitate health.
- Co-production can be even more powerful when people form alliances to the benefit of all.
- All QI projects should aim to co-produce the project with the people involved—patients and families, and providers including leaders, managers and clinical staff.

In ➲ Chapter 8, the challenge of co-production is discussed in detail.

Further reading

Batalden, P. (2018). Getting more health from healthcare: quality improvement must acknowledge patient coproduction—an essay by Paul Batalden. BMJ, p. k3617. doi: 10.1136/bmj.k3617

Batalden, M., Batalden, P., Margolis, P., et al. (2015). Coproduction of healthcare service. BMJ Quality and Safety, 25(7), pp. 509–17. doi: 10.1136/bmjqs-2015-004315.

Holland-Hart, D.M., Addis, S.M., Edwards, A., Kenkre, J.E., and Wood, F. (2018). Coproduction and health: public and clinicians' perceptions of the barriers and facilitators. Health Expectations, 22(1), pp. 93–101. doi: 10.1111/hex.12834.

Reference

Elwyn, G., Nelson, E., Hager, A. and Price, A. (2020). Coproduction: when users define quality. BMJ Quality and Safety, 29(9), pp. 711–16. doi: 10.1136/bmjqs-2019-009830.

The challenge to integrate care

The design of the modern healthcare system has resulted in care being delivered in silos. People have to traverse different systems to receive what they need within healthcare (e.g. primary, secondary, and tertiary care) and between healthcare and other systems such as social care.

Integrated care can be viewed from four perspectives (Goodwin, 2016) (Table 2.2).

Table 2.2 Integrated care

Care	To provide a continuum of care to an individual across different components of a system
Management	Managerial integration is required to create a common infrastructure for different stakeholders
Society	A social science approach is needed to integrate all aspects of care from policy, funding, and administrative and organizational structures to service delivery at clinical levels
Individual	At an individual level, care should be integrated around the person receiving care delivered by an integrated care team

Integration of care can be:
- *Horizontal* across different services (i.e. social care, health, education);
- *Vertical* across primary, secondary, or tertiary care for an individual with a chronic condition;
- At *different levels*, focused on the individual or a group of individuals or the community as a whole;
- As an *integrated care pathway*, which is a multidisciplinary care plan detailing each step needed to deliver the care required.

Models of integrated care include the Chronic Care Model developed for people with diabetes, which can be used for any long-term condition (Berwick, 2019; Bodenheimer et al., 2002) In all forms of integration, co-production and empowerment of people are essential to designing an integrated model (see ➲ Chapters 8, 10, and 11).

The International Foundation for Integrated Care has proposed nine evidence-informed ingredients or pillars 'to create the conditions for successful integrated care implementation irrespective of the model or scope chosen' (Table 2.3). These can be applied at different levels within and across systems.

In any improvement project, focus on how the care can be integrated around the wants and needs of the person and family should be considered.

Table 2.3 The nine pillars for integrated care

Pillar	Description
Vision	Developing a shared vision across communities and with the people delivering and receiving care for integration of care at individual and community levels
Population health	Viewing healthcare within the context of population health needs and the local context
Partnerships	Working with people as partners in health and their care to empower them to develop integration
Resilience	Building resilient communities that can respond to challenges such as a pandemic
Workforce	Developing the workforce capability to integrate care and the capacity to deliver integrated care
Governance	Establishing system-wide approaches to governance and leadership, including across different systems with which the person may need to engage
Digital solutions	Using digital solutions to enable and facilitate integrated care within and across systems
Finance	Aligning payment systems to facilitate integration rather than siloed working
Transparency	Being transparent with all that we do, including the results achieved and the impact on the system and people

Signposting

International Foundation for Integrated Care. Available at: https://integratedcarefoundation.org/ (accessed 10 September 2023).

References

Berwick, D.M. (2019). Reflections on the chronic care model—23 years later. *The Milbank Quarterly*, 97(3), pp. 665–8. doi: 10.1111/1468-0009.12414.

Bodenheimer, T., Wagner, E.H., and Grumbach, K. (2002). Improving primary care for patients with chronic illness. *JAMA*, 288(15), p. 1909. doi: 10.1001/jama.288.15.1909.

Goodwin, N. (2016). Understanding integrated care. *International Journal of Integrated Care*, 16(4), p. 6. doi: 10.5334/ijic.2530.

International Foundation for Integrated Care. *Nine pillars of integrated care*. Available at: https://integratedcarefoundation.org/nine-pillars-of-integrated-care (accessed 10 September 2023).

The challenge of training in quality improvement

Most graduates in healthcare have to learn how to improve the processes on the job. Inclusion of the new sciences of improvement and implementation would go a long way to improving healthcare, as demonstrated in the case study in Box 2.6.

Box 2.6 Case study of a nurse practitioner in training

Patrick is a nurse in his final year of postgraduate training as a nurse practitioner and needs to complete a QI project for his e-portfolio. His current job in gastroenterology endoscopy is very busy. He is concerned that some patients are discharged without appropriate follow-up, prescriptions, and/or discharge letters. He wants to introduce a simple 5-point 'sign-out' to be completed by all team members at discharge. However, he has no idea of how to go about this, where to go to gain support, or if it is even worthwhile.

Patrick is curious about improvement and decides to ask a colleague who seems to know more about QI with his project. His colleague points him to online learning modules on QI, which provide him with the basic training. This allows Patrick to design a solution with his fellow nurses and the doctors in training, and to test the solutions. This is the first step on his QI journey and his curiosity of how to improve has been ignited. On reflection, he wishes this had been part of his postgraduate training/ nursing school training.

'As practise makes perfect, I cannot but make progress, each drawing one makes, each study one paints is a step forward.'

Van Gogh

Why should we integrate safety and QI into healthcare professional training?

Healthcare professionals cannot practise QI if they are not taught how to improve.
- Those in training are on the front line and hold insights into processes and system failures that are endemic on the ground.
- There is a need to change how and when we teach theory in order to embed practice of QI and teach skills to trainees.
- Training in the formative years can develop and foster learning for a progressive healthcare professional.
- By embedding QI skills earlier, we can equip all healthcare professionals with skills to enrich patient care, improve outcomes, better population health, and encourage practice of sustainable, equitable, and environmentally conscious care (see ➔ Chapters 5 and 6).

How do we do this?

The design and implementation of a training programme needs faculty, time, goals, funding, and measurable outcomes, and should be sustainable.

- Firstly, by educating current healthcare professionals, a faculty and repository of mentors can be established.
- The next step involves developing a core curriculum to be introduced during medical training, ideally during foundation years.
- The framework is then expanded to slowly incorporate the theory of QI through lectures, small group learning, and problem-based learning, as shown in Figure 2.2.
- The provision of mentorship and support can facilitate the clinical application of QI in supported projects for those on clinical placement.

Pre-clinical years UGMT

Core curriculum
Introduction
Basic principles
Concepts
Lectures
Small group learning

Problem-based learning
Problem identification
Teamwork
Leader roles
Toolkit of QI

Clinical years UGMT

Problem finding
First patient encounters
Introduce themes
Patient safety
Timely and effective care

Develop themes
Efficient care,
Patient-centred,
Equitable

Introduction to health service
Error reporting
Systems

Problem finding in clinical practice

First year PGMT

QI in practice
Problem
identification
Assist on project
Handover
Safety huddles
Adverse event
reporting

Second year PGMT

QI project
Leadership
Sustaining change
Support and Research

Figure 2.2 Example framework for integration of quality improvement principles and practices into undergraduate and postgraduate medical training. PGMT, postgraduate medical training; QI, quality improvement; UGMT, undergraduate medical training.

Based on Davey, Thakore, and Tully (2022).

- QI projects and use of a structured guide to good practice in reporting the project should be encouraged.
- Trainees should present their work (locally and nationally) and ideally submit for publication.
- A similar programme can be adapted for nurses and other health professionals in training.

Further reading

Jones, A.C., Shipman, S.A., and Ogrinc, G. (2015). Key characteristics of successful quality improvement curricula in physician education: a realist review. *BMJ Quality and Safety*, 24(1), pp. 77–88. doi: 10.1136/bmjqs-2014-002846.

Jones, B. and Chatfield, C. (2022). Lessons in quality improvement. *BMJ*, 376, p. o475. doi: 10.1136/bmj.o475.

Reference

Davey, P., Thakore, S., and Tully, V. (2022). How to embed quality improvement into medical training. *BMJ*, 376, p. e055084. doi: 10.1136/bmj-2020-055084.

Top tips

- In an improvement project, ask what really matters to the people involved, as it is often more than sorting out the processes.
- Do not assume improvement will have an impact on everyone's equity—always consider the equity challenge.
- All improvements must consider safety as part of the challenge to be addressed.
- Always ask what the environmental impact of the project will be.
- A key outcome should be decreasing unwarranted variation.
- Person-centred care is the foundation of a project, and the outcomes must promote an integrated approach and address what really matters using the power of co-production.

Summary

The QI methodology initially addresses the defects in the system. As we move to Quality 3.0 and the next phase of improvement, we need to go beyond the initial focus of sorting our defects and address the challenges we have discussed in this chapter:

- The COVID-19 pandemic has exposed the SDHs of health as never before.
- Safety will always be important in every way.
- The challenge of climate change is compelling and urgent.
- Unwarranted variation is costly and unsafe, and needs to be addressed.
- Person-centred care is fragile and must be protected, and health co-produced.
- Integrated care is a response to the complexity of healthcare and how care is organized.
- Healthcare professionals need QI to be integrated in their training.

In the following chapters, we will address each of these challenges in greater detail, so that an improvement project can be designed to take all these complex challenges into account. New challenges will always become apparent and as one develops the ability to apply the methodology, we can add these challenges to those discussed in this chapter.

Improvement Science

Key points
- The Science of Improvement has evolved through the twentieth century.
- The theories of change can be applied to healthcare settings and can result in successful implementation of improvement initiatives.
- Quality must be planned, controlled, managed, and improved.
- Outcomes are the result of an interplay of systems and processes.
- Application of the Science of Improvement requires an understanding of the *Lenses of Profound Knowledge*:
  - *System*: appreciation of how the system works;
  - *Variation*: studying variation of processes within a system;
  - *Psychology*: understanding the beliefs of people;
  - *Knowledge*: having a theory of change.
- Statistical process control charts provide a way to understand how the system is working.
- Continuous improvement uses the Plan–Do–Study–Act (PDSA) cycle to test changes.
- Total quality management and quality systems bring the theories together in a systematic way for an organization to drive quality.

Introduction

> 'It is not enough to do your best,
> you must know what to do, and then do your best.'
>
> W. Edwards Deming ℘ www.deming.org

The Science of Improvement, a relatively new body of knowledge, has evolved over the course of the twentieth century. The theories of change and how to ensure successful implementation of improvement initiatives were developed in other industries, primarily by psychologists, engineers, sociologists, and statisticians. Most of the improvement methods have been derived from the work of Donabedian, Shewhart, Juran, Gilbreth, and Deming.

In this chapter, we will discuss the core theories and methods that have been introduced into healthcare. These can be applied in both improvement and clinical work. In subsequent chapters, the methods derived from the theories discussed in this chapter will be presented.

The message of this chapter is that when one develops an improvement programme one must:

- Understand the system and processes undertaken to get work done;
- Institute quality planning in all activities;
- Establish measurement of the processes and outcomes;
- Involve the people in the system—both healthcare providers and patients—in improvement work and to make continuous improvement an integral part of day-to-day work;
- Co-produce and co-design change with all involved, including patients and their families.

Further reading

Langley, G.L., Nolan, K.M., Nolan, T.W., et al. (2009). The Improvement Guide: A Practical Approach to Enhancing Organizational Performance, 2nd edition. San Francisco, CA: Jossey-Bass Publishers.

Parry, G.J. (2014). A brief history of quality improvement. Journal of Oncology Practice, 10(3), pp. 196–9. Doi: 10.1200/jop.2014.001436.

The Donabedian theory

'Systems awareness and systems design are important for health professionals, but they are not enough. They are enabling mechanisms only. It is the ethical dimensions of individuals that are essential to a system's success.'

Avedis Donabedian

What is the theory?

Donabedian, a physician who was a pioneer in the improvement movement, introduced a framework to evaluate the quality of healthcare. To achieve good outcomes, we need to have structures and processes in place, as well as the culture to improve (Figure 3.1).

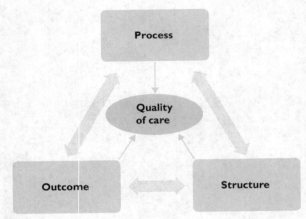

Figure 3.1 The Donabedian model.

The model provides a useful approach to analysing why an outcome has been achieved, as shown in Table 3.1.

The categories are sequential, as a good structure increases the likelihood of effective processes and, in turn, increases the likelihood of good outcomes. Drawing the connections between processes and outcomes can be difficult. It may require large sample populations, adjustments by case mix, and long-term follow-up data (Donabedian, 2003).

How does one use the theory to improve clinical care?

The Donabedian model can be applied to all healthcare settings, using the categories to obtain information for assessing whether the quality of care is poor, fair, or good. For example, the Systems Engineering Initiative for Patient Safety (SEIPS) model (see ⊙ Chapters 12 and 14) integrates the theory with human factors.

Table 3.1 Applied Donabedian model

Category	Components	Examples
Structure	**How work is organized**	
	Organizational structure	There are sufficient staff to do the work
		The way shifts are organized to ensure staff are not overworked
	Human resources	Staff have the expertise to undertake the tasks
	Material resources	Equipment is available to diagnose and treat the conditions with which people present
		All equipment is functioning
		Good supply chains
		One example is supply of protective equipment during a pandemic
Process	**How work is done**	
	Information about the process can be obtained from: • Medical records • Interviews with patients and practitioners • Direct observations of healthcare visits	Practitioner activities, for example: • Diagnosis • Treatment • Prevention • Education Patient activities, for example: • Preventive activities (e.g. exercise, smoking cessation) • Taking medications
Outcomes	Outcome of work organization and process	Impact of care on health status of patients and populations, either desirable or detrimental

Data from Donabedian, A. (1988).

In Box 3.1 the practical application of the model is demonstrated in a case study.

The Donabedian model has gained widespread acceptance. However, critics of this model describe it as too linear of a framework that does not recognize how the three categories influence and interact with one another. Adding culture to the three parts of the model addresses this concern.

• Another criticism is that patient characteristics and environmental factors are not incorporated into the model, factors which are important in the evaluation of quality of care.

• Donabedian believed that culture is an essential component and the beliefs of the people in the system impact the outcomes achieved.

Box 3.1 Case study of the application of the
Donabedian Model

Jane B is a 68-year-old woman who wanted to receive her influenza vaccination. She attended the general practice. However, on arrival, the
waiting room was dirty, packed, and cold and the nurse was rude to her
and dismissed her when she checked in. She left after waiting for an hour
without receiving the influenza vaccination. She subsequently did not receive the vaccine that year. She contracted influenza that winter and was
hospitalized.

- *Structure*: the environment was unpleasant.
- *Process*: there was no clear process for patient flow.
- *Outcome*: Jane B was placed at higher risk of influenza.
- *Equity*: all people should have equal access.
- *Sustainability*: the facilities should be maintained in a clean way.
- *Person-centredness*: the practice should consider the wants of
  service users.

Further reading

Carayon, P., Schoofs Hundt, A., Karsh, B.-T., et al. (2006). Work system design for patient
    safety: the SEIPS model. *Quality and Safety in Health Care*, 15(suppl 1), pp. i50–8. doi: 10.1136/
    qshc.2005.015842.
Coyle, Y. and Battles, J. (1999). Using antecedents of medical care to develop valid quality of care
    measures. *International Journal for Quality in Health Care*, 11(1), pp. 5–12. doi: 10.1093/intqhc/
    11.1.5.

References

Donabedian, A. (1988). The quality of care. How can it be assessed? *JAMA*, 260(12), pp. 1743–8.
    doi: 10.1001/jama.260.12.1743.
Donabedian, A. (2003). *An Introduction to Quality Assurance in Health Care*, 1st edition, volume 1.
    New York, NY: Oxford University Press.

The Juran Trilogy

'All improvement happens project by project and in no other way.'
Joseph M. Juran ♒ https://www.juran.com/

What is the quality issue?

Quality improvement is about making sense of a complex system, so that we can improve outcomes. These include patient safety, person satisfaction and experience, and efficiency. One must decide what is important and what needs to be improved, and then have a clear pathway to improve care. Most of the issues in quality result from poor process design without any measures to study the process.

The Juran Trilogy provides a framework to approach complex issues and develop a quality system to manage the improvement of care.

Why is the theory important?

Improvement is an essential part of the management process, and the Juran Trilogy provides staff, managers, and leaders with a framework with which to make changes to improve care

What is the theory?

- Josef Juran was an engineer who provided a stepwise process to have continual improvement. He proposed that to improve, one requires a guiding principle that would be the basis for improvement.
- The Juran Trilogy is the foundation for achieving excellence in performance and consists of three actions:
  - Planning for quality;
  - Establishing controls for measurement;
  - Quality improvement with a feedback loop for learning.

The three stages are illustrated in Figure 3.2.

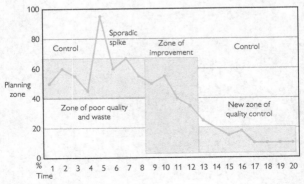

Figure 3.2 The Juran Trilogy.

The three stages provide a framework for continual improvement. Kaizen (in Japanese *Kei* means change and *Zen* means good) is the philosophy underlying continual improvement and focuses on eliminating wastes inherent to any system. Waste can be categorized into seven types (Table 3.2).

Kaizen incorporates continuous incremental improvement involving everyone in the system, for example, clinicians and managers. A Kaizen event is an organized improvement activity to solve a problem. These principles align with the methods of Lean Six Sigma and the reliability theory (see ◉ Chapter 14).

Table 3.2 Seven wastes to be eliminated or minimized

Waste	Example
Overproduction	Doing more than is needed (e.g. delayed discharge means treating a person when it is not required)
	Need to repeat an intervention (e.g. a blood result lost)
Transportation	Moving patients around a health facility unnecessarily
	Bringing people into outpatients when not required
Motion	Equipment not available and you have to look for it (e.g. when taking blood tests)
Overprocessing	Repeating blood tests that are not needed
Waiting	People waiting in the emergency department to be seen
Inventory	Overordering of equipment due to poor supply chains (e.g. storing of extra cannulae)
Defects	Hospital-acquired infections, adverse events

How does one use the theory to improve clinical care?

All improvement consists of a series of projects that need to fit into a common purpose. When you undertake an improvement project, it should be part of an overall quality strategy and have defined measures and a defined improvement process. Requirements for a successful improvement process include:

- Improving the customer or patient experience;
- Creating opportunities for improvement by staff with appropriate methods;
- Leadership at all levels to make the changes.

In Box 3.2 the practical application of the Juran Trilogy is demonstrated in a case study.

Tips and summary

- Always include relevant stakeholders in the planning.
- Make the measurement or control process easy to do.
- Ensure that the feedback loop is designed into the process and is not onerous.

The pharmacy manager has established that pharmacists spend a lot of their time on correcting prescriptions that are incorrectly filled with either missing data or wrong completed data. This could cause harm to patients and is a major risk.

Planning

The pharmacists decided to adopt Juran's approach and start to plan an improvement process, that is, a Kaizen event. To do this, they would need to demonstrate the problem and start thinking of ways to design solutions. They opted to take a human factors approach.

Control

The pharmacists started to record all the different errors for each script while correcting dispensing. Hence, they would have the evidence to plan the intervention, that is, to study the current errors of prescribing.

They arranged the errors using the *Pareto Principle* (see ➲ Chapter 13), so that they would be able to concentrate on the frequent errors. Measures included the number of errors, the types of errors, and the time spent on correction of prescriptions (waste).

Improvement

Once they had the data, they approached the consultant of the medical ward and the clinical staff. They explained the problem and then over the next few months, they worked with the clinical team to design interventions to decrease the error rate and have a safer system of prescribing.

Using the *SEIPS human factors model* (see ➲ Chapters 12 and 14), they studied the work system and designed a 'sterile cockpit' for prescribing, which contained all the tools for the prescribing process. All prescribing was now to be performed within the designated prescribing area. They redesigned prescribing forms to be user-friendly. They also provided regular feedback to the clinical staff, rewarding successful prescribers.

Equity

This project aimed to ensure that the system was reliable, so that every person had an equal chance of a correct prescription.

Sustainable healthcare

The decrease in wasteful movement and repeat scripts ensured there was a saving of consumables which could be measured.

Person-centred care

Getting it right the first time every time ensured that patients' needs for safe care were met.

Signposting

Juran,J.M. (2019). *The Juran Trilogy: quality planning*. Available at: ⚲ https://www.juran.com/blog/the-juran-trilogy-quality-planning/ (accessed 10 September 2023).

Further reading

Carayon, P., Schoofs Hundt, A., Karsh, B.-T., et al. (2006). Work system design for patient safety: the SEIPS model. *Quality and Safety in Health Care*, 15(suppl 1), pp. i50–8. doi: 10.1136/qshc.2005.015842.

Juran, J.M. (1988). *Quality Control Handbook*. New York, NY: McGraw Hill.

The Lenses of Profound Knowledge

'Without theory, experience has no meaning. Without theory, one has no questions to ask. Hence, without theory, there is no learning.'

W. E. Deming in *Out of the Crisis*

What is the theory?

William Edward Deming, a statistician, developed the underlying philosophy of quality as outlined in his *'System of Profound Knowledge'*. This comprises four key elements, or lenses, through which a problem can be analysed (Figure 3.3; Table 3.3).

Deming's theory is a synthesis of research in the fields of psychology, human behaviour, systems, statistics, and sociology. Deming provides the theoretical framework we will use in this book, as well as the foundation for the methods of change you will learn.

Every improvement project can be analysed and implemented using the four improvement lenses. Deming called this *'Profound Knowledge'* because of the complexity of systems and change. While we may never fully understand why they act as they do, we will be continually learning and thereby continually improving.

When he was a patient following an injury, Deming was admitted to intensive care and required a blood transfusion. He gained insight into a poorly designed health system with unwanted variation.

- Despite hardworking staff in the unit, Deming noted that this unwanted variation could only be improved by leadership and that *'management's job is to optimize the whole system'*.

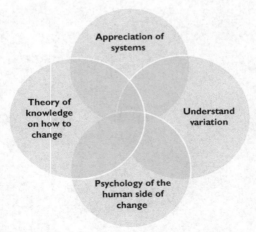

Figure 3.3 Lenses of Profound or Improvement Knowledge.

Table 3.3 System of Profound Knowledge

Improvement lens	What does this mean?
Appreciation for a system	We all work within a system, and the system in healthcare is made up of people and processes involving tasks and technology within an environment that may be complex and changing (see ➲ Chapter 12)
Understanding variation	Deming said that we have to study variation and the types of variation within the process; for example, do we do what has been agreed reliably or does it vary as to which team is on or the time of day? (see ➲ Chapter 13)
Understanding psychology and human behaviour	The beliefs and attitudes of the people in the system, whether they are providers of care or the people receiving care, are an essential part of improvement. Success in an improvement programme depends on the heart and mind more than on the technical skills (see ➲ Chapter 10)
Theory of knowledge	Improvement requires a theory and a method if it is to be successful, and Deming proposed a method of continual learning using prediction and testing against that prediction (see ➲ Chapters 14 and 17)

- He believed that a system will achieve results due to its design and that workers within that system should not be blamed for poor results.
- Poorly performing systems should be redesigned by managers by implementing key steps to improve quality and job satisfaction and to reduce waste.

In Box 3.3 examples of system challenges are demonstrated in a case study.

Box 3.3 Case study of a poorly designed system in healthcare

Waiting for something to happen is a feature of most healthcare systems. For example, in an outpatient clinic:
- Patients wait for doctors;
- Doctors wait for patients;
- All patients may arrive at the start of the clinic and wait to be seen;
- Clinics start late;
- Clinics overrun;
- There are not enough clinical staff to see the patients;
- Each consultation is based on an average time to see a patient, so some will take up more time and some less.

All of the above contribute to a poorly run system, with wide variation in processes, and the outcomes may not be to the benefit of either the staff or the patients.

How does one use the theory to improve clinical care?

Deming's '*System of Profound Knowledge*' can be applied by using the essentials required for quality improvement, summarized in the '14 points of management', which can be applied to healthcare (Table 3.4). These principles are embodied in many of the approaches to teamworking discussed in subsequent chapters.

In Box 3.4 the practical application of the Lenses of Profound Knowledge is demonstrated in a case study.

Table 3.4 Deming's 14 points of management

Principle	Application to healthcare
Create constancy of purpose for improving products and services	Leaders at every level set a vision that defines activities—see the microsystem theory (see ➲ Chapters 12 and 17)
Adopt the new philosophy of improvement	Organizations that have achieved high-quality care and reliability have adopted a new way of thinking in the way they manage their operations
Cease dependence on inspection to achieve quality	In healthcare, we have relied on inspection (see ➲ Chapter 9) as a way to measure quality. It is proposed that a continually improving process will have self-inspection that will facilitate continual improvement
End the practice of awarding business on price alone; instead, minimize total cost by working with a single supplier	In healthcare, we often use many suppliers for items; it is better to standardize, where possible, so that there is reliability in operations (see ➲ Chapter 13)
Improve constantly and forever every process for planning, production, and service	This is the core value of quality improvement and has now been adopted for teams in healthcare (see ➲ Chapter 11)
Institute training on the job	This is a foundation of healthcare; we need to add quality and safety to clinical training (see ➲ Chapter 2)
Adopt and institute leadership	Leadership for quality and safety has been highlighted as an essential component of delivering a quality service (see ➲ Chapter 1)
Drive out fear	A fundamental part of psychological safety is not allowing fear to be part of the culture of safety (see ➲ Chapter 10)
Break down barriers between staff areas	Healthcare is often delivered in silos; integrated care is the way to ensure that care is person-centred (see ➲ Chapter 8)
Eliminate slogans, exhortations, and targets for the workforce	Healthcare has adopted targets as a way to improve; this has produced short-term gain (e.g. 4-hour waits in emergency departments), but not long-term sustainable change—the system needs to change (see ➲ Chapter 11)

Table 3.4 (Contd.)

Principle	Application to healthcare
Eliminate numerical quotas for the workforce and numerical goals for management	Targets are often used in healthcare and these can be detrimental. They should be realistic goals that the system can deliver (e.g. eliminating infections)
Remove barriers that rob people of pride of workmanship, and eliminate the annual rating or merit system	In England, ranking of hospitals has been a favoured approach, but its benefits have not been sustained. An alternative approach is to build agency, a sense of belonging and pride, that will promote and produce good quality (see ➲ Chapters 10 and 11)
Institute a vigorous programme of education and self-improvement for everyone	This is the basis of continuous medical education, which should include Improvement Science (see ➲ Chapter 2)
Put everybody in the company to work to accomplish the transformation	Once one has a shared vision, quality and safety become an integral part of day-to-day work and it is everybody's responsibility to improve care

Box 3.4 Case study to illustrate the Lenses of Profound Knowledge

A 72-year-old man was admitted for a laparoscopic cholecystectomy. His day-case procedure was uncomplicated and required simple analgesia during the afternoon prior to discharge. On discharge, he was given a prescription for oral morphine in error. He was found unresponsive at home and despite resuscitative efforts, he died two days later in hospital.

Appreciation for a system

This is an interdependent group of people or processes working together. In this case, the intern who prescribed the medication was on his first day and the pharmacist who dispensed the medication had never dispensed morphine before and did not realize that there was a protocol in place.

Understanding variation

There is variation in everything we can measure or observe. The intern had not realized there were prefilled day-case simple analgesic prescriptions following laparoscopic cholecystectomy, and used a new prescription pad.

Theory of knowledge

The more knowledge someone has about how a system functions, the more likely a change will result in improvement. Following a similar incident 4 years previously, which was recognized prior to discharge, the clinical director had implemented specific changes in the department, including the discharge prefilled prescription and discharge instructions letter to all patients, unless the surgeon who carried out the procedure prescribed any other medications required. A follow-up audit showed

(Continued)

Box 3.4 (Contd.)

that 100% of patients received the prefilled prescription and letter the month following implementation.

Understanding psychology and human behaviour
Understand how people interact with each other and with a system. The intern had not attended the induction training on the unit, as he felt that it was not applicable to him.

Equity
This project aimed to ensure that the system was reliable, so that every person had an equal chance of a correct prescription.

Sustainable healthcare
The decrease in wasteful movement and repeat scripts ensured there was a saving of consumables, which could be measured.

Person-centred care
Getting it right the first time every time ensured that patients' needs for safe care were met.

Tips and summary

- Develop an appreciation and understanding for the system in which you work.
- Learn how your system functions, so that you can maximize improvements through changes you make.
- Variation is common. By studying variation in the process, you will discover opportunities to improve.
- Minimize unwanted variation in your practice to improve outcomes.
- Try to understand how people interact with each other and with your system to improve quality and job satisfaction and to reduce waste.

Signposting

The Deming Institute. Available at: ℵ https://deming.org/ (accessed 10 September 2023).

Further reading

Best, M. (2005). W Edwards Deming: father of quality management, patient and composer. *Quality and Safety in Health Care*, 14(4), pp. 310–12. doi: 10.1136/qshc.2005.015289.
Perla, R.J. and Parry, G.J. (2011). The epistemology of quality improvement: it's all Greek. *BMJ Quality and Safety*, 20(Suppl 1), pp. i24–7. doi: 10.1136/bmjqs.2010.046557.
Provost, L.P. (2011). Analytical studies: a framework for quality improvement design and analysis. *BMJ Quality and Safety*, 20(Suppl_1), pp. i92–6. doi: 10.1136/bmjqs.2011.051557.

Measuring variation and testing changes

Assignable causes of variation may be found and eliminated.

Walter Shewhart, *Economic Control of Quality of Manufactured Product*. p. 8, 1931.

Walter Shewhart provided the foundation for all quality improvement work with the statistical control chart and the Plan–Do–Study–Act (PDSA) cycle, also known as the Shewhart cycle, which he developed in the 1920s.

Statistical process control

As indicated by the lenses of Deming's Profound Knowledge, much of quality improvement depends on understanding the variation that exists within the system and the process of care.

- For example, if we want to decrease waiting times in the emergency department, we will need to understand the arrival patterns of people needing care, that is, the variation in this pattern and the variation in meeting this demand for care.
- Without a deep understanding of variation, we would not solve this problem.
- This applies to every process within the healthcare system.

Statistical process control (SPC) provides the gold standard for measuring improvement over time.

- SPC is an effective and powerful analysis tool which can provide ongoing assessment of system functioning and enables an improvement team to assess the impact of applied intervention and external forces on the system.
- Importantly, it involves a key understanding of the variation in the data over time.
- Operational definitions of measures are important to ensure the measures are valid and can be understood by all in the process.

Shewhart defined two forms of variation:

- *Common cause variation*, which is inherent in the system—every system has processes that will produce variation, and to address the common cause variation, we will need to change the way in which the system works.
- *Special cause variation*, which can be attributed to an event that is not part of the system—or may be as a result of a change in the way in which the system operates.

In Box 3.5 the practical application of the types of variation is demonstrated in a case study.

Shewhart charts will be discussed in Chapter 13.

People arrive at the emergency department randomly. Nonetheless there are several factors that can influence this pattern, for example, common epidemiological events such as the influenza season which causes seasonal variation.

Random arrival is called *common cause variation*. To change the pattern of arrival time, one would study the causes of the variation and have an improvement programme to address the causes.

Special cause variation is when there is an event, for example, a motor vehicle accident involving a bus which will cause a spike in the arrivals outside the predicted variation. COVID-19 created a special cause in admissions to hospital and presentations to the emergency department.

A study of the demand for services would be the first step in understanding how to develop the supply side, that is, the service required to meet the demand.

The Shewhart cycle: Plan–Do–Study (Check)–Act

To measure continuous improvement, Shewhart adapted the scientific method used in laboratories for iterative research and developed the methodology of small cycles to test change. The PDSA cycle is fundamental to many methods in quality improvement, including Model for Improvement (MFI) and Lean Six Sigma.

- The PDSA is aimed at learning and testing whether an idea will work in practice and whether one's prediction is correct.
- As the PDSA is a learning cycle, after each cycle, you will change and adapt according to the learning.
- These PDSA cycles involve:
  - Planning what will be done and predicting what will happen;
  - Prediction of what will happen in the cycle;
  - Doing (i.e. implementing the idea or change);
  - Studying what happened and testing whether the prediction was correct;
  - Acting to apply the learning from the testing and studying phase, so that changes can be made before one enters the next cycle (Figure 3.4).
- Each PDSA cycle begins with theories or ideas.
- With each short cycle, knowledge is obtained, which can inform action and can result in positive outcomes.
- Following a PDSA cycle, the process is repeated with the knowledge gained from the previous cycle.
- A PDSA cycle can never be too small, often starting with one idea, one patient, and one clinician.
- However, PDSA cycles can be too large and not be able to test the change or the prediction.
- Like any test in a laboratory, PDSA cycles require rigour in application and measurement of outcomes.
- To ensure that a quality improvement project can be replicated, the application of PDSA must be done carefully, recording the prediction and how it was applied.

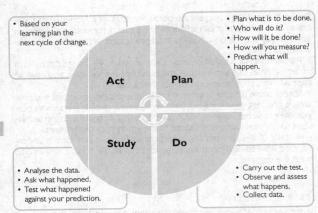

Figure 3.4 Plan–Do–Study (Check)–Act (PDSA).

Further reading

Benneyan, J.C., Lloyd, R.C., and Plsek, P.E. (2003). Statistical process control as a tool for research and healthcare improvement. *Quality and Safety in Health Care*, 12(6), pp. 458–64. doi: 10.1136/qhc.12.6.458.

Perla, R.J., Provost, S.M., Parry, G.J., Little, K., and Provost, L.P. (2021). Understanding variation in reported covid-19 deaths with a novel Shewhart chart application. *International Journal for Quality in Health Care*, 33(1), p. mzaa069. doi: 10.1093/intqhc/mzaa069.

Reed, J.E. and Card, A.J. (2016). The problem with Plan–Do–Study–Act cycles. *BMJ Quality and Safety*, 25(3), pp. 147–52. doi: 10.1136/bmjqs-2015-005076.

Taylor, M.J., McNicholas, C., Nicolay, C., Darzi, A., Bell, D., and Reed, J.E. (2014). Systematic review of the application of the plan–do–study–act method to improve quality in healthcare. *BMJ Quality and Safety*, 23(4), pp. 290–8. doi: 10.1136/bmjqs-2013-001862.

Reference

Shewhart, W.A. (1931). *Economic Control of Quality of Manufactured Product*. New York, NY: D. Van Nostrand Company (reprinted by ASQC Quality Press, 1980).

Total quality management

Total quality management

> 'The basic managerial idea introduced by systems thinking, is that to manage a system effectively, you might focus on the interactions of the parts rather than their behavior taken separately.'
>
> Russell L. Ackoff and Fred Emery (1972) On purposeful systems, cited in: Lloyd Dobyns, Clare Crawford-Mason (1994) Thinking about quality: progress, wisdom, and the Deming philosophy. p. 40

What is the theory?

The term total quality management (TQM) covers the philosophy of taking a broad and system-wide approach to quality and encompasses the theories that were developed by Shewhart Juran and Deming, among others. It aims to improve the competitiveness of an organization by establishing quality pillars and concepts. This has moved on to the concept of developing a quality management system, which governs how quality is delivered by an organization or a clinical team.

In healthcare, TQM systems have been established to prevent clinical and administrative problems, reduce costs, increase patient satisfaction, improve organizational processes, and provide high-quality patient care. The principles of TQM are illustrated in Figure 3.5.

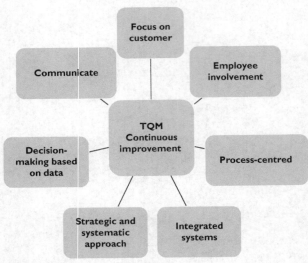

Figure 3.5 Principles of total quality management.

How does one use the theory to improve clinical care?

Application of the TQM principles to a healthcare organization can result in significant improvement in clinical care (Table 3.5). Many organizations have adopted this approach to develop learning health systems (see ➔ Chapter 12).

For sustainable change and continual improvement in a team or organization, developing a quality system using the principles of TQM is a good way to approach the challenge.

In Box 3.6 the practical application of the TQM is demonstrated in a case study.

Table 3.5 Focus of total quality management applied to healthcare

Focus	Action required
Focus on the customer (can be the patient, another clinician, etc.)	Healthcare depends on their patients, just as other organizations depend on their customers. It is crucial to understand the patient's current and future needs to ensure that their requirements are met and expectations are exceeded
Employee involvement (i.e. all involved in delivering care)	Leaders within a healthcare setting can establish common purpose and direction to create and maintain a positive working environment. This allows employee engagement and a sense of belonging, which facilitates attainment of the objectives of the healthcare organization
Process-centred	Processes are a set of interrelated or interacting healthcare activities (i.e. how work is done to achieve outcomes). Decreasing variation in processes and continually improving processes make healthcare more efficient and reduce pressure on healthcare professionals
Integrated system	A healthcare organization consists of many different departments. These are often organized into vertically siloed departments. Highly performing systems integrate processes to achieve outcomes
Strategic and systematic approach	A strategic and systematic approach can contribute to the healthcare organization's effectiveness and efficiency in achieving its objectives
Decision-making based on facts and data	Quality improvement is dependent on the use of data to drive change. Accurate, timely, and objective data are essential to improving quality
Communication and transparency	Transparent communication with and among all healthcare organization staff, suppliers, patients, and their families is a fundamental component of a quality system
Continuous improvement	Use of Plan–Do–Study–Act (PDSA) cycles for continuous improvement is the foundation of a quality system

Signposting

Healthcare Improvement Scotland (2022). *Moving from quality improvement to quality management*. Available at: ℬ https://ihub.scot/media/9012/qitoqms-vfinal.pdf (accessed 10 September 2023).

Virginia Mason Medical Institute in Seattle in the United States is one of the exemplar organizations in the delivery of high-quality care. The organization has adopted Lean, as it underlies quality philosophy and methodology within the context of development of a total quality management system. The organization incorporates the theories discussed in the chapter. The National Health Service (NHS) linked with the Virginia Mason Institute to test the ideas at five NHS organizations. The key learning from this initiative was that to develop a quality management system, the following is required:

- A strong culture of peer learning and knowledge sharing in which communication is a vital component of change, so that all members of staff feel they belong in the improvement process and in the way in which the organization is run;
- Leadership at every level is committed to improvement and is sustained, even when there are challenges (e.g. during the COVID-19 pandemic);
- Leadership is shared, so all are involved and belong, including clinicians and middle managers;
- Improvement is focused and aligned with organizational strategies and priorities, in turn aligned with regional and national priorities to improvement programmes;
- Continuous improvement is part of the culture of organizations;
- Priority setting is important;
- Measurement capability of organizations and systems to provide data for improvement is essential.

In summary, a total management system approach is required, based on values, developing the infrastructure, and making improvement part of the business strategy and process of the organization.

Burgess, Nicola, Currie, Graeme, Crump, Bernard and Dawson, Alexander (2022). Leading change across a healthcare system: how to build improvement capability and foster a culture of continuous improvement: lessons from an evaluation of the NHS-VMI partnership. Coventry: Warwick Business School. Available at: ✍ https://warwick.ac.uk/fac/soc/wbs/research/vmi-nhs/reports/ (accessed 10 September 2023).

Jones, B. (2022). Building an organisational culture of continuous improvement. The Health Foundation, London. Available at: ✍ https://www.health.org.uk/publications/long-reads/building-an-organisational-culture-of-continuous-improvement (accessed 10 September 2023).

Further reading

Alzoubi, M.M., Hayati, K.S., Rosliza, A.M., Ahmad, A.A., and Al-Hamdan, Z.M. (2019). Total quality management in the health-care industry: integrating the literature and directing future research. *Risk Management and Healthcare Policy*, 12, pp. 167–77. doi: 10.2147/rmhp.s197038.

Talib, F., Rahman, Z., and Azam, M. (2010). Total quality management implementation in the healthcare industry: a proposed framework. Available at: ✍ https://papers.ssrn.com/sol3/papers.cfm?abstract_id=2729808 (accessed 10 September 2023).

Talib, F., Rahman, Z., and Azam, M. (2011). Best practices of total quality management implementation in health care settings. *Health Marketing Quarterly*, 28(3), pp. 232–52. doi: 10.1080/07359683.2011.595643.

Top tips

- Understand your own system and processes within your organization to maximize the work you can get done.
- Institute quality planning.
- Set up objective measurement systems of the processes and outcomes.
- Engage the people in the system—both healthcare providers and patients. Co-produce and co-design outcomes.

Summary

The Science of Improvement is a relatively new body of knowledge in healthcare. Improvement Science is grounded in the following concepts:

- The systems theory informs the way in which we understand improvement. Donabedian proposed that one needs to consider how systems operate and the processes within the systems to achieve outcomes.
- Juran proposed that there is a trilogy of quality planning, control, and improvement.
- Deming's *Lenses of Profound Knowledge*, that is, systems, variation, psychology, and knowledge, are the basis for assessing and then improving quality.
- We need to be pragmatic in the process of improvement in different contexts and make choices based on our learning (conceptual pragmatism).
- Beliefs and attitudes of people in the system are important. This is a combination of psychology and logic when making decisions.
- Appreciation of context is essential in the process of discovering solutions.
- Operational definitions are essential components of defining the measures.
- Shewhart's statistical control is essential to ensuring there is only common cause variation kept in control.
- Change and learning are based on testing and learning cycles, that is, PDSA.
- Develop a quality management system to deliver quality as the business strategy of the organization or clinical team.

Further reading

Perla, R.J., Provost, L.P., and Parry, G.J. (2013). Seven propositions of the science of improvement. *Quality Management in Health Care*, 22(3), pp. 170–86. doi: 10.1097/qmh.0b013e31829a6a15.

Implementation Science and quality improvement

Key points

- Improvement Science provides the construct for testing new ideas and proving fidelity.
- Implementation Science provides you with the methods and tools to apply to enhance the successful implementation of your project.
- It focuses on the implementation of what is known to work and how it can be implemented in different contexts and environments.
- Implementation Science assesses the effectiveness of the clinical intervention and the success of the implementation activity or strategy.
- Implementation Science frameworks can provide rigour to the implementation part of the improvement process.
- Assessment of readiness, adaptability, fidelity, and appropriateness of the intervention can guide actions to take to improve the uptake of the intervention.

Introduction

In its broadest sense, science is the endeavour of knowledge discovery. This discovery can be made by using many different approaches. New knowledge is key to improving health and care. In ➔ Chapter 3, the principles of Improvement Science were explored. This chapter moves onto Implementation Science.

The Health Foundation describes the goal of Improvement Science as follows:

> 'The overriding goal of improvement science is to ensure that quality improvement efforts are based as much on evidence as the best practices they seek to implement. Improvement science is about finding out how to improve and make changes in the most effective way. It is about systematically examining the methods and factors that best work to facilitate quality improvement.'

Health Foundation, 2011.

The foundations of the improvement approach are laid out in Deming's synthesis of many theorists in his System of Profound Knowledge (see ➔ Chapter 3). This approach is underpinned by the generation of knowledge through the exploration of how different factors come together. The cornerstone is learning by predicting and testing in biased, messy, moving, real-world situations. Changes and new approaches emerge progressively as they are tested, first locally and then adapted at scale to differing contexts.

As noted in ➔ Chapter 1, the challenge for improvers is to be able to test and prove efficacy and fidelity, that is, the extent to which the results of an intervention can be attributed to what was done. Then they need to implement in different contexts and environments, that is, implementation adaptability. As improvement often fails to be transferred to, or sustained in, new contexts, the improvement approach has been called into question as a science (Dixon-Woods, 2019).

Implementation Science has a focus on the analysis and understanding of not only if something works, but also why, where, when, for whom, and how. It is founded on the theories of operations research, management science, epidemiology, behavioural economics, anthropology, sociology, and ethics. The scope of Implementation Science is broad and includes:

- Identification of strategies to promote implementation;
- Concepts for planning implementation;
- Frameworks to guide implementation;
- Approaches to analyse the fidelity of implementation;
- Methods to evaluate the structures, processes, and outcomes of implementation;
- Ways to explore the relationship between intervention and context.

The research question or implementation concern is the starting point for inquiry and determines the research method to be used. Implementation Science aims to explore, describe, influence, explain, and predict, with the ultimate goal of influencing improvement. The Implementation Science process is guided by implementation theories and conceptual frameworks.

In this chapter, we discuss selected tools from Implementation Science that can be useful in generating a broader knowledge for improvement, especially when faced with the challenges of spread, scale-up, and sustainability of tested change ideas (Box 4.1).

Box 4.1 Programme spread, scale-up, and sustainability

- *Spread* is a horizontal process that is better for complex problems (e.g. changing behaviour), generally built bottom–up at grassroots or frontline level. It will develop over time and usually requires customization to the local context (Shaw et al., 2018).
- *Scale-up* is better for complicated problems and is usually top–down, takes place more rapidly, and needs leadership from the top to ensure take-up. Commonalities across sites allow for a more singular approach rather than contextualization (Shaw et al., 2018).
- *Sustainability* is the extent to which an intervention or improvement is sustained over time once funding or the project has ended (Chamber et al., 2013).

Further reading

Rabin, B.A., Brownson, R.C., Haire-Joshu, D., Kreuter, M.W., and Weaver, N.L. (2008). A glossary for dissemination and implementation research in health. *Journal of Public Health Management and Practice*, 14(2), pp. 117–23. doi: 10.1097/01.phh.0000311888.06252.bb.

References

Chambers, D.A., Glasgow, R.E., and Stange, K.C. (2013). The dynamic sustainability framework: addressing the paradox of sustainment amid ongoing change. *Implementation Science*, 8(1), p. 117. doi: 10.1186/1748-5908-8-117.

Dixon-Woods, M. (2019). How to improve healthcare improvement—an essay by Mary Dixon-Woods. *BMJ*, 367, p. l5514. doi: https://doi.org/10.1136/bmj.l5514.

Health Foundation (2001). *Evidence scan: improvement science*. Available at: https://www.health.org.uk/sites/default/files/ImprovementScience.pdf (accessed 10 September 2023).

Shaw, J., Tepper, J., and Martin, D. (2018). From pilot project to system solution: innovation, spread and scale for health system leaders. *BMJ Leader*, 2(3), pp. 87–90. doi: 10.1136/leader-2017-000055.

What is Implementation Science?

What is the quality issue?

Fast and reliable implementation of evidence-based interventions and care has been a challenge for all in healthcare. This is evident in many of the attempts to scale up what works, for example, in patient safety. The theories, methods, and approaches of Implementation Science can assist us in addressing this problem.

Definition of Implementation Science

Bauer et al. (2015) defined Implementation Science as '*the scientific study of methods to promote the systematic uptake of research findings and other Evidence Based Practice into routine practice, and, hence, to improve the quality and effectiveness of health services.*'

One could argue that Implementation Science is more focused on the research of how best to implement at scale and then define it as '*the scientific study of methods to promote the systematic uptake of research findings and other evidence-based practices into routine practice, and, hence, to improve the quality and effectiveness of health services and care*' (Eccles and Mittman, 2006).

Implementation Science is increasingly being applied as action-based research, with ongoing implementation research embedded in change programmes to inform optimization of change initiatives as they progress. This is summarized in Figure 4.1.

Implementation research includes the study of factors affecting implementation, that is, the process of implementation and the results of implementation as they pertain to policies, programmes, or individual practice. This includes factors such as professional behaviour, the environment, organizational culture, resources, and structural characteristics.

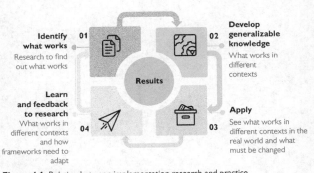

Identify what works 01
Research to find out what works

Develop generalizable knowledge 02
What works in different contexts

Results

Learn and feedback to research 04
What works in different contexts and how frameworks need to adapt

Apply 03
See what works in different contexts in the real world and what must be changed

Figure 4.1 Relation between implementation research and practice.

Based on Ramaswamy, R., Mosnier, J., Reed, K., Powell, B. J., & Schenck, A. P (2019). Building capacity for Public Health 3.0: introducing implementation science into an MPH curriculum. *Implementation Science: IS, 14*(1), 18. ⌀ https://doi.org/10.1186/s13012-019-0866-6.

A simple description of Implementation Science

Curran (2020) describes Implementation Science as shown in Box 4.2.

As we look at the scope of Implementation Science and how it can assist in improvement projects, it is clear that the approach is to continually learn about how one can implement a proven intervention in different contexts and environments.

Box 4.2 Implementation Science made simple

- The intervention is THE THING.
- Effectiveness research is about whether THE THING works.
- Implementation research looks at how best to help people or places do THE THING.
- Implementation strategies are the stuff we do to try and help people or places do THE THING.
- The main implementation outcomes are HOW MUCH and HOW WELL they do THE THING.

Adapted from Curran G. M (2020). Implementation science made too simple: a teaching tool. *Implementation Science Communications*, 1, 27. ℗ https://doi.org/10.1186/s43058-020-00001-z.

References

Bauer, M.S., Damschroder, L., Hagedorn, H., Smith, J., and Kilbourne, A.M. (2015). An introduction to implementation science for the non-specialist. *BMC Psychology*, 3(1), p. 32. doi: 10.1186/s40359-015-0089-9.

Curran, G.M. (2020). Implementation science made too simple: a teaching tool. *Implementation Science Communications*, 1, p. 27. doi: 10.1186/s43058-020-00001-z.

Eccles, M.P. and Mittman, B.S. (2006). Welcome to implementation science. *Implementation Science*, 1, p. 1. doi: 10.1186/1748-5908-1-1.

Ramaswamy, R., Mosnier, J., Reed, K., Powell, B.J., and Schenck, A.P. (2019). Building capacity for Public Health 3.0: introducing implementation science into an MPH curriculum. *Implementation Science*, 14(1), p. 18. doi: 10.1186/s13012-019-0866-6.

Integrating Methodologies for Improvement

Quality improvement has many examples of successful projects in one context or environment, and failure in spread of the intervention to different contexts. A good example is the Matching Michigan programme in England, which failed to transfer what appeared to be a simple intervention to a different environment (Box 4.3).

Box 4.3 Case study: Matching Michigan

The Michigan Keystone project applied an improvement approach to reduce central venous catheter (CVC) bloodstream infections in over 100 Michigan intensive care units (ICUs). It was lauded as an exemplar of how Improvement Science can achieve large-scale improvement through iterative testing and reliable adoption of a checklist for CVC insertion. In a bid to replicate the success of this checklist approach, the National Health Service (NHS) and UK National Patient Safety Agency launched *Matching Michigan* across 200 ICUs in England from 2009 to 2011. Disappointingly, *Matching Michigan* failed to produce improvements in this new setting over and above trends that were already occurring in ICUs across England.

A study of the reasons for this lack of success showed there was more to the success in Michigan than the checklist. Through the lens of Implementation Science, a review of the original Michigan Keystone initiative suggests that the following features were also key contributors to its success:

- A self-sustaining desire among participating organizations to conform to this new group norm;
- The establishment of a strong network and community around this quality issue, facilitated by regular communication;
- Characteristics of a social movement, with CVC-related infections reframed as a solvable social or behavioural issue;
- Use of multiple interventions that shaped a culture of commitment to doing better;
- Systematic collection of data and their use to influence change;
- A mostly softer approach to persuasion with firm edges (e.g. strict programme rules on data submission).

For *Matching Michigan*, the following factors have been recognized as likely impediments to success:

- Many ICUs were already performing well and this programme failed to respect their good performance as a starting point;
- This was not novel—it had been subject to considerable focus through prior initiatives;
- Staff were resentful of previous centrally led efforts at data-driven performance management;
- The programme was run by a central regulatory body, as opposed to emerging from within a professional group and its will for improvement;
- The programme included the same components but did not adequately support network formation, with relatively little ongoing communication between sites.

Based on: Dixon-Woods, M., Leslie, M., Tarrant, C., & Bion, J (2013). Explaining Matching Michigan: an ethnographic study of a patient safety program. *Implementation Science: IS*, 8, 70. https://doi.org/10.1186/1748-5908-8-70.

Matching Michigan illustrated that improvement involves many factors. It demonstrated that a review of the contextual factors, as well as the process, individual, and intervention characteristics, is required to modulate the success of improvement.

Reference

Dixon-Woods, M., Leslie, M., Tarrant, C., and Bion, J. (2013). Explaining Matching Michigan: an ethnographic study of a patient safety program. *Implementation Science*, 8, p. 70. doi: 10.1186/1748-5908-8-70.

Comparing Improvement and Implementation Science

What is the theory?

Implementation and Improvement Sciences have many similarities and areas of overlap, particularly in spreading improvement at scale.

- Quality improvement usually starts with a problem, for which solutions are progressively generated within that unique context.
- Implementation Science usually starts with a research question and method, with the aim of generating knowledge that can lead to closure of the 'know–do' gap.

The similarities and differences are shown in Table 4.1.

Table 4.1 Similarities and differences

	Improvement Science	Both	Implementation Science
Taxonomy or classification	Different		Different
Systems	Systems-level work at the frontline to test interventions	Shared definitions of systems	Work on uptake of Evidence Based (EB) interventions
Problem addressed	Direct quality problems and variation in quality		Problem is poor uptake of EB solutions (fidelity, process, or relationship with context)
Aim	To improve care quality rapidly in a real-world context	To improve health and care	To understand factors impacting successful implementation in order to inform effective improvement
Methods	MFI PDSA Lean Six Sigma DMAIC TQM	Process mapping Staff engagement Patient engagement Measurement	Uses implementation frameworks and strategies, including QI approaches Rapid PDSAs Audit and feedback
Outcomes	Measures of quality	Spread Sustainability Cost benefit	Quantitative and qualitative research findings on use of EB and factors that influence use

EB, evidence-based; MFI, Model for Improvement; PDSA, Plan–Do–Study–Act; DMAIC, Define, Measure, Analyse, Improve, and Control; TQM, total quality management; QI, quality improvement. Table based on Øvretveit, J., et al. (2017 and 2021) and Koczwara, B. et al. (2018).

Further reading

Øvretveit, J. (2011). Understanding the conditions for improvement: research to discover which context influences affect improvement success. *BMJ Quality and Safety*, 20(Suppl 1), pp. i18–23. doi: 10.1136/bmjqs.2010.045955.

References

Koczwara, B., Stover, A.M., Davies, L., *et al.* (2018). Harnessing the synergy between improvement science and implementation science in cancer: a call to action. *Journal of Oncology Practice*, 14(6), pp. 335–40. doi: 10.1200/jop.17.00083.

Øvretveit, J., Mittman, B., Rubenstein, L., and Ganz, D.A. (2017). Using implementation tools to design and conduct quality improvement projects for faster and more effective improvement. *International Journal of Health Care Quality Assurance*, 30(8), pp. 755–68. doi: 10.1108/ijhcqa-01-2017-0019.

Ovretveit, J., Mittman, B. S., Rubenstein, L. V., & Ganz, D. A. (2021). Combining Improvement and Implementation Sciences and Practices for the Post COVID-19 Era. *Journal of general internal medicine*, 36(11), 3503–3510.

Expert Recommendations for Implementing Change

The Expert Recommendations for Implementing Change (ERIC) is an expert-driven taxonomy consensus on a range of implementation strategies and how they may be defined. The ERIC compiles 73 separate strategies, including many strategies commonly employed in quality improvement. These strategies are analogous to building blocks for implementing change (Powell *et al.*, 2015).

The strategies can be grouped into nine categories or clusters (Waltz *et al.*, 2015):

- Evaluation and iteration of improvement and implementation strategies;
- How to adapt and tailor an intervention to different contexts;
- How to train and educate people to undertake improvement and implementation;
- How to engage consumers involved in projects;
- How to change the infrastructure to enable projects;
- How to provide interactive assistance to people involved in a project;
- How to develop relationships among stakeholders;
- How to support clinicians with implementation of their intervention;
- How to use financial strategies to facilitate implementation.

References

Powell, B.J., Waltz, T.J., Chinman, M.J., *et al.* (2015). A refined compilation of implementation strategies: results from the Expert Recommendations for Implementing Change (ERIC) project. *Implementation Science*, 10(1), p. 21. doi: 10.1186/s13012-015-0209-1.

Waltz, T.J., Powell, B.J., Matthieu, M.M., *et al.* (2015). Use of concept mapping to characterize relationships among implementation strategies and assess their feasibility and importance: results from the Expert Recommendations for Implementing Change (ERIC) study. *Implementation Science*, 10(1), p. 109. doi: 10.1186/s13012-015-0295-0.

Introduction to Implementation Science frameworks

One of the features of Implementation Science is that it provides several frameworks and theories that are used to help identify the theoretical bases of implementation and understand the mechanisms by which implementation is likely to succeed.

Nilsen (2015) categorizes the frameworks into five distinct entities (Table 4.2).

Table 4.2 Types of frameworks

Type	Description	Examples
Process models	How to translate research into practice	Evidence-based practice intervention model (EPIS) (Aarons, Hurlburt and Horwitz, 2010)
		Practical, Robust Implementation, and Sustainability Model (PRISM) (Feldstein and Glasgow, 2008)
		The Quality Implementation Framework (Meyers, Durlak and Wandersman, 2012)
Determinant frameworks	Assess the different variables—dependent and independent—which could be enablers of, or barriers to, implementation	Consolidated Framework for Implementation Research (CFIR) (Damschroder et al., 2022)
		Promoting Action on Research Implementation in Health Services (PARIHS) framework (Helfrich et al., 2010)
		Theoretical domains (Michie et al, 2005)
Classic theories	These involve theories from sociology and psychology that may influence implementation	Organizational theory (Birken et al., 2017)
		Diffusion of innovation (Dearing and Cox, 2018)
		Behavioural theories (Glanz and National Cancer Institute (U.S, 2005)
Implementation theories	These are *de novo* theories to understand implementation	Readiness for change (Weiner, 2009)
		Normalization process theory (Murray et al., 2010)
		Implementation climate (Weiner et al., 2011)
Evaluation frameworks	To assess the success of implementation	RE-AIM framework to guide planning and evaluation of programmes (RE-AIM, 2023)
		Proctor outcomes for implementation research (Proctor et al., 2011)

Reference

Nilsen, P. (2015). Making sense of implementation theories, models and frameworks. *Implementation Science*, 10(1), p. 53. doi: 10.1186/s13012-015-0242-0.

Process models

Aarons, G.A., Hurlburt, M. and Horwitz, S.M. (2010). Advancing a Conceptual Model of Evidence-Based Practice Implementation in Public Service Sectors. *Administration and Policy in Mental Health and Mental Health Services Research*, [online] 38(1), pp. 4–23. doi.org/10.1007/s10488-010-0327-7.

Feldstein, A.C. and Glasgow, R.E. (2008). A Practical, Robust Implementation and Sustainability Model (PRISM) for Integrating Research Findings into Practice. *The Joint Commission Journal on Quality and Patient Safety*, 34(4), pp. 228–243. doi.org/10.1016/s1553-7250(08)34030-6.

Meyers, D.C., Durlak, J.A. and Wandersman, A. (2012). The Quality Implementation Framework: A Synthesis of Critical Steps in the Implementation Process. *American Journal of Community Psychology*, 50(3-4), pp. 462–480. doi.org/10.1007/s10464-012-9522-x.

Determinant frameworks

Damschroder, L.J., Reardon, C.M., Widerquist, M.A.O. and Lowery, J. (2022). The updated Consolidated Framework for Implementation Research based on user feedback. *Implementation Science*, 17(1). doi.org/10.1186/s13012-022-01245-0.

Helfrich, C.D., Damschroder, L.J., Hagedorn, H.J., Daggett, G.S., Sahay, A., Ritchie, M., Damush, T., Guihan, M., Ullrich, P.M. and Stetler, C.B. (2010). A critical synthesis of literature on the promoting action on research implementation in health services (PARIHS) framework. *Implementation Science*, 5(1). doi.org/10.1186/1748-5908-5-82.

Michie, S., Johnston, M., Abraham, C., Lawton, R., Parker, D., Walker, A., & "Psychological Theory" Group (2005). Making psychological theory useful for implementing evidence based practice: a consensus approach. *Quality & safety in health care*, 14(1), pp. 26–33. doi.org/10.1136/qshc.2004.011155.

Classic theories

Birken, S.A., Bunger, A.C., Powell, B.J., Turner, K., Clary, A.S., Klaman, S.L., Yu, Y., Whitaker, D.J., Self, S.R., Rostad, W.L., Chatham, J.R.S., Kirk, M.A., Shea, C.M., Haines, E. and Weiner, B.J. (2017). Organizational theory for dissemination and implementation research. *Implementation Science*, 12(1). doi.org/10.1186/s13012-017-0592-x.

Dearing, J.W. and Cox, J.G. (2018). Diffusion of Innovations Theory, Principles, and Practice. *Health Affairs*, 37(2), pp. 183–190. doi.org/10.1377/hlthaff.2017.1104

Glanz, K. and National Cancer Institute (U.S (2005). *Theory at a glance : a guide for health promotion practice*. Bethesda? Md.: U.S. Dept. Of Health And Human Services, National Cancer Institute. https://cancercontrol.cancer.gov/sites/default/files/2020-06/theory.pdf. Accessed 10 September 2006.

Implementation theory

Murray, E., Treweek, S., Pope, C., MacFarlane, A., Ballini, L., Dowrick, C., Finch, T., Kennedy, A., Mair, F., O'Donnell, C., Ong, B.N., Rapley, T., Rogers, A. and May, C. (2010). Normalisation process theory: a framework for developing, evaluating and implementing complex interventions. *BMC Medicine*, 8( ). doi.org/10.1186/1741-7015-8-63.

Weiner, B.J., Belden, C.M., Bergmire, D.M. and Johnston, M. (2011). The meaning and measurement of implementation climate. *Implementation Science*, 6(1). doi.org/10.1186/1748-5908-6-78.

Weiner, B.J. (2009). A theory of organizational readiness for change. *Implementation Science*, [online] 4(1). doi.org/10.1186/1748-5908-4-67.

Evaluation Framework

Proctor, E., Silmere, H., Raghavan, R., Hovmand, P., Aarons, G., Bunger, A., Griffey, R. and Hensley, M. (2011). Outcomes for implementation research: Conceptual distinctions, measurement challenges, and research agenda. *Administration and Policy in Mental Health and Mental Health Services Research*, [online] 38(2), pp.65–76. doi.org/10.1007/s10488-010-0319-7.

RE-AIM. (2023). *RE-AIM – Home – Reach Effectiveness Adoption Implementation Maintenance*. [online] Available at: https://re-aim.org/. (accessed 10 September 2023)

Useful Implementation Science frameworks

The Quality Implementation Framework

Meyers et al. (2012) synthesized over 25 frameworks into one that could conceptually be used by quality improvement teams in a realistic way. This framework can add value to your improvement project. The framework aligns with the diffusion of innovation theory postulated by Rogers (2003), in which there are five stages of innovation:

- Dissemination of the concept;
- Early adoption of the intervention to try it;
- Implementation of the intervention;
- Evaluation of its impact; and then
- Institutionalization into how work is routinely undertaken.

The Quality Implementation Framework assumes the first two stages have been completed and that these fall into the area of quality improvement testing. An adapted version of the framework is shown in Figure 4.2. It is in keeping with the Plan–Do–Study–Act (PDSA) cycles discussed in ➲ Chapters 3 and 18.

Implementation has a number of steps, and the framework provides the improver with a logical way to implement the improvement intervention at scale. Each phase is continuous once it commences.

1. *Phase one* deals with context, which is a critical aspect of implementation, as noted by Øvretveit (2011). Context is all of the critical conditions required for implementation which are not part of the intervention itself. These include capacity, resources (both physical and human), training, and environment, much like is indicated in the work system of microsystems and the Systems Engineering Initiative for Patient Safety (SEIPS) model (see ➲ Chapters 12 and 14). An assessment of readiness for implementation can be undertaken using a readiness model (Wandersman Center's Readiness Thinking Tool; Weiner, 2009).

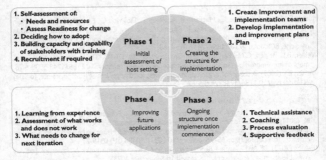

Figure 4.2 Adapted Quality Implementation Framework.
Adapted from Meyers, D. C., Durlak, J. A., & Wandersman, A. (2012).

2. *Phase two* involves creating the will for change and the implementation team, which may be different from the team involved with improvement. Here the strategy for implementation and the plan is developed (see ➔ Chapter 11).
3. *Phase three* is where implementation takes place, and is evaluated in real time and supported at every stage.
4. *Phase four* is one of reflection and learning, so that lessons from implementation can be learnt (i.e. what worked and what did not).

When planning for any implementation, it can be valuable to ask several questions that assist in generating an implementation plan (Box 4.4).

Box 4.4 Implementation questions to ask

When implementing your project, there are 10 questions to ask:
1. Is the intervention *acceptable* to the context and people—that is, do they believe it has value?
2. Can the intervention be *adopted* within the given context?
3. Is the intervention *appropriate* for the problem to be addressed and the context?
4. Is the intervention *feasible*—that is, are there resources to allow for successful implementation?
5. Will the implementation be *cost-effective*, with a cost benefit? (See ➔ Chapter 7)
6. How will the intervention *penetrate* the intended population to achieve the desired outcome?
7. How will you measure the *fidelity* of the intervention—that is, can outcome be attributed to the intervention? (See ➔ Chapter 15)
8. Will the intervention have an impact on the *environment*? (See ➔ Chapter 5)
9. Will the outcome of the intervention be *equitable*? (See ➔ Chapter 6)
10. Will the intervention be *sustained*, and will the change be *'hardwired'* into the system? (See ➔ Chapter 12)
11. Will the implementation be *co-designed* and/or *co-produced* to ensure person-centredness? (See ➔ Chapters 8 and 14)

Proctor's Conceptual Model

This model seeks to distinguish 'implementation outcomes' from quality and patient outcomes. The proposed taxonomy of implementation outcomes includes acceptability, adoption, appropriateness, feasibility, fidelity, cost, penetration, and sustainability. The purpose of the model is to provide guidance for conceptualization and measurement in implementation research.

RE-AIM

RE-AIM stands for Reach, Efficacy, Adoption, Implementation, and Maintenance. It is a framework designed to assist in assessing and reporting factors that impact on the external validity of research findings, particularly in public health and policy. Its purpose is to assist in building an understanding of how an intervention works in a particular setting, such that it may be spread or scaled.

Promoting Action on Research Implementation in Health Services Framework (PARIHS)

This framework proposes that successful implementation is a function of three interacting domains:

- Nature and type of evidence (including research, clinical and patient experience, and local information);
- Qualities of the context (including culture, leadership, and evaluation);
- Facilitation (who is facilitating change and how facilitation is approached).

This framework was designed to broaden focus on the key elements required when seeking to implement research into practice.

Consolidated Framework for Implementation Research (CFIR)

The CFIR brings together many different constructs and integrates them, as shown in Figure 4.3. The framework integrates characteristics of the intervention, individual, and process with the internal and external settings, that is, all the factors that may have an impact on implementation.

The framework is broadly categorized into three categories:

1. Describing and/or guiding the process of translating research into practice;
2. Understanding and/or explaining what influences implementation outcomes; and
3. Evaluating implementation (Nilsen, 2015).

Implementation Science and research seek to close the gap between what needs to be done and what is done.

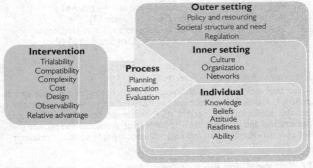

Figure 4.3 Implementation Science: the characteristics involved.
Adapted from Damschroder LJ, Aron DC, Keith RE, Kirsh SR, Alexander JA, Lowery JC. (2009) Fostering implementation of health services research findings into practice: a consolidated framework for advancing implementation science. *Implement Sci.* 2009;4:50. DOI: 10.1186/1748-5908-4-50.

In Box 4.5, a case study shows how the framework can be incorporated in an improvement programme.

Box 4.5 Case study: early palliative care implementation research using improvement approaches

The problem

The American Society of Clinical Oncology (ASCO) recommends the use of ' ... *combined standard oncology care and palliative care ... early in the course of illness for any patient with metastatic cancer and/or high symptom burden.*'

Unfortunately, early palliative care is not routinely incorporated into treatment plans at the onset of an advanced diagnosis, thereby depriving patients of the potential quality of life benefits, especially in low-access populations such as minorities and rural-dwellers. Further, little is known about how to best assist health systems that want to integrate early palliative care services into their usual oncology care.

The intervention

Virtual learning collaboratives (VLCs), composed of multiple health systems working together (virtually) on a common goal to implement an evidence-based practice, offer a potential solution. VLC features include formation of quality improvement or implementation teams, group problem-solving and learning, and data reporting/feedback. Despite widespread use of VLCs in healthcare, few studies have evaluated their effectiveness.

The implementation design

To address this gap, an implementation-effectiveness trial is to be conducted to test the effectiveness of a VLC implementation strategy compared to a typical technical assistance (TA) approach to integrate an early concurrent oncology palliative care programme. ENABLE (Educate, Nurture, Advise, Before Life Ends) is an evidence-based, scalable early palliative care programme promoted by the National Cancer Institute (NCI) Research Tested Intervention Program.

Frameworks used

This cluster randomized controlled trial in community oncology practices is guided by the RE-AIM framework and uses Proctor's Outcomes for Implementation Research Model to implement the ENABLE programme and evaluate implementation, service, and patient outcomes.

Outcomes

Key outcomes include effectiveness of VLC versus TA on ENABLE programme uptake, ENABLE programme implementation, and patient and caregiver outcomes (e.g. quality of life, mood). The *long-term goal* of this study is to: (1) generate knowledge about methods to improve adoption, adaptation, integration, and scalability of evidence-based practices; and (2) improve integration of the evidence-based ENABLE programme in oncology practices for advanced cancer patients. Study results will fill a knowledge gap on VLC effectiveness and enhance the rigour and reproducibility of implementation strategies to adopt evidence-based palliative care.

(With permission Research Funding: reference NCI R01CA229197; NCI UG1CA189961)

Signposting

University of Washington (n.d.). *Implementation Science at UW: theories, models, and frameworks.* Available at: 🔗 https://impsciuw.org/implementation-science/research/frameworks/ (accessed 10 September 2023).

Reference

Øvretveit, J. (2011). Understanding the conditions for improvement: research to discover which context influences affect improvement success. *BMJ Quality & Safety*, 20(Suppl 1), pp. i18–i23. doi:https://doi.org/10.1136/bmjqs.2010.045955.

Further reading

PARIHS framework

Bergström, A., Ehrenberg, A., Eldh, A.C., et al. (2020). The use of the PARIHS framework in implementation research and practice: a citation analysis of the literature. *Implementation Science*, 15(1), p. 68. doi: 10.1186/s13012-020-01003-0.

Proctor Conceptual Model

Proctor, E., Silmere, H., Raghavan, R., et al. (2011). Outcomes for implementation research: conceptual distinctions, measurement challenges, and research agenda. *Administration and Policy in Mental Health and Mental Health Services Research*, 38(2), pp. 65–76. doi: 10.1007/s10488-010-0319-7.

RE-AIM framework

Glasgow, R.E., Harden. S.M., Gaglio, B., et al. (2019). RE-AIM Planning and Evaluation Framework: adapting to new science and practice with a 20-year review. *Frontiers in Public Health*, 7, p. 64. doi: 10.3389/fpubh.2019.00064.

References

Meyers, D.C., Durlak, J.A., and Wandersman, A. (2012). The Quality Implementation Framework: a synthesis of critical steps in the implementation process. *American Journal of Community Psychology*, 50(3–4), pp. 462–80. doi: 10.1007/s10464-012-9522-x.

Nilsen, P. (2015). Making sense of implementation theories, models and frameworks. *Implementation Science*, 10(1), p. 53. doi: 10.1186/s13012-015-0242-0.

Rogers, E.M. (2003). *Diffusion of Innovations*, 5th edition. New York, NY: Free Press.

Wandersman Center. *The Readiness Thinking Tool.* Available at: 🔗 https://www.wandersmancenter.org/using-readiness.html (accessed 10 September 2023).

Weiner, B.J. (2009). A theory of organizational readiness for change. *Implementation Science*, 4, p. 67. doi: 10.1186/1748-5908-4-67.

Integrating the theory and method

In this chapter, the concepts in Implementation Science have been discussed with the aim of improving your improvement project. The methods of improvement and implementation are complementary and as an improver, you will move from one to the other, so that you can achieve, sustain, and spread improvement.

Figure 4.4 summarizes how Improvement and Implementation Sciences can be combined for optimal improvement.

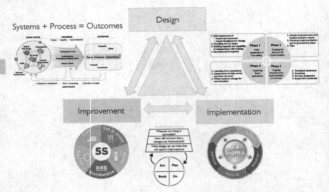

Figure 4.4 Integration of design, improvement, and implementation theory and methods.

Adapted from Ramaswamy, R., Mosnier, J., Reed, K., Powell, B.J. and Schenck, A.P. (2019). Building capacity for Public Health 3.0: introducing implementation science into an MPH curriculum. *Implementation Science*, 14(1). doi: 10.1186/s13012-019-0866-6.

- All improvement includes a design phase, an improvement phase, and an implementation phase, using a wide range of methods.
- Human-centred design, which aims to bring together what is technically possible and human or person-centred, has synergy with Implementation Science (Chen et al., 2021).
- Improvement Science methods can empower clinical improvement teams to achieve their outcomes (Wandersman et al., 2015).
- Improvement and implementation have been shown in the coronavirus disease 2019 (COVID-19) pandemic to be essential and compatible theories and methods that, if used together, can make an impact on achieving desired outcomes (Øvretveit et al., 2021).

To achieve the best possible change, knowledge generated through Improvement and Implementation Science approaches can be integrated to maximize impact.

References

Chen, E., Neta, G., and Roberts, M.C. (2021). Complementary approaches to problem solving in healthcare and public health: implementation science and human-centered design. *Translational Behavioral Medicine*, 11(5), pp. 1115–21. doi: 10.1093/tbm/ibaa079.

Øvretveit, J., Mittman, B.S., Rubenstein, L.V., and Ganz, D.A. (2021). Combining Improvement and Implementation Sciences and Practices for the post COVID-19 era. *Journal of General Internal Medicine*, 36(11), pp. 3503–10. doi: 10.1007/s11606-020-06373-1.

Ramaswamy, R., Mosnier, J., Reed, K., Powell, B.J., and Schenck, A.P. (2019). Building capacity for Public Health 3.0: introducing implementation science into an MPH curriculum. *Implementation Science*, 14(1), p. 18. doi: 10.1186/s13012-019-0866-6.

Wandersman, A., Alia, K.A., Cook, B., and Ramaswamy, R. (2015). Integrating empowerment evaluation and quality improvement to achieve healthcare improvement outcomes. *BMJ Quality and Safety*, 24(10), pp. 645–52. doi: 10.1136/bmjqs-2014-003525.

Top tips

- Appreciate the complexity of the 'know–do' implementation gap.
- Use Implementation Science frameworks to assess the contextual factors that may modulate the success of a change intervention.
- Use Implementation Science questions to guide strategy and planning.
- Consider the resources required for successful implementation.
- Consider the use of implementation research to rigorously evaluate your improvement approach.

Steps to take in implementation

For the purpose of the improver, one needs to have practical steps to take to ensure that the implementation process is planned in a way that it has a high chance of success The steps to be taken are to:

- Identify opportunities where there are gaps;
- Identify barriers of, and facilitators to, consistent use of evidence-based interventions;
- Review evidence on implementation interventions;
- Develop interventions to improve performance;
- Implement the interventions;
- Evaluate how implementation has progressed;
- Evaluate the outcomes of the interventions.

Summary

- Improvement and Implementation Sciences can work together to optimize uptake of interventions.
- Improvement Science allows for rapid testing of change ideas and adaptation to context.
- Implementation Science provides methods, frameworks, and rigour to ensure that implementation can be successfully repeated and the outcomes are sustained.

Signposting

Implementation Science is a journal with papers on theory and methodology. Available at: ℜ https://implementationscience.biomedcentral.com/ (accessed 10 September 2023).

Implementation Science Communications. Available at: ℜ https://implementationsciencecomms.biomedcentral.com/ (accessed 10 September 2023).

Further reading

Wilson, P. and Kislov, R. (2022). *Implementation Science*. Cambridge: Cambridge University Press. doi: 10.1017/9781009237055.

Equity and quality improvement

Key points
- Equity is a critical domain of quality that has long been neglected.
- Equity can refer to different population groups such as those defined by ethnicity, gender, age, ability, or sexual orientation.
- Quality improvement projects can increase disparities if not designed to ensure that this does not occur.
- Cultural competence and addressing implicit biases are the key steps to addressing inequity.
- Measurement of outcomes in a quality improvement project should be stratified to ensure that one understands the impact on diverse populations.

The challenge of equity in healthcare

'Of all the forms of inequality, injustice in health is the most shocking and inhuman.'
Martin Luther King

What is the equity challenge?

In ⊃ Chapter 2, inequity in healthcare delivery and resultant outcomes was highlighted as one of the key challenges and gaps in quality improvement. Despite the progress made in most of the original six domains of quality, equity has been the most challenging domain to address and, as such, has been neglected until recently. A reason for this is that the majority of factors that impact the achievement of health and the provision of equitable healthcare extend beyond healthcare itself. In addition, the assessment of equity is not consistently included in quality improvement projects.

The coronavirus disease 2019 (COVID-19) pandemic exposed the enormity of the equity challenge due to the way we have historically designed healthcare systems, as well as inbuilt societal injustices and disparities. Nundy *et al.* (2022) proposed that equity be added to the *Quadruple Aim* to create the *Quintuple Aim* of better health, better experience, healthcare worker well-being, and equitable care at lower per capita cost (Figure 5.1).

Inequity is an issue in most healthcare systems. For example, in the United States, there are wide disparities in health services and outcomes (O'Kane *et al.*, 2021). In the United Kingdom, despite universal health coverage, there is widespread inequity at every level for people from different ethnic backgrounds, gender, sexuality, and physical and intellectual ability (Kapadia *et al.*, 2022).

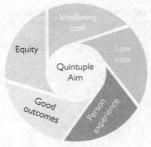

Figure 5.1 The Quintuple Aim.

Why is this important for quality of health and healthcare?

The separation of the various domains of quality is artificial, and in all our quality improvement projects, we must ensure that the outcome will be equitable for all. If there is inequity in the target population, one must design programmes that will mitigate against this, and there may be improvement projects that will focus on inequity itself. In a quality improvement project or programme, one should include equity in every project by asking three questions:

- Can I identify a disparity that may exist before implementation of the improvement programme?
- Will all those who will benefit from the project/programme benefit equally?
- Will the design of the project/programme allow the equity gap to be closed, or will the design widen the gap or make no difference?

In this chapter, we will discuss the concept of equity, the challenges inequity brings to us as clinicians, and the moral imperative to include achievement of equity at the core of every quality improvement project. The aim is to guide you to ways in which your improvement project can improve equity, even if it is focused on one of the other domains of quality. In addition, you will learn how to consider equity within every clinical encounter with people who receive care.

Although published literature focuses largely on ethnicity and the social construct of race, we will consider all forms of inequity within the approach to addressing the equity challenge. We offer a step-by-step process that will assist you in including equity in every project that you undertake. In Box 5.1 a case study example of being curious about equity is provided.

Box 5.1 Case study: being curious about equity

John is a new intern on the medical ward. He notices that the ward has patients from many different backgrounds. He also notices that the length of stay for some patients is longer than for others, even when they have the same clinical condition. He asks the consultant on the ward whether there can be a reason for this. After all, the care is the same and the diagnosis is the same. They discuss every patient equally and provide what they perceive to be standardized care. He wonders whether there is something more to this and if they could design an improvement project to ensure that everyone has an equal chance of going home as soon as possible. He realizes this will need an integrated approach to care, involving all who are part of the wider care for the people on the ward.

Signposting

Health Improvement Scotland (Scotland). *Equity, health inequality and quality improvement.* Available at: ℘ https://ihub.scot/media/7605/inequalities-and-quality-improvement.pdf (accessed 10 September 2023).

Health Service Executive (Ireland). *Diversity, equality and inclusion.* Available at: ℘ https://health service.hse.ie/staff/procedures-guidelines/diversity-equality-and-inclusion/ (accessed 10 September 2023).

Institute for Healthcare Improvement (United States). *Health equity.* Available at: ℘ https://www.ihi.org/Topics/Health-Equity/Pages/default.aspx (accessed 10 September 2023).

NHS England (England). *The equality and health inequalities hub.* Available at: ℘ https://www.engl and.nhs.uk/about/equality/equality-hub/ (accessed 10 September 2023).

Further reading

Stokes, J. (2022). Inequalities exacerbated: an all-too-familiar story. *BMJ Quality and Safety*, 31(8), pp. 561–4. doi: 10.1136/bmjqs-2021-014422.

Van Daalen, K.R., Kaiser, J., Kebede, S., et al. (2022). Racial discrimination and adverse pregnancy outcomes: a systematic review and meta-analysis. *BMJ Global Health*, 7(8), p. e009227. doi: 10.1136/bmjgh-2022-009227.

Warner, M., Burn, S., Stoye, G., Aylin, P.P., Bottle, A., and Propper, C. (2021). Socioeconomic deprivation and ethnicity inequalities in disruption to NHS hospital admissions during the COVID-19 pandemic: a national observational study. *BMJ Quality and Safety*, 31(8), pp. 590–8. doi: 10.1136/bmjqs-2021-013942.

References

Kapadia, D., Zhang, J., Salway, S., et al. (2022). *Ethnic inequalities in healthcare: a rapid evidence review*. Available at: 🔗 https://www.nhsrho.org/publications/ethnic-inequalities-in-healthcare-a-rapid-evidence-review/ (accessed 10 September 2023).

Nundy, S., Cooper, L.A., and Mate, K.S. (2022). The Quintuple Aim for health care improvement. *JAMA*, 327(6), pp. 521–2. doi: 10.1001/jama.2021.25181.

O'Kane, M., Agrawal, S., Binder, L., et al. (2021). An equity agenda for the field of health care quality improvement. *NAM Perspectives*, 2021, p. 10.31478/202109b. doi: 10.31478/202109b.

What is health equity?

What is the theory?

We do not live in a society where everyone has equal opportunities, even when healthcare is free at the point of contact, as in the United Kingdom. Health equity has been defined as follows:

> 'Health equity means that everyone has a fair and just opportunity to be as healthy as possible. This requires removing obstacles to health such as poverty and discrimination and their consequences, including powerlessness and lack of access to good jobs with fair pay, quality education and housing, safe environments, and health care. For the purposes of measurement, health equity means reducing and ultimately eliminating disparities in health and its determinants that adversely affect excluded or marginalised groups.'
>
> Braveman et al., 2017, p. 2

In Table 5.1, the risk factors contributing to health equity are outlined.

Equality does not mean that care is equitable, as shown in Figure 5.2. In the United Kingdom, all citizens have equal access to healthcare in that it is free at the point of contact. However, care is not equitable in that it depends on where one lives as to what care is on offer.

The challenge is wider than the design of healthcare itself, as inequity is rooted across society, such as in education, the social and community context, the neighbourhood and built environment, economic stability, and education—the social determinants of health. Therefore, every improvement project will need to consider how these determinants will impact the outcome of the project.

Table 5.1 Factors contributing to health inequity

Poverty	Poverty contributes to lower health access and worse health outcomes
Race and ethnicity	Implicit bias, discrimination, and prejudice against people of a certain race or ethnic group increase inequity
Refugees	In most countries, refugees are disadvantaged in healthcare
Gender	Bias against women is evident in many healthcare systems
Sexual identity	The LGBTQ+ community has historically been discriminated against
Age	The elderly may be impacted by ageism, with decisions made on the basis of age, and not on individual need. The cost benefit of treating an elderly person may be raised, which is a potential bias
Intellectual, learning, and/or physical disability	People with intellectual, learning, and/or physical disabilities face challenges with access and coordination of healthcare/
Location	Historically, people in inner city or rural communities have had inequitable access to care

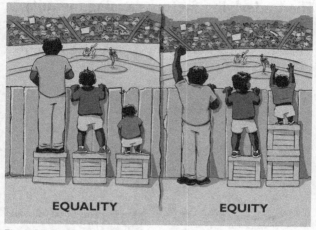

Figure 5.2 Difference between equality and equity.

Reproduced with permission of Interaction Institute for Social Change | Artist: Angus Maguire. ℘ interactioninstitute.org and ℘ madewithangus.com.

Further reading

Cecil, E. (2021). How equitable is the NHS really for children? *Archives of Disease in Childhood*, 107(1), pp. 1–2. doi: 10.1136/archdischild-2021-323191.

Cerdeña, J.P., Plaisime, M.V., and Tsai, J. (2020). From race-based to race-conscious medicine: how anti-racist uprisings call us to act. *The Lancet*, 396(10257), pp. 1125–8. doi: 10.1016/S0140-6736(20)32076-6.

Green, A.R., Tan-McGrory, A., Cervantes, M.C., and Betancourt, J.R. (2010). Leveraging quality improvement to achieve equity in health care. *The Joint Commission Journal on Quality and Patient Safety*, 36(10), pp. 435–42. doi: 10.1016/s1553-7250(10)36065-x.

References

Braveman, P., Arkin, E., Orleans, T., Proctor, D., and Plough, A. (2017). *What Is Health Equity? And What Difference Does a Definition Make?* Princeton, NJ: Robert Wood Johnson Foundation.

The underlying factors causing inequity

'Healers are called to heal. When the fabric of communities upon which health depends is torn, then healers are called to mend it. The moral law insists so. Improving the social determinants of health will be brought at last to a boil only by the heat of the moral determinants of health.'

Berwick, 2020

While the health system may state that there is equal access, the reality is that one needs to do more than provide equal access to ensure equity.

Several factors impact the delivery of equitable care and the achievement of equitable outcomes (Figure 5.3).

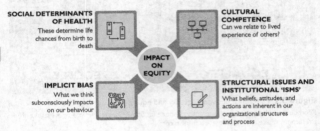

SOCIAL DETERMINANTS OF HEALTH
These determine life chances from birth to death

CULTURAL COMPETENCE
Can we relate to lived experience of others?

IMPACT ON EQUITY

IMPLICIT BIAS
What we think subconsciously impacts on our behaviour

STRUCTURAL ISSUES AND INSTITUTIONAL 'ISMS'
What beliefs, attitudes, and actions are inherent in our organizational structures and process

Figure 5.3 Determinants of equity.

Social determinants of health

- Michael Marmot introduced the concept of the social determinants of health (SDHs), stating that health outcomes are determined by '*the conditions in which people are born, grow, live, work and age*' (Marmot, 2005).
- For children and adults, social determinants influence life opportunities, disease profiles, health outcomes, and life expectancy. These SDHs include lack of power, poor access to jobs with fair wages, inadequate education, suboptimal or lack of housing, and poor healthcare.
- Despite the identification of social determinants, the way in which healthcare has been designed has had limited effect on alleviating their impact.
- Institutional and structural racism and societal prejudices continue to impede actions that are required to address SDHs.
- In a review in 2020, Marmot concluded that social and economic status determines health outcomes, and the lower the socio-economic status, the worse the outcome. In many countries, there have been similar reviews conducted in which social determinants have been documented to have a severe adverse impact on people (Marmot, 2020).
- The COVID-19 pandemic highlighted the significance of SDHs. For example, people of colour had significantly higher hospitalization rates and mortality for COVID-19, exacerbated by disparities in access to care.

Cultural competence barriers

- We live in a diverse society, and to meet the needs and what matters to our patients, we need to understand their priorities and their cultures, beliefs, and attitudes to health.
- The concept of cultural competence, that is, the appreciation and understanding of people from diverse cultures and backgrounds and the ability to interact in a positive way, requires one to have respect for values, beliefs, attitudes, and behaviours that may differ from one's own.
- While it is challenging to obtain a comprehensive understanding of every culture, the core principles of listening, hearing, and respecting the other person and finding out what really matters to them can help in providing care that is more than the technical, so it also meets the cultural needs of the individual.
- Some organizations offer training in cultural competence, though respect for all reflects the overall culture of the organization.

In Box 5.2 the challenge of addressing LGPTQ+ equity is illustrated.

Box 5.2 Cultural competence and LGBTQ+ communities

The challenge for people adversely affected due to lack of cultural competence by healthcare workers is exemplified by the way lesbian, gay, bisexual, and trans+ (LGBTQ+) people are treated.

In many countries, the civil rights for LGBTQ+ people are newly acquired, fragile, and not widely accepted. In other countries, there are no rights at all and therefore, LGBTQ+ people are marginalized.

As a result of these inequities, LGBTQ+ people report poorer health outcomes than the general population, and worse experiences of healthcare, particularly in cancer, palliative/end-of-life, dementia, and mental health provision, (Westwood et al., 2020). Mental health issues, especially in the adolescent age group, are high, as are risk-taking behaviours. (Hafeez et al., 2017)

Healthcare workers may not have the cultural competence to be able to address the needs of LGBTQ+ individuals and this is an area that requires improvement. Improvement programmes can acknowledge this challenge and aim to address the inequity that exists.

Implicit bias

- All healthcare workers are members of a wider community and research has demonstrated that, like the wider community, healthcare workers, including physicians, nurses, and allied professionals, may have subconscious or implicit biases that could influence decision-making and interactions with colleagues and patients (Box 5.3).
- These could be stereotyped perceptions, for example, that a particular population group has greater pain tolerance, that neonates do not suffer pain, that a person with specific pre-existing conditions should not be intubated, or that a person above a certain age should not have surgery.

Box 5.3 Case study: implicit bias and pain control

Despite a lack of racial differences in perception of pain or in pain management preferences, people of colour are less likely to receive appropriate and adequate analgesics, compared to 'white' patients. Practice differences stem from conscious or unconscious racial biases of healthcare providers and erroneous beliefs that there are racial differences in pain tolerance or there is a likelihood of misusing prescription opioids. (Morden et al., 2021)

This disturbing difference contributes to unnecessary suffering due to untreated or undertreated pain in specific patient populations. (Hoffman et al., 2016)

A quality improvement project to improve pain assessment and management must therefore collect and track data by differences in race and ethnicity to reduce disparities, as well as to avoid worsening existing disparities.

- These unconscious or implicit associations can influence how we speak, our non-verbal actions, and how we make decisions.
- One can have biases against providers and receivers of healthcare.

In Box 5.3 the way implicit bias impacts on pain management is demonstrated.

Structural issues and institutional 'isms'

- The structure of healthcare has not been designed to deliver equitable care.
- Historically, healthcare has been 'white male'-dominated, built on traditions and hierarchies.
- While the National Health Service (NHS) in the United Kingdom may have the overall principle of free access at the point of delivery, the distribution of resources may not be equitable, and within the organizational structure, there may be structural racism, sexism, homophobia, ageism, etc.
- In many countries, healthcare has inbuilt structural racism, which, in addition to the social determinants, results in inequitable care and poorer outcomes, as the healthcare system has been built on historical divisions and power distribution.
- Structural racism and ageism played major parts in the health outcomes of specific communities during the COVID-19 pandemic. In Figure 5.4, the processes involved in implicit bias and structural 'isms' are demonstrated.
- Many people will have a combination of biases and 'isms', for example, racism, sexism, and ageism.

In Box 5.4 the challenge of gender inequity is demonstrated.

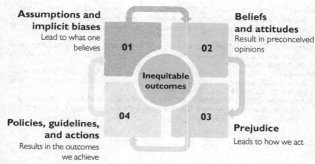

Assumptions and implicit biases
Lead to what one believes

01

Beliefs and attitudes
Result in preconceived opinions

02

Inequitable outcomes

04

03

Policies, guidelines, and actions
Results in the outcomes we achieve

Prejudice
Leads to how we act

Figure 5.4 Structural 'isms'.

Box 5.4 Case study: gender inequality

There have been numerous reports on the difficulty women have when attempting to receive the care they need and want, when compared to the care that is received by men.

In 2021, a House of Lords Health Committee reported that there are several areas where women do not receive equal treatment—from mental health to childbirth to menopause (Winchester, 2021). A 2018 BMA report indicated that there are wide disparities in health outcomes and gender is a key factor. These varied at different stages of a woman's life (Allen and Sesti, 2018).

For example, a 2016 study demonstrated that women with dementia received worse treatment than men, despite living longer (Cooper et al., 2017).

Gender inequity is a major challenge to be addressed and if combined with ethnicity, race, or disability, the impact is more severe.

References

Allen, J. and Sesti, F. (2018). *Health inequalities and women—addressing unmet needs*. Available at: https://www.bma.org.uk/media/2116/bma-womens-health-inequalities-report-aug-2018.pdf (accessed 10 September 2023).

Berwick, D.M. (2020). The moral determinants of health. *JAMA*. 324(3), pp. 225–6. doi: 10.1001/jama.2020.11129.

Cooper, C., Lodwick, R., Walters, K., et al. (2017). Inequalities in receipt of mental and physical healthcare in people with dementia in the UK. *Age and Ageing*, 46(3), pp. 393–400. doi: 10.1093/ageing/afw208.

Hafeez, H., Zeshan, M., Tahir, M.A., Jahan, N., and Naveed, S. (2017). Health care disparities among lesbian, gay, bisexual, and transgender youth: a literature review. *Cureus*, 9(4), p. e1184. doi: 10.7759/cureus.1184.

Hoffman, K.M., Trawalter, S., Axt, J.R., and Oliver, M.N. (2016). Racial bias in pain assessment and treatment recommendations, and false beliefs about biological differences between blacks and whites. *Proceedings of the National Academy of Sciences of the United States of America*, 113(16), pp. 4296–301. doi: 10.1073/pnas.1516047113.

Marmot, M. (2005). Social determinants of health inequalities. *The Lancet*, 365(9464), pp. 1099–104. doi: 10.1016/s0140-6736(05)74234-3.

Marmot, M., Allen, J., Boyce, T., Goldblatt, P., and Morrison, J. (2020). *Health equity in England: the Marmot review 10 years on*. London: The Health Foundation. Available at: 🔗 http://www.instituteofhealthequity.org/resources-reports/marmot-review-10-years-on (accessed 10 September 2023).

Morden, N.E., Chyn, D., Wood, A., and Meara, E. (2021). Racial inequality in prescription opioid receipt: role of individual health systems. *New England Journal of Medicine*, 385(4), pp. 342–51. doi: 10.1056/nejmsa2034159.

Westwood, S., Willis, P., Fish, J., Hafford-Letchfield, T., et al. (2020). Older LGBT+ health inequalities in the UK: setting a research agenda. *Journal of Epidemiology and Community Health*, 74(5), pp. 408–11. doi: 10.1136/jech-2019-213068.

Winchester, N. (2021). *Women's health outcomes: is there a gender gap?* Available at: 🔗 https://lordslibrary.parliament.uk/womens-health-outcomes-is-there-a-gender-gap/ (accessed 10 September 2023).

Leadership for equity

In all domains of quality, leadership is a vital component to achieve improved outcomes. For equity, this is essential, given the inbuilt structural barriers to equity and the complexity of the issue.

Addressing inequity needs to be a strategic objective at every level in an organization, from the board to the executive team to the frontline staff. Equity is the responsibility of everyone. Although most of the focus has been on inequity of healthcare due to the impact of structural racism, this applies to every other type of inequity.

- At the board level, the commitment to addressing all forms of inequity must be a priority and this includes both in the management of patients and their families and for just and fair employment practices.
- The executive must have equity as a strategic objective, with clear measurable objectives and outcomes.
- Many organizations will have a Chief Equity Officer, the equivalent of a Patient Safety Officer, whose responsibility is to oversee equity programmes.
- At middle management level, equity must be as important as financial management.
- At clinical levels, every team member must place equity at the core of their clinical work.

The main role of leadership is to ensure that:
- Inequity is not acceptable and is regarded as a serious event;
- Linkages are made across sectors to integrate the response to inequity;
- Structures and funding are provided to address inequity;
- A psychologically safe environment is fostered that allows people to call out incidents of inequity;
- Solutions are co-produced with the communities that are impacted by structural inequity;
- Data on access and outcomes are segmented to enable assessment of the current state and progress made;
- All improvement projects include equity as an outcome.

To address inequity, a culture of equity must be developed and nurtured, as indicated in Box 5.5.

Box 5.5 Essential ingredients for a culture of equity

1. Make healthcare equity a strategic priority for organizational leaders
2. Measure and track health inequities and disparities
3. Develop processes supported by organizational or team structures to deliver equitable outcomes
4. Address institutional workplace practices to ensure that they are equitable
5. Address institutional 'isms', such as racism, sexism, and ageism, within teams and the organization to support the workforce
6. Focus on health as a shared value which requires integrated work across teams, organizations, and sectors
7. Co-produce solutions with communities, so that their perspectives, preferences, needs, and goals are addressed.

Further reading

Chin, M.H., Clarke, A.R., Nocon, R.S., et al. (2012). A roadmap and best practices for organizations to reduce racial and ethnic disparities in health care. *Journal of General Internal Medicine*, 27(8), pp. 992–1000. doi: 10.1007/s11606-012-2082-9.

Dougall, D. and Buck, D. (2021). *My role in tackling health inequalities: a framework for allied health professionals*. London: Kings Fund. Available at: ℘ https://www.kingsfund.org.uk/publications/tackling-health-inequalities-framework-allied-health-professionals (accessed 10 September 2023).

Gebreyes, K., Rabinowitz, D., Ferguson, N., and Gerhardt, W. (2021). *Mobilizing toward health equity: action steps for health care organizations*. Deloitte Insights. Available at: ℘ https://www2.deloitte.com/us/en/insights/industry/health-care/health-care-equity-steps.html# (accessed 10 September 2023).

Health Improvement Scotland (2020). *Equity, health inequality and quality improvement*. Available at: ℘ https://ihub.scot/media/7605/inequalities-and-quality-improvement.pdf (accessed 10 September 2023).

Marks, A.K., Regenstein, M., Heinrich, P., and Mutha, S. (2012). *Bringing equity into QI: practical steps for undertaking improvement*. San Francisco, CA: Center for the Health Professions, University of California. Available at: ℘ https://healthforce.ucsf.edu/sites/healthforce.ucsf.edu/files/publication-pdf/6.2%20Part%202_Equity%20into%20QI.pdf (accessed 10 September 2023).

Mutha, S., Marks, A., Bau, I., and Regenstein, M. (2012). *Bringing equity into quality improvement: an overview and opportunities ahead*. San Francisco, CA: Center for the Health Professions, University of California. Available at: ℘ https://healthforce.ucsf.edu/sites/healthforce.ucsf.edu/files/publication-pdf/6.1%20Part%201%20_Equity%20into%20QI.pdf (accessed 10 September 2023).

Poynter, P., Hamblin, R., Shuker, C., and Jadria Cincotta, J. (2017). *Quality improvement: no quality without equity?* Wellington: Health Quality and Safety Commission. Available at: ℘ https://thehub.swa.govt.nz/resources/quality-improvement-no-quality-without-equity/ (accessed 10 September 2023).

Wyatt, R., Laderman, M., Botwinick, L., Mate, K., and Whittington J. (2016). *Achieving health equity: a guide for health care irganizations*. IHI White Paper. Cambridge, MA: Institute for Healthcare Improvement. Available at: ℘ https://www.ihi.org (accessed 10 September 2023).

Integrating models of care to decrease inequity

In ⏵ Chapter 12, the concept of complex adaptive systems will be introduced—that is, healthcare is a series of systems that interact in a dynamic way to deliver outcomes, both desired and undesired. When considering equity, one needs to consider more layers of complexity as the wider society as a whole is involved—social determinants, in addition to widespread beliefs, attitudes, and prejudices that may impact how services are designed and delivered.

- Care is siloed and the links between education, social care, and healthcare are complicated.
- People are falling through the cracks, especially those at the margins
- Funding is not integrated and the different interventions are not coordinated.

Integration of care is now a focus of quality improvement and needs to go further than managing disease when addressing equity.

- A systems approach is required, with a focus on health and prevention of disease.
- Interventions need to be made across sectors, as was demonstrated in the response to the COVID-19 pandemic.
- Social determinants require a multisectoral approach with integrated thinking.
- Communities need to co-produce solutions with providers aiming to increase the value of services (see ⏵ Chapter 8).

In one's improvement project, consider how the project can play a role in integrating the different elements that could decrease inequity. In Box 5.6, an example of integration of services to decrease inequity is shown.

> **Box 5.6 Integrating care to decrease inequity**
>
> In the NHS, there have been several initiatives to decrease inequity by integrating the way healthcare, social care, and education are delivered.
>
> In Scotland, the Early Years programme aims to work across sectors to give every child a start in life that will improve their life chances and decrease future inequity. The programme works closely with parents and families, and uses improvement methodology to develop solutions and scale them up (Early Years Scotland, n.d.).
>
> In England, the Born in Bradford programme aims to integrate care in a similar way in a deprived area with high levels of inequity. The programme aims to improve the outcomes for children and their families by working across sectors. It includes education and addressing environmental factors such as air pollution, as well as interventions to improve health (Born in Bradford, n.d.).
>
> NHS England has several programmes aimed at integrating care to decrease inequity, with a focus on prevention (NHS England, n.d.).

Further reading

NHS England (2019). *Integrated care in action—health inequalities*. Available at: ℘ https://www.england.nhs.uk/publication/integrated-care-in-action-health-inequalities/ (accessed 10 September 2023).

UCL Institute of Health Equity (2018). *Reducing health inequalities through new models of care: a resource for new care homes*. Available at: ℘ https://www.instituteofhealthequity.org/resources-reports/reducing-health-inequalities-through-new-models-of-care-a-resource-for-new-care-models/reducing-health-inequalities-through-new-models-of-care-a-resource-for-new-care-models.pdf (accessed 10 September 2023).

References

Born in Bradford (n.d.). *Born in Bradford*. Available at: ℘ https://borninbradford.nhs.uk (accessed 10 September 2023).

Early Years Scotland (n.d.). *Early Years Scotland: investing in our youngest children*. Available at: ℘ https://earlyyearsscotland.org/ (accessed 10 September 2023).

NHS England (n.d.). *Integrated care*. Available at: ℘ https://www.england.nhs.uk/integratedcare/ (accessed 10 September 2023).

Measuring to address equity

What is the theory for the measurement of equity?

A crucial step in addressing equity is to ask whether the data collected can be stratified to assess and track disparities and whether the improvement effort benefits all and closes disparities. (Kapadia et al., 2022) Ideally, these data are embedded into quality dashboards (O'Kane et al., 2021).

Hirschorn et al. (2021) recommend that one needs to look beyond the usual quantitative metrics and use a mixed measurement of qualitative and quantitative measures to ensure that the lived experience is captured. One needs to identify disparities and then implement programmes to ensure that these gaps are closed, and not widened.

Be aware of ways that improvement interventions could unintention- ally reinforce or exacerbate disparities. For example, artificial intelligence is being used to develop predictive algorithms to assess patients' risks for conditions and make treatment decisions. However, some algorithms, such as those that adjust for race, may reinforce historical patterns and further contribute to bias (Vyas et al., 2020).

How does one measure to improve equity?

To achieve measurement for equity, one needs to (adapted from Wyatt et al., 2016):

- Combine and stratify measures to show comparisons;
- Measure disparities in absolute terms to show differences in ratios or relative terms, to demonstrate changes over time;
- Show both favourable and adverse events to demonstrate comparisons of health indicators.

One needs to recognize that an improvement programme can have three effects on equity, as demonstrated in Figure 5.5. This is often termed the 'rising tide' impact of improvement—that is, all improve, but the disparity remains. In some cases, the disparity may increase.

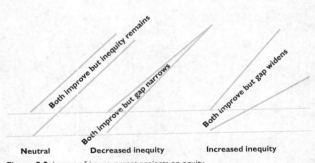

Figure 5.5 Impact of improvement projects on equity.

In Box 5.5 the potential of telehealth to increase inequity is illustrated.

Adapted from ⌕ https://www.solvingdisparities.org/tools/roadmap/linking-quality-and-equity.

Box 5.7 Case study: COVID-19 and telehealth

The COVID-19 pandemic led to a rapid acceleration of the adoption of telehealth in medicine. This increase in the use of telehealth increased healthcare access and reduced transmission of COVID-19 in healthcare settings. However, disparities in use of telehealth by patients with lack of access to technology and limited digital literacy were exacerbated. (Nouri et al., 2020)

These differences were especially problematic for rural populations, older adults, specific racial or ethnic groups, people with low income, and individuals with limited English proficiency. (Hsueh et al., 2021) Quality improvement efforts to increase telehealth use must address these technology-driven disparities during the design of interventions and collect data to track and reduce these disparities.

Further reading

Green, A.R., Tan-McGrory, A., Cervantes, M.C., and Betancourt, J.R. (2010). Leveraging quality improvement to achieve equity in health care. The Joint Commission Journal on Quality and Patient Safety, 36(10), pp. 435–42. doi: 10.1016/s1553-7250(10)36065-x.

References

Hirschhorn, L.R., Magge, H., and Kiflie, A. (2021). Aiming beyond equality to reach equity: the promise and challenge of quality improvement. BMJ, 374, p. n939. doi: 10.1136/bmj.n939.

Hsueh, L., Huang, J., Millman, A.K., et al. (2021). Disparities in use of video telemedicine among patients with limited English proficiency during the COVID-19 pandemic. JAMA Network Open, 4(11), p. e2133129. doi: 10.1001/jamanetworkopen.2021.33129.

Kapadia, D., Zhang, J., Salway, S., et al. (2022). Ethnic inequalities in healthcare: a rapid evidence review. Available at: https://www.nhsrho.org/publications/ethnic-inequalities-in-healthcare-a-rapid-evidence-review/ (accessed 10 September 2023).

Nouri, R., Khoong, E.C., Lyles, C.R., and Karliner, L. (2020). Addressing equity in telemedicine for chronic disease management during the COVID-19 pandemic. NEJM Catalyst Innovations in Care Delivery, 1(3). Available at: https://catalyst.nejm.org/doi/full/10.1056/CAT.20.0123 (accessed 10 September 2023).

O'Kane, M., Agrawal, S., Binder, L., et al. (2021). An equity agenda for the field of healthcare quality improvement. NAM Perspectives, 2021, p. 10.31478/202109b. doi: 10.31478/202109b.

Vyas, D.A., Eisenstein, L.G., and Jones, D.S. (2020). Hidden in plain sight—reconsidering the use of race correction in clinical algorithms. Obstetrical and Gynecological Survey, 76(1), pp. 5–7. doi: 10.1097/01.ogx.0000725672.30764.f7.

Wyatt, R., Laderman, M., Botwinick, L., Mate, K., and Whittington, J. (2016). Achieving health equity: a guide for health care organizations. IHI White Paper. Cambridge, MA: Institute for Healthcare Improvement. Available at: https://www.ihi.org/resources/Pages/IHIWhitePapers/Achieving-Health-Equity.aspx (accessed 10 September 2023).

Ye, S., Kronish, I., Fleck, E., et al. (2021). Telemedicine expansion during the COVID-19 pandemic and the potential for technology-driven disparities. Journal of General Internal Medicine, 36(1), pp. 256–8. doi: 10.1007/s11606-020-06322-y.

Quality improvement and equity

Translating the theory into practice can be a challenge. To address this problem, when you design your improvement project, the 10 steps in Box 5.8 can assist in your conceptual thinking.

Box 5.8 Designing an improvement project for equity

1. Recognize the problem.
2. Examine and reflect on possible inherent implicit biases that may impact on decision-making.
3. Consider the culture of the organization/team.
4. Reflect on the causes of the problem—both upstream (society) and downstream in the organization or team:
   a. The social determinants;
   b. The culture, system, and language used;
   c. The processes of care;
   d. The context;
   e. The wider community factors.
5. Consider the lived experience of all, especially those disadvantaged by the system and processes of care.
6. Segment, stratify, and analyse your data to demonstrate the problem.
7. Build trust with people, their families, and their caregivers.
8. Co-produce and share the solution with people providing and those receiving care.
9. Track and report data to demonstrate improvement from an equity perspective.
10. Continually ask if you are solving the equity challenge.

When you start your project, engage healthcare staff and patients and their families during the design and implementation phases, to ask them for their views and understand their lived experiences of delivering and receiving care.

This approach of '*what really matters*' will help you design, implement, and sustain a person-centred care project (see ➲ Chapter 8).

The key is to integrate equity into every quality improvement aim statement, driver diagram, and measurement plan. Co-production of solutions with people directly affected by inequity can ensure that equity as a domain of quality is not ignored and that solutions are realistic, effective, and sustainable.

The following two case studies are examples of how one can apply these principles. Inequity in quality improvement is often a problem of design, as indicated in the case study in Box 5.9.

In Box 5.10, there is an example of disparities in childbirth and how one can implement changes to address inequity.

Box 5.9 Missed opportunities

Diabetes is a growing problem in many communities and is disproportionally higher among the socially disadvantaged. A systematic review of quality improvement projects aimed at improving outcomes in diabetes found that only 95 out of 278 programmes that met the inclusion criteria included equity-relevant considerations (Lu et al., 2018).

This demonstrated the need for better definitions of the challenges, improved data collection, and analysis of the SDHs that impact outcomes for people with diabetes.

Box 5.10 Case study: decreasing disparities in childbirth

In many countries, maternal death in black and ethnic minorities is much higher than in the general population. In the United States, it is 3–4 times higher, and in the United Kingdom, it is five times higher than in the general population (MBRRACE-UK, n.d.).

Addressing this disparity requires interventions at different levels (Bingham et al., 2019):

- A systems approach looking at the SDHs or at a socio-ecological model from the individual to the community and the support systems;
- Acknowledging and addressing inherent systemic racism and inherent biases;
- Application of quality improvement methodologies, for example, with a cause-and-effect analysis (fishbone diagram) and stratified measurement;
- Applying continual improvement programmes aimed at decreasing and eliminating the disparity.

An understanding of these factors can help mitigate potential risk factors.

References

Bingham, D., Jones, D.K., and Howell, E.A. (2019). Quality improvement approach to eliminate disparities in perinatal morbidity and mortality. *Obstetrics and Gynecology Clinics of North America*, 46(2), pp. 227–38. doi: 10.1016/j.ogc.2019.01.00.

Lu, J.B., Danko, K.J., Elfassy, M.D., Welch, V., Grimshaw, J.M., and Ivers, N.M. (2018). Do quality improvement initiatives for diabetes care address social inequities? Secondary analysis of a systematic review. *BMJ Open*, 8(2), p. e018826. doi: 10.1136/bmjopen-2017-018826.

MBRRACE-UK (Mothers and Babies: Reducing Risk through Audits and Confidential Enquiries across the UK) (n.d.). Available at: ℘ https://www.npeu.ox.ac.uk/mbrrace-uk/reports (accessed 10 September 2023).

Top tips for SQUARE DEALS

As you approach the challenge of equity, this acronym may help us to give all: SQUARE DEALS (Table 5.2).

Table 5.2 SQUARE DEALS

Systems	Reassess healthcare delivery and financing systems and infrastructures to address structural inequities
Quantify and measure	Collect, report, and disseminate data on disparities to decision-makers and the public
Unify and integrate	Consider how integrated models of care can address inequity
Acknowledge	Be aware of potential biases and ensure cultural competency
Recognize	Raise consciousness of potential biases against those who may be vulnerable to any form of inequity. Consider how quality improvement interventions affect diverse groups
Engage	People, their families, and communities are essential partners in the design of improvement projects and programmes
Define	Call out inequities and disparities
Engage and co-produce	Engage and partner with communities, stakeholders, and patients to co-design solutions
Ask and be curious	Always be curious about inequity—if you do not look or ask, you will not find it
Lead	Leadership for equity at every level, from the board to frontline clinical teams, promotes psychological safety and investment in eliminating inequities
Study and analyse	Analyse and track data through an equity lens, and integrate equity into quality dashboards

Summary

Of all the domains of quality, equity has been the most difficult to address and is often neglected in an improvement initiative.

This may be due to the complexity of the domain, the SDHs, and the in-built structures in society that may facilitate and promote inequitable care.

The first step to take is to acknowledge that inequity exists and that all quality improvement programmes need to include equity as a core outcome.

The second step is to measure inequity to demonstrate what needs to be done.

The third step is to ensure that the quality improvement programme delivers the SQUARE DEALS.

Signposting

Advancing Health Equity. Available at: ℘ https://advancinghealthequity.org/roadmap-to-ahe/ (accessed 10 September 2023).

National Equity Project. Available at: ℘ https://www.nationalequityproject.org (accessed 10 September 2023).

NHS Race and Health Observatory. Available at: ℘ https://www.nhsrho.org (accessed 10 September 2023).

Further reading

Definitions

Cerdeña, J.P., Plaisime, M.V., and Tsai, J. (2020). From race-based to race-conscious medicine: how anti-racist uprisings call us to act. The Lancet, 396(10257), pp. 1125–8. doi: 10.1016/S0140-6736(20)32076-6.

Green, A.R., Tan-McGrory, A., Cervantes, M.C., and Betancourt, J.R. (2010). Leveraging quality improvement to achieve equity in health care. The Joint Commission Journal on Quality and Patient Safety, 36(10), pp. 435–42. doi: 10.1016/s1553-7250(10)36065-x.

Social determinants of health

Boozary, A.S. and Shojania, K.G. (2018). Pathology of poverty: the need for quality improvement efforts to address social determinants of health. BMJ Quality and Safety, 27(6), pp. 421–4. doi: 10.1136/bmjqs-2017-007552.

Chauhan, A., Walton, M., Manias, E., et al. (2020). The safety of health care for ethnic minority patients: a systematic review. International Journal for Equity in Health, 19(1), p. 118. doi: 10.1186/s12939-020-01223-2.

Lachman, P. (2021). Where to make a difference: research and the social determinants in pediatrics and child health in the COVID-19 era. Pediatric Research, 89(2), pp. 259–62. doi: 10.1038/s41390-020-01253-0.

Paremoer, L., Nandi, S., Serag, H., and Baum, F. (2021). Covid-19 pandemic and the social determinants of health. BMJ, 372(129), p. n129. doi: 10.1136/bmj.n129.

Robertson, R., Williams, E., Buck, D., and Breckwoldt, J. (2021). Ethnic health inequalities and the NHS: driving progress in a changing system. London: The King's Fund and NHS Race and Health Observatory. Available at: ℘ https://www.nhsrho.org/wp-content/uploads/2021/06/Ethnic-Health-Inequalities-Kings-Fund-Report.pdf (accessed 10 September 2023).

Singh, G., Zhu, H., and Cheung, C.R. (2021). Public health for paediatricians: fifteen-minute consultation on addressing child poverty in clinical practice. Archives of Disease in Childhood: Education and Practice, 106(6), pp. 326–32. doi: 10.1136/archdischild-2020-319636.

Tinson, A. (2020). Living in poverty was bad for your health before COVID-19. London: The Health Foundation. Available at: ℘ https://www.health.org.uk/publications/long-reads/living-in-poverty-was-bad-for-your-health-long-before-COVID-19 (accessed 10 September 2023).

Cultural competence

Horvat, L., Horey, D., Romios, P., and Kis-Rigo, J. (2014). Cultural competence education for health professionals. Cochrane Database of Systematic Reviews, 5, p. CD009405. doi: 10.1002/14651858.cd009405.pub2.

Saha, S., Beach, M.C., and Cooper, L.A. (2008). Patient centeredness, cultural competence and healthcare quality. *Journal of the National Medical Association*, 100(11). pp. 1275–85. doi: 10.1016/s0027-9684(15)31505-4.

Shepherd, S.M., Willis-Esqueda, C., Newton, D., Sivasubramaniam, D., and Paradies, Y. (2019). The challenge of cultural competence in the workplace: perspectives of healthcare providers. *BMC Health Services Research*, 19(1), pp. 1–11. doi: 10.1186/s12913-019-3959-7.

Implicit bias

FitzGerald, C. and Hurst, S. (2017). Implicit bias in healthcare professionals: a systematic review. *BMC Medical Ethics*, 18(1), p. 19. doi: 10.1186/s12910-017-0179-8.

Greenwald, A.G. and Banaji, M.R. (1995). Implicit social cognition: attitudes, self-esteem, and stereotypes. *Psychological Review*, 102(1), pp. 4–27. doi: 10.1037//0033-295x.102.1.4.

Marcelin, J.R., Siraj, D.S., Victor, R., Kotadia, S., and Maldonado, Y.A. (2019). The impact of unconscious bias in healthcare: how to recognize and mitigate it. *Journal of Infectious Diseases*, 220(2), pp. 62–73. doi: 10.1093/infdis/jiz214.

Raphael, J.L. and Oyeku, S.O. (2020). Implicit bias in pediatrics: an emerging focus in health equity research. *Pediatrics*, 145(5), p. e20200512. doi: 10.1542/peds.2020-0512.

Equity and quality improvement

Alfred, M. and Tully, K.P. (2022). Improving health equity through clinical innovation. *BMJ Quality and Safety*, p. bmjqs-2021-014540. doi: 10.1136/bmjqs-2021-014540.

Davidson, C., Denning, S., Thorp, K., *et al.* (2022). Examining the effect of quality improvement initiatives on decreasing racial disparities in maternal morbidity. *BMJ quality & safety*, 31(9), 670–678. doi.org/10.1136/bmjqs-2021-014225.

Glover, W. and Vogus, T. (2022). Beyond the equity project: grounding equity in all quality improvement efforts. *BMJ quality & safety*, 32(3), 129–132. doi: 10.1136/bmjqs-2022-015858.

Kumar, B., Mosher, H., Farag, A., and Swee, M. (2022). How can we champion diversity, equity and inclusion within Lean Six Sigma? Practical suggestions for quality improvement. *BMJ Quality and Safety*, 32(5), 296–300. doi: 10.1136/bmjqs-2022-014892.

Equity and patient safety

Chauhan, A., Walton, M., Manias, E., *et al.* (2020). The safety of health care for ethnic minority patients: a systematic review. *International Journal for Equity in Health*, 19(1), p. 118. doi: 10.1186/s12939-020-01223-2.

Chin, M.H. (2020). Advancing health equity in patient safety: a reckoning, challenge and opportunity. *BMJ Quality and Safety*, 30, 356–361. doi: 10.1136/bmjqs-2020-012599.

Research

Lion, K.C. and Raphael, J.L. (2015). Partnering health disparities research with quality improvement science in pediatrics. *Pediatrics*, 135(2), pp. 354–61. doi: 10.1542/peds.2014-2982.

Quality improvement and equity

Alfred, M. and Tully, K.P. (2022). Improving health equity through clinical innovation. *BMJ Quality and Safety*, 31, 634-637 doi: 10.1136/bmjqs-2021-014540.

Bingham, D., Jones, D.K., and Howell, E.A. (2019). Quality improvement approach to eliminate disparities in perinatal morbidity and mortality. *Obstetrics and Gynecology Clinics of North America*, 46(2), pp. 227–38. doi: 10.1016/j.ogc.2019.01.006.

Davidson, C., Denning, S., Thorp, K., *et al.* (2022). Examining the effect of quality improvement initiatives on decreasing racial disparities in maternal morbidity. *BMJ Quality and Safety*, 31(9), 670–678. doi: 10.1136/bmjqs-2021-014225.

Donaghy, G. and Pawlik, D. (2019). *What can be done to leverage quality improvement practice to increase its contribution to equity (and prevent increase in inequity)?* Available at: ✎ https://q.health.org.uk/document/what-can-be-done-to-leverage-quality-improvement-practice-to-increase-its-contribution-to-equity-and-prevent-increase-in-inequity/ (accessed 10 September 2023).

McHugh, S., Riordan, F., and Shelton, R.C. (2022). Breaking the quality–equity cycle when implementing prevention programmes. *BMJ Quality and Safety*, 32(5), 247–250. doi: 10.1136/bmjqs-2022-015558.

Reichman, V., Brachio, S.S., Madu, C.R., Montoya-Williams, D., and Peña, M.-M. (2021). Using rising tides to lift all boats: equity-focused quality improvement as a tool to reduce neonatal health disparities. *Seminars in Fetal and Neonatal Medicine*, 26(1), p. 101198. doi: 10.1016/j.siny.2021.101198.

Training

Aysola, J. and Myers, J.S. (2018). Integrating training in quality improvement and health equity in graduate medical education. *Academic Medicine*, 93(1), pp. 31–4. doi: 10.1097/acm.0000000000002021.

Parsons, A., Unaka, N.I., Stewart, C., et al. (2021). Seven practices for pursuing equity through learning health systems: notes from the field. *Learning Health Systems*, 5(3), p. e10279. doi: 10.1002/lrh2.10279.

Case study

Hadebe, R., Seed, P.T., Essien, D., et al. (2021). Can birth outcome inequality be reduced using targeted caseload midwifery in a deprived diverse inner city population? A retrospective cohort study, London, UK. *BMJ Open*, 11(11), p. e049991. doi: 10.1136/bmjopen-2021-049991.

Sustainable
quality improvement

Key points

- The climate emergency is a health emergency—now is the time to act!
- Healthcare is a major contributor to greenhouse gas emissions, air pollution, and single-use plastic consumption.
- Health professionals can create positive change and improve sustainability of the healthcare system through thoughtful design and quality improvement interventions.
- The Sustainability in Quality Improvement (SusQI) framework outlines an approach to integrating sustainability into quality improvement projects.
- Sustainability can be considered at every stage of your quality improvement project.
- Effective quality improvement projects can maximize value by improving health outcomes, while reducing negative environmental, social, and financial negative impacts.

What is the problem?

The climate emergency is a health emergency. The World Health Organization (WHO) has determined that climate change is the greatest threat of the twenty-first century to human health (Roland *et al.*, 2020). The time for action is now and the responsibility for change lies with us all. The impact of climate change and destruction of ecosystems influences public health in interconnected ways, as shown in Figure 6.1.

- The climate crisis disproportionately affects the health of vulnerable and economically disadvantaged populations who already suffer from health inequity.
- The WHO attributed 13.7 million deaths in 2016 to environmental factors.
- Although health systems endeavour to improve the health of populations, they are a significant contributor to carbon emissions (Eurostat, 2019).
- Healthcare in the world's largest economies accounts for 4.4% of the world's carbon emissions.

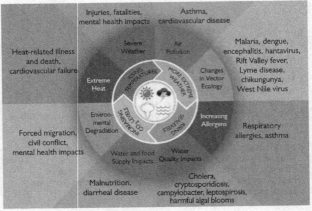

Figure 6.1 Impact of climate change on healthcare.

Reproduced with permission from Centers for Disease Control and Prevention (Climate Effects on Health | CDC, 2020).

Signposting

Centers for Disease Control and Prevention (2022). *Climate effects on health*. Available at: https://www.cdc.gov/climateandhealth/effects/default.htm (accessed 10 September 2023).

World Health Organization (n.d.). *Climate change*. Available at: https://www.who.int/health-topics/climate-change#tab=tab_1 (accessed 10 September 2023).

References

Eurostat (2019). *Healthcare expenditure statistics: statistics explained*. Available at: ℜ https://ec.eur opa.eu/eurostat/statistics-explained/index.php?title=Healthcare_expenditure_statistics (accessed 10 September 2023).

Roland, J., Kurek, N., and Nabarro, D. (2020). *Health in the climate crisis: a guide for health leaders*. Doha, Qatar: World Innovation Summit for Health. Available at: ℜ https://2020.wish.org.qa/ app/uploads/2020/09/IMPJ7849-01-Climate-Change-and-Health-WISH2020-201030-WEB. pdf (accessed 10 September 2023).

What can we do in healthcare?

We all have the responsibility and duty to actively make a difference in both our personal and work lives. We can reduce the risk to health through collaborative and decisive actions in reducing emissions, contributing to global efforts to limit the temperature increase to below 1.5°C.

- Mitigation activities against climate change can deliver health benefits (Box 6.1).
- Innovative leadership and mindful design can forge a more resilient, sustainable, high-quality healthcare system.

Box 6.1 Potential health benefits of actions on climate change

By decreasing air pollution
We can reduce the risk of:
- Sudden cardiac death
- Childhood respiratory diseases
- Prevalence and exacerbation of chronic obstructive pulmonary disease

By decreasing animal source fat and meat consumption and by increasing plant-based consumption
We can reduce the risk and prevalence of:
- Cardiovascular disease
- Type 2 diabetes
- We can decrease methane production in the dairy and beef industry

By increasing physical activity
We can decrease risk and prevalence of:
- Diabetes
- Cancer such as breast and colonic carcinomas
- We can improve mental well-being

Data from Remais et al., 2014.

Reference

Remais, J.V., Hess, J.J., Ebi, K.L., et al. (2014). Estimating the health effects of greenhouse gas mitigation strategies: addressing parametric, model, and valuation challenges. *Environmental Health Perspectives*, 122(5), pp. 447–55. doi: 10.1289/ehp.1306744.

What are sustainability and quality?

It is not possible to isolate quality improvement (QI) from the changes in climate (and their impacts on healthcare demand and health service delivery) and from the imperative for sustainable healthcare.

- High-quality healthcare involves delivering the right care to the right patient at the right time.
- Domains of quality include: safety, timeliness, effectiveness, efficiency, equity, and patient-centredness (Institute of Medicine, 2001).
- Sustainability has been established as a central domain of quality, with a focus on improving care for the patients of today without jeopardizing the health or care of patients of the future (Atkinson et al., 2010).
- Sustainable value in healthcare is maximized by assessing health outcomes of patients and populations against a triple bottom line of environmental, social, and financial sustainability.

$$Sustainable\ value = \frac{Outcomes\ for\ patients\ and\ populations}{Environment + societal + financial\ impact}$$

(re-created from Mortimer, Isherwood, and Wilkinson 2018, with permission)

- The cost of delivering healthcare relates not only to economic costs, but also to environmental and societal costs—a 'triple bottom line' (Mortimer et al., 2018). Societal and environmental costs are additions to the usual assessment (also see ➲ Chapter 7).
- Value may be increased by reducing waste, for example, through thoughtfully streamlining processes (see ➲ Chapter 13).
- Consideration of environmental and social sustainability is central to any QI intervention.

Further reading

Elley, C.R., Kerse, N., Arroll, B., and Robinson, E. (2003). Effectiveness of counselling patients on physical activity in general practice: cluster randomised controlled trial. BMJ, 326(7393), pp. 793. doi: 10.1136/bmj.326.7393.793.

Institute of Medicine (2001). Crossing the Quality Chasm: A New Health System for the 21st Century. Washington, DC: National Academy Press.

References

Atkinson, S., Ingham, J., Cheshire, M., and Went, S. (2010). Defining quality and quality improvement. Clinical Medicine, 10(6), pp. 537–9. doi: 10.7861/clinmedicine.10-6-537.

Institute of Medicine (2001). Crossing the Quality Chasm: A New Health System for the 21st Century. Washington, DC: National Academy Press.

Mortimer, F., Isherwood, J., Wilkinson, A., and Vaux, E. (2018). Sustainability in quality improvement: redefining value. Future Healthcare Journal, 5(2), pp. 88–93. doi: 10.7861/futurehosp.5-2-88.

Sustainable quality improvement

When setting goals for a QI project, the overall aim should be to increase the sustainable value of the service, process, or pathway on which you are working, using the sustainable value equation given above. The Sustainability in Quality Improvement (SusQI) framework provides a guideline on how to approach sustainable QI in your project (Table 6.1). This can be part of your planning and is incorporated in the analysis of a system (see ⊃ Chapter 12).

Table 6.1 The 'SusQI' framework

Setting goals	Actions
Studying the system (see ⊃ Chapter 12)	1. When undertaking your process map (see ⊃ Chapter 13), identify where environmental, social, and financial resources are being used at each step. This will help you identify waste and carbon 'hotspots', as well as unnecessary or low-value steps in a process. Hotspots can be defined as areas of intense production of greenhouse gases.
	a. Environmental resources might include: energy use, waste disposal, medical equipment, and patient/carer travel.
	b. Social resources might include: patient/carer or staff time, well-being, or other costs (e.g. time off work or school).
	2. Process mapping (see ⊃ Chapter 13) enables the identification of waste from resource mismanagement, overuse or over-reliance on resources, unnecessary steps in a process, and overuse of low-value steps/interventions. This can highlight potential assets.
	3. The environmental impact of a step or process can be measured in a number of ways, most commonly as carbon emissions.
	4. Carbon emissions (or carbon equivalent for non-carbon greenhouse gases) associated with various healthcare activities have already been estimated in many cases (Academy of Royal Medical Colleges, 2014).
	5. Include questions in the problem assessment on wasteful use of resources and the amount of carbon used at each step.
Designing the improvement project	Sustainable clinical practice aims first to minimize the need for healthcare activity in the first place and then to reduce the environmental impact of this activity. By using the principles of sustainable healthcare to generate improvement ideas, quality improvement projects can maximize sustainable value for healthcare.
	The principles of sustainable healthcare, listed in descending order of importance, are:
	1. Prevention of avoidable disease and complications;
	2. Patient empowerment and self-care to reduce reliance on health services;
	3. Lean systems and pathways (see ⊃ Chapter 14);
	4. Preferential use of technologies and interventions with lower environmental impact.

Table 6.1 *(Contd.)*

Setting goals	Actions
Measuring the impact	Employ the 'triple bottom line' approach and expand analysis of outcomes to capture: • Environmental impacts (e.g. reduced carbon emissions from decreased patient journeys); • Social benefits (e.g. staff well-being, time savings, increased productivity); • Financial costs (see ➲ Chapter 7).

Data from Mortimer *et al.*, 2018.

References

Academy of Royal Medical Colleges (2014). *Protecting resources, promoting value: a doctor's guide to cutting waste in clinical care.* Available at: ℘ https://www.aomrc.org.uk/wp-content/uploads/2016/05/Protecting_Resources_Promoting_Value_1114.pdf (accessed 10 September 2023).

Mortimer, F., Isherwood, J., Wilkinson, A., and Vaux, E. (2018). Sustainability in quality improvement: redefining value. *Future Healthcare Journal*, 5(2), pp. 88–93. doi: 10.7861/futurehosp.5-2-88.

How to calculate the carbon footprint in your project

The carbon impact of individual projects, services, and procedures is not routinely measured. However, in line with the commitments of the National Health Service (NHS) to reduce direct carbon emissions to net zero by 2040, those working in the NHS will be asked increasingly to understand, measure, and reduce the environmental impact of the work they do. It is therefore important for clinicians doing quality improvement projects and quality improvement managers to become carbon-literate. This is an essential skill for evaluating the impact of a quality improvement project in terms of its sustainable value across the triple bottom line.

A carbon footprint can be understood by using this equation:

Carbon footprint ($kg\ CO_2\ e$) = Activity or resource used $\times$ greenhouse gas emission factors

(Source: SUSQI https://www.susqi.org/)

- The carbon footprint of a process or pathway can be calculated by working out the amount of resources used or activity undertaken at each step, and multiplying by the greenhouse gas (GHG) emission factor.
- Working out the carbon footprint of an entire process can help to identify 'carbon hotspots'.
- These are areas with the highest carbon footprint, and identifying these can help you to find a project focus.
- When calculating the carbon savings made by your improvement idea, you only need to calculate the carbon footprint of the parts of the process that are affected by your improvement (Box 6.2).

Follow these steps for calculating the carbon footprint of a process:
1. Specify each step with a process map (see ⊃ Chapter 13).
2. Using the equation given above, measure the carbon emissions (or carbon equivalent) associated with each step of the process by quantifying the amount of resource used or activity undertaken and multiplying by the emission factor.
3. Emission factors can be found on the SusQI website.
4. Introduce the change idea and measure the change in resource use or activity data (e.g. a 10% reduction in the number of patient journeys).
5. Multiply the change by the relevant carbon emission factor to get the carbon savings.

- It is important to note that you do not always need to work out a carbon footprint to get an idea of the environmental impact of a process, pathway, or intervention. Calculating the overall use of a particular resource is a simple way to quantify the environmental impact, and can be achieved by measuring the amount of resource that is used, wasted, or disposed of for each part of a process (e.g. the amount of water used by a haemodialysis machine per use, or the number of non-sterile gloves used by a hospital department in 1 month).
- It is also important to have in mind that there are other environmental impacts of the healthcare system such as water, soil, or air pollution. The impact of this pollution may not be best captured with a carbon footprint but should still be considered as an important area of the healthcare system's negative environmental impact.

Box 6.2 Calculating the carbon footprint

Ali's quality improvement idea reduces the number of duplicate prescriptions for pressurized metered-dose inhalers (PMDIs) prescribed to
patients with asthma on his respiratory ward. Ali is aware that PMDIs
have a significant carbon footprint of 24kg per inhaler (Green Inhaler,
n.d.).

**Before the intervention per
3 months:**

50 duplicate prescriptions	$= 24kgCO_2e$ per inhaler
PMDI inhaler emission factors	$= 50 \times 24 = 1200kgCO_2e$
Carbon footprint	

After the intervention:

25 duplicate prescriptions	$=$ change of 50%
50% of $1200kgCO_2e$	$= 600kgCO_2e$
Carbon savings per 3 months	$= 600kgCO_2e$
	$= 2500km$ driven in a small petrol car
	$=$ Lighting the Eiffel tower for 8 days
	$= 20$ adult trees absorbing carbon dioxide over a year

Signposting

NHS England (2020). *Delivering a net zero NHS*. Available at: ℘ https://www.england.nhs.uk/gre
enernhs/publication/delivering-a-net-zero-national-health-service/ (accessed 10 September
2023).

Further reading

Tennison, I., Roschnik, S., Ashby, B., et al. (2021). Health care's response to climate change: a carbon
footprint assessment of the NHS in England. *The Lancet Planetary Health*, 5(2), pp. e84–92.
doi: 10.1016/S2542-5196(20)30271-0.

References

Green Inhaler (n.d.). *The problem with inhalers*. Available at: ℘ https://greeninhaler.org/the-prob
lem-with-inhalers/ (accessed 10 September 2023).
The Centre for Sustainable Healthcare (n.d.). *Measuring environmental impact* (calculation of emission factors). Available at: ℘ https://www.susqi.org/_files/ugd/f57abc_5da876a6470d491a9
23a1af69f2c64a9.pdf (accessed 10 September 2023).

How to measure the social impacts of your project

The social impacts of a project are understood in terms of impacts on patients and their carers/relatives, staff, the wider community, and vulnerable groups (e.g. those with disabilities or deprived groups).

- Social impacts refer to the social determinants of health—the conditions in which a person lives that determine their experience of health and disease (education, satisfaction and well-being, financial security, community networks) (see ⮑ Chapter 5).
- For example, if a patient's pathway involves many trips to the hospital for appointments, tests, or investigations, then this can negatively impact on the patient's employment (need to take days off work) or education (need to take days off school).
- Social impacts can be more difficult to quantify but can follow a similar process to calculating the carbon footprint of your project.
- You need to measure:
  - The social impacts of your current process, pathway, step, or procedure on patients and their carers/relatives, staff, the wider community, and specific vulnerable groups; and
    - How improvement idea positively or negatively changes the social impact.
- You can measure social impacts using qualitative data (e.g. staff or patient feedback via surveys) or quantitative data (e.g. number of schooldays missed). This might include proxy measures; for example, staff sickness days can be an indicator of staff stress, burnout, or low satisfaction.

Signposting

Centre for Sustainable Healthcare. *Measure the impact*. Available at: ⌖ https://www.susqi.org/measuring-impact (accessed 10 September 2023).

Further reading

Mortimer, F., Isherwood, J., Pearce, M., Kenward, C., and Vaux, E. (2018). Sustainability in quality improvement: measuring impact. *Future Healthcare Journal*, 5(2), pp. 94–7. doi: 10.7861/futurehosp.5-2-94.

Intervention ideas for sustainable quality improvement

We can generate high-value change ideas by using the principles of sustainable healthcare, as indicated in Box 6.3.

You can also break down the impact of healthcare on the environment to define areas where an impact can be made, as shown below.

Box 6.3 Intervention ideas

1. *Prevention strategies*
- Prevention of avoidable illness and disease (e.g. increased referrals to smoking cessation services).

2. *Patient empowerment*
- Introducing programmes of shared decision-making and self-management for people who have long-term conditions, thereby decreasing their dependence on healthcare providers.

Consider how your service engages with patients and families (see ➔ Chapter 8)

3. *Lean pathways*
(See ➔ p. 59 and ➔ Chapter 14 p. 308.)
- Applying lean methodologies to reduce steps in a process that do not add value, for example, setting up an integrated process for people with a chronic multiorgan condition, thereby reducing the number of clinics they need to attend, including the introduction of telemedicine where possible.

Work with other clinicians to integrate services around the patient.

4. *Low carbon alternatives (e.g. interventions that can decrease carbon waste)*
- Reviewing and changing the use of higher-carbon inhalers to lower-carbon versions (e.g. from salbutamol to salamol in all clinics).
  Consider all the clinics in which you can reduce your carbon footprint.
- Decreasing the waste of energy; for example, staff turning off equipment and machines at night and weekends could create significant energy savings (e.g. a hospital could save 120 000kWh and €9100 per annum).

Consider all your activities to see how you can save carbon and reduce the use of consumables.

Challenge of healthcare waste

Healthcare produces substantial waste, which requires careful consideration, so that we can move to a more rational utilization of resources. The focus can be on recycling and reusing where possible, but more importantly on asking whether there is any need to use the item in the first place.

The coronavirus disease 2019 (COVID-19) pandemic increased the amount of single-use personal protective equipment (PPE). As PPE reduces transmission and protects staff and patients, we need to ensure rational use of PPE and that unnecessary use is decreased. A WHO (2022) report on PPE and waste in COVID-19 showed that 75% of waste could be prevented by rational use and safe reuse. In addition, a move from single-use to recyclable PPE may be possible (Rizan et al., 2021). Reduction in the use of PPE, as well as reuse and recycling, is essential, along with local manufacturing to decrease transport (Uddin et al., 2021).

In Box 6.4 an example of how to decrease the carbon footprint is given.

Box 6.4 Case study: decreasing carbon footprint by waste prevention and diversion of recyclables

Healthcare risk waste (HCRW), due to its potentially infectious nature, must be disposed of correctly. In Ireland, the Green Healthcare Programme found that only 66% of the waste in HCRW bins was, in fact, risk waste (Green Healthcare, n.d.). The cost differential between incineration of HCRW at €2123 per tonne versus general waste at €130–200 per tonne and recycling at €0–170 per tonne is sizeable. The co-benefits of prioritizing sustainability in healthcare are apparent, as correct waste classification is economically efficient, as well as environmentally preferable.

What can you do?
- Develop or review your facility's waste classification policy.
- Raise awareness and train staff on segregation policies.
- Remove HCRW bins from inappropriate areas to avoid incorrect disposal of waste.
- Risk waste benchmarking allows hospitals to identify if they produce more or less waste than the national average.

Quality improvement project example
Roger recently learnt of the price differential between various types of hospital waste. He had noticed inappropriate waste being placed in the sharps containers for years, but now was the time to act! Over the course of 2 weeks, he assessed the waste in the sharps containers and made an estimate of their weight. He presented his findings at the next ward meeting and educated his colleagues on the impact of incorrectly disposing of waste. He created an infographic and, in consultation with the ward manager, attached it to the wall above the bins. He piloted this intervention on one ward initially. After 1 month, he assessed the contents of the sharps containers. He extended his project to a number of other wards thereafter.

Challenge of greenhouse gas emissions from activities in healthcare

Greenhouse gas emissions remain a problem in healthcare activities. Examples include:
- Embedded emissions from the manufacture and processing of healthcare products through supply;
- Energy use in care facilities;

- Use of water in facilities, as well as for cooling equipment;
- Detergents used in laundries impacting on water quality;
- Unnecessary travel for staff and patients.

In Box 6.5 an example of how to decrease carbon footprint using telemedicine is described.

> **Box 6.5 Case study: decreasing carbon footprint by using telemedicine and digital health to decrease unnecessary travel**
>
> Telemedicine signifies a viable mitigation strategy to lower carbon emissions associated with transportation when compared to the traditional model (NHS Sustainable Development Unit, 2012). The acceleration in adoption of telemedicine across various specialties due to the COVID-19 pandemic has created a unique opportunity for change. The carbon footprint savings range between 0.70 and 372kgCO$_2$e per consultation (Holmner et al., 2014).
>
> *Benefits for patients*
> - Decreased transportation cost
> - High patient satisfaction
> - Lower rates of outpatient non-attendance
> - Rural access to healthcare
>
> *What can you do?*
> Carbon emissions within the domain of telemedicine are also variable; for example, videoconferencing has a higher energy consumption vs phone consultation. As with any other sustainable project, it is important to scrutinize carbon expenditure at each step of the process. Further important considerations include patient safety, equity, and effectiveness.
>
> *Quality improvement project example*
> Conor is a dermatology trainee. During the COVID-19 pandemic, his department adopted telemedicine to improve access to care. He has moved to a new department and is eager to introduce telemedicine as a mechanism to promote sustainable healthcare. Conor creates a 'driver diagram' (see ⟳ Chapter 18) and organizes a meeting with the key stakeholders: consultants, administrators, the IT department, and hospital management. Conor creates a process map to outline each step of the new service development and assign tasks. Training is organized for doctors and administrators in the operation of the telemedicine software. After the new service is introduced, Conor would like to know if the dermatology patients are satisfied. He disseminates an online questionnaire and asks for feedback. Some patients preferred to have face-to-face contact, so more preference options were introduced whereby particular patients who would benefit from face-to-face consultations were still seen, thereby enhancing person-centred care.

Introducing lean pathways to decrease overuse or misuse of different aspects of care

This is a common problem, and one in which we all can play a part in reducing its impact:
- Medications prescribed when not needed, and not stopped when indicated;

- Diagnostic processes being overused;
- Interventions and procedures that do not add diagnostic or therapeutic value;
- Unplanned or unnecessary admissions to a facility for treatment when it could be ambulatory.

In Box 6.6 an example of decreasing the carbon footprint in a laboratory is provided.

Box 6.6 Case study: decreasing carbon footprint in laboratories

The carbon footprint of laboratory investigations is primarily associated with sample collection (e.g. plastic in phlebotomy tubes and vials), rather than with reagent use or power consumption. It is estimated that 12–44% of pathology tests ordered are not clinically indicated (McAlister et al., 2020). The main opportunity to decrease carbon emissions is through change in physicians' behaviour to avoid and reduce unnecessary testing.

What can you do?
- Order tests that are clinically appropriate (e.g. when the outcome will inform clinical decision-making and patient care).
- Create evidence-based investigation protocols.
- Co-produce solutions with patients to decrease the need for tests.

Quality improvement project example
Paul is a new registrar on the neurology ward. He is concerned about the carbon used in the processes for blood testing. He decides to try to reduce the carbon footprint. He studied the process for routine blood testing and noticed that every week, routine SMAC blood test was undertaken on every patient on the ward, even if it was not indicated. He decided to work out how much carbon was used per blood test. He broke down the analysis into:
- The needles and plastic packaging;
- The sterile pack;
- Other consumables on the ward.

He then went to the laboratory and, with the technique, worked out the carbon footprint of the actual test (e.g. energy expenditure, water use, reagents, waste). Once he had the baseline data, he then approached the consultant and nursing team with an improvement plan to reduce the carbon footprint of blood testing. The aim was to decrease the number of inappropriate tests over the next 6 months, and one of the outcome measures was a decrease in carbon footprint.

Empowering people to make changes

For meaningful progress to be made, all clinicians need to make sustainable healthcare a core part of their daily work processes, with clear outcomes. In ⊃ Chapter 10, ways to empower people are discussed, with strategies used to bring people together on the improvement and sustainability journey and to bring about a culture change:

- Adopting a systems approach to assess the way in which the microsystem works (see ➔ Chapter 12);
- Assessing all processes of care to see opportunities for change;
- Starting with the processes that are within your control;
- Collaborating with different teams, wards, and specialties, acting as an agent of change (Box 6.7);
- Joining the Green Impact Team/Green Champions or reaching out to the Sustainability Officer/Sustainability Team to see how you can be involved.

Box 6.7 Case study: doctors as agents of change

Prescribing

Pharmaceuticals contribute to approximately 20% of NHS England's carbon footprint. This is a major carbon hotspot for primary care, contributing to 40% of its total emissions and metered dose inhalers to 22%. It has been estimated that £300 m of medication remains unused in England annually, creating downstream economic and environmental impacts (Tennison *et al.*, 2021).

What can you do?

- Employ evidence-based prescribing.
- Prescribe generic medication when available.
- Promote medication adherence through patient education.
- Avoid overprescribing and overmedicalization—see 'Too Much Medicine' available at https://www.bmj.com/too-much-medicine (accessed 10 September 2023) ; and 'Choosing Wisely', available at: ℅ https://www.choosingwisely.org (accessed 10 September 2023).

Quality improvement project example

Amira has recently become interested in sustainable healthcare but is unsure of how she can make a difference as a junior doctor. While reflecting on her daily tasks as a surgical trainee, she noted the high volume of post-operative discharge prescriptions that she completed. First, Amira wondered whether her prescriptions for analgesia were evidence-based and whether there was an up-to-date protocol.

She wanted to reduce waste in her practice and also examine whether unnecessary opiate medication, in particular, was being prescribed for post-operative use. Applying the Plan–Do–Study–Act (PDSA) strategy (see ➔ Chapters 3, 14 and 18), she retrospectively reviewed the prescribing practices on the ward. She then wondered how many opiate medications had been prescribed in excess of pain requirements. To investigate this further, she developed a questionnaire for dissemination at patients' first post-operative outpatient visit.

Amira's interventions included:

- Adding a visual pain analogue scale to the chart;
- Dissemination of the WHO analgesic ladder to colleagues;
- Practising person-centred care by discussing opiate use with patients prior to discharge;
- Developing a patient information leaflet on post-operative analgesia.

The aim was to reduce unnecessary prescribing, with the co-benefit of increasing awareness of potential opiate dependence.

Signposting

World Health Organization (2022). *Global analysis of health care waste in the context of COVID-19: status, impacts and recommendations*. Geneva: World Health Organization. Available at: ℘ https://www.who.int/publications/i/item/9789240039612 (accessed 10 September 2023).

Further reading

Born, K. B., Levinson, W., and Vaux, E. (2023). Choosing wisely and the climate crisis: a role for clinicians. *BMJ Quality and Safety*. Doi: 10.1136/bmjqs-2023-015928.

References

Green Healthcare (n.d.). Risk waste. Available at: ℘ https://greenhealthcare.ie/topics/risk-waste/ (accessed 10 September 2023).

Holmner, Å., Ebi, K.L., Lazuardi, L., and Nilsson, M. (2014). Carbon footprint of telemedicine solutions: unexplored opportunity for reducing carbon emissions in the health sector. *PloS One*, 9(9), p. e105040. doi: 10.1371/journal.pone.0105040.

McAlister, S., Barratt, A.L., and McGain, F. (2020). The carbon footprint of pathology testing. *Medical Journal of Australia*, 213(10), p. 477. doi: 10.5694/mja2.50839.

Rizan, C., Reed, M., and Bhutta, M.F. (2021). Environmental impact of personal protective equipment distributed for use by health and social care services in England in the first six months of the COVID-19 pandemic. *Journal of the Royal Society of Medicine*, 114(5), p. 014107682110015. doi: 10.1177/01410768211001583.

Tennison, I., Roschnik, S., Ashby, B., *et al*. (2021). Health care's response to climate change: a carbon footprint assessment of the NHS in England. *The Lancet Planetary Health*, 5(2), pp. e84–92. doi: 10.1016/S2542-5196(20)30271-0.

Uddin, M.A., Afroj, S., Hasan, T., *et al*. (2021). Environmental impacts of personal protective clothing used to combat COVID-19. *Advanced Sustainable Systems*, p. 2100176. doi: 10.1002/adsu.202100176.

Benefits of sustainable healthcare

All quality improvement projects can incorporate the principles of sustainable healthcare. On a system-wide level, there needs to be a strategic decision to include green healthcare at the core of all decisions—in how we plan, deliver, and measure healthcare quality.

The WHO (2016) has identified the following benefits from making sustainable healthcare a strategic objective. Sustainable healthcare can:

- Reduce the negative environmental impacts of health system activities;
- Provide environmental benefits from reducing negative, and strengthening positive, impacts;
- Facilitate financial benefits such as through more efficient use of energy and other resources;
- Lead to health benefits such as through improved management of waste materials;
- Improve access/quality benefits such as through use of telehealth technologies to reduce the need for patient travel;
- Ensure workforce benefits such as increased levels of employee engagement and improvements in recruitment and retention;
- Improve climate resilience such as better preparedness for extreme weather events.

In Box 6.8 co-benefits of sustainable healthcare are described.

> ### Box 6.8 Case study: co-benefits of sustainable healthcare
>
> *Green space projects (e.g. NHS Forest)*
> *Walks in green spaces represent a more holistic approach to patient care. Nature-based activities and exercise have many therapeutic benefits for physical and mental health.*
>
> Investment in green spaces is an excellent model for sustainable healthcare; the intervention benefits current disease and acts as a preventative strategy towards future disease. A positive externality of this health production is also carbon absorption and conservation. Through green space projects (e.g. NHS Forest, available at: ℘ https://nhsforest.org), patients, staff, and the wider community can reconnect with nature and enjoy the health benefits.
>
> *What can you do?*
> Healthcare providers can write 'green prescriptions' by prescribing physical activity in green space. For every 10 green prescriptions written, it has been shown that a 20–30% risk reduction in all-cause mortality can be achieved (Elley et al., 2003).
>
> Green walking applies the principle of sustainable clinical practice. Mental health sustainable value may be achieved through (adapted from Centre for Sustainable Healthcare, n.d.):
> - Prioritizing prevention to decrease the need for future use of healthcare;
> - Improving resilience by empowering people and their kin using shared decision-making and self-management, as well as social networks;
> - Delivering reliable care—right intervention, right person, right time— by the right person to the right person.

Box 6.8 (Contd.)

Quality improvement project example

Aoife is a new general practice registrar with an interest in health promotion and disease prevention. She wanted to introduce the concept of 'green prescription' to her current practice. Before embarking on her quality improvement project, she set out her SMART aims (see ➲ Chapter 18):

- To introduce green prescriptions to the Orchard General Practice, aiming for an increase from the baseline measure of 10% to 25% within the next 6 months (i.e. by December 2023).

The project is relevant, as green prescriptions can achieve a risk reduction in all-cause mortality and are achievable over the study period, based on the number of prescriptions currently issued.

Once she had identified the key stakeholders, she presented the evidence surrounding 'green prescribing' and discussed her quality improvement project at a practice meeting. In collaboration with the practice manager, practice nurse, community development officer, and community walker, they developed a physical activity programme.

Clients could enter the programme via self-referral or through green prescribing by a health professional. A number of routes for outdoor walking and running were established.

References

Centre for Sustainable Healthcare (n.d.). Available at: ⅏ https://sustainablehealthcare.org.uk (accessed 10 September 2023).

Elley, C.R., Kerse, N., Arroll, B., and Robinson, E. (2003). Effectiveness of counselling patients on physical activity in general practice: cluster randomized controlled trial. *BMJ*, 326(7393), pp. 793. doi: 10.1136/bmj.326.7393.793.

World Health Organization (2016). *Towards environmentally sustainable health systems in Europe: a review of the evidence*. Geneva: World Health Organization. Available at: ⅏ https://apps.who.int/iris/bitstream/handle/10665/340377/WHO-EURO-2017-2242-41997-57725-eng.pdf?sequence=3&isAllowed=y (accessed 10 September 2023).

Top tips

Think about sustainability at all stages of your work and in your improvement project.

In your day-to-day work

1. Be an agent of change and ask the following:
    a. Is this investigation clinically indicated?
    b. Is my prescription evidence-based?
    c. Can I reduce waste (e.g. packaging)?
    d. Does the patient need to come to the clinic or hospital?
    e. Can I decrease the use of water and energy?
2. Incentivize clinical engagement:
    a. Hold Green Ward competitions.
    b. Make sustainable healthcare a daily priority on the ward round or in your clinic.
    c. Measure the use of carbon in every clinical process we undertake.
3. In your improvement project:
    a. Be curious and ask how you can decrease the use of carbon.
    b. Study your clinical processes and assess the use of carbon and other environmental, social, and financial resources.
    c. When designing your QI project, ask what impact your intervention will have from a sustainable health perspective.
    d. Consider a QI project with a focus on improving sustainability.
    e. Discover the potential co-benefits of QI and sustainable health.
    f. Co-design and co-produce solutions with patients and frontline staff (see ➲ Chapter 8)

Summary

- Nurturing a culture of environmental sustainability in healthcare systems can introduce many benefits, including health promotion, enhanced efficiency, and financial savings.
- Thoughtful design of QI projects which focus on sustainability will produce benefits for patient and population health, as well as reduce costs and decrease negative environmental and social impacts.
- Sustainable QI places focus on maximizing high-value interventions and minimizing those which offer lower value to patients and the wider healthcare system.
- Health professionals can be agents of change by considering sustainability in their everyday work and encouraging colleagues and patients to act sustainably.

Signposting

Centre for Sustainable Healthcare. Available at: ℘ https://sustainablehealthcare.org.uk (accessed 10 September 2023).

Choosing Wisely (promotes patient–physician conversations about overuse in healthcare). Available at: ℘ https://www.choosingwisely.org (accessed 10 September 2023).

NHS England. *Greener NHS*. Available at: ℘ https://www.england.nhs.uk/greenernhs/ (accessed 10 September 2023).

Further reading

The challenges of climate change

This chapter is focused on QI and sustainable health. The references provide background reading on the challenge and impact of climate change for health and healthcare.

Lenzen, M., Malik, A., Li, M., *et al.* (2020). The environmental footprint of health care: a global assessment. *The Lancet Planetary Health*, 4(7), pp. e271–9. doi: 10.1016/s2542-5196(20)30121-2.

Romanello, M., McGushin, A., Di Napoli, C., *et al.* (2021). The 2021 report of the Lancet Countdown on health and climate change: code red for a healthy future. *The Lancet*, 398(10311), pp. 1619–62. doi: 10.1016/S0140-6736(21)01787-6.

Salas, R.N., Shultz, J.M., and Solomon, C.G. (2020). The climate crisis and Covid-19: a major threat to the pandemic response. New England *Journal of Medicine*. 383(11), p. e70. doi: 10.1056/nejmp2022011.

Sampath, B., Jensen, M., Lenoci-Edwards, J., Little, K., Singh, H., and Sherman, J.D. (2022). *Reducing healthcare carbon emissions: a primer on measures and actions for healthcare organizations to mitigate climate change.* (Prepared by Institute for Healthcare Improvement under Contract No. 75Q80122P00007.) AHRQ Publication No. 22-M011. Rockville, MD: Agency for Healthcare Research and Quality. Available at: ℘ https://www.ahrq.gov/healthsystemsresearch/decarbonization/index.html (accessed 10 September 2023).

Singh, H., Eckelman, M., Berwick, D.M., and Sherman, J.D. (2022). Mandatory reporting of emissions to achieve net-zero health care. *New England Journal of Medicine*, 387(26), pp. 2469–76. doi: 10.1056/nejmsb2210022.

Watts, N., Amann, M., Arnell, N., *et al.* The 2018 report of the Lancet Countdown on health and climate change: shaping the health of nations for centuries to come. *The Lancet*, 392(10163), pp. 2479–514. doi: 10.1016/s0140-6736(18)32594-7.

Economics of quality improvement

Key points

- Healthcare cost is an important element of quality. High-quality healthcare should be cost-effective and provide 'value for money'.
- Quality improvement (QI) initiatives may:
  - Reduce resource use and costs by making healthcare delivery more efficient;
  - Avoid unnecessary resource use and costs by reducing the risk of adverse events and poor outcomes;
  - Justify additional resources by improving healthcare delivery and outcomes.
- Health economic evaluation provides a framework for the assessment of costs and outcomes of QI initiatives:
  - The assessment of costs and effects without a comparison to an alternative is considered a partial evaluation.
  - In a full evaluation, cost-effectiveness is established by comparing the relationship between incremental costs and incremental outcomes of new initiatives compared with current practice.
  - The cost-effectiveness plane is a useful tool to illustrate and interpret the results of health economic evaluations.
- The costs and outcomes of QI initiatives should be assessed. At a minimum, consider the:
  - Costs of conducting the QI initiative;
  - Changes in targeted resource use, process, and health outcomes;
  - Consequential savings and avoided costs.
- Health economic benefits, such as costs saved, may not be realized as explicit financial savings but may generate capacity for use elsewhere.

Introduction

The resources available for healthcare are finite, and yet up to 30% of healthcare budgets are spent on wasteful processes (Shrank et al., 2019). Quality improvement (QI) activities can reduce waste and improve care and outcomes. However, the cost and value of these improved outcomes are not routinely measured or reported (Ko et al., 2022; McCarthy et al., 2021). This represents a missed opportunity to quantify the economic value of QI.

Health economics provides tools to appraise 'value for money'. A health economic evaluation assesses the relationship between health outcomes and costs. These evaluations can be applied to all interventions designed to improve quality.

In this chapter, you will learn:

● About the costs and outcomes of QI initiatives and how these can be assessed;

● How to use health economic evaluation of QI to support decisions about the most effective use of resources;

● Top tips for applying health economic evaluation in practice.

References

Ko, C.Y., Shah, T., Nathens, A., et al. (2022). How well is surgical improvement being conducted? Evaluation of 50 local surgery-related improvement efforts. *Journal of the American College of Surgeons*, 235(4), pp. 573–80.

McCarthy, S.E., Jabakhanji, S.B., Martin, J., Flynn, M.A., and Sørensen, J. (2021). Reporting standards, outcomes and costs of quality improvement studies in Ireland: a scoping review. *BMJ Open Quality*, 10(3), p. e001319.

Shrank, W.H., Rogstad, T.L., and Parekh, N. (2019). Waste in the US health care system: estimated costs and potential for savings. *JAMA*, 322(15), pp. 1501–9.

Terms used in the chapter

Terms used in the chapter are described in Table 7.1.

Table 7.1 Terms used in the chapter

Term	Definition
Partial health economic evaluation	Measures costs and/or health outcomes but does not have a comparator and does not relate costs to outcomes
Full health economic evaluation	Compares the costs, resource use, and effects of an intervention to a comparator and relates the costs to the effects in a summary metric
Unit cost	The cost of one unit of resource use
Opportunity cost	The potential benefit of a foregone alternative
Cost savings	The quantity of resource use and costs (i.e. the value of resource use) saved
Costs avoided	Costs of an event that are avoided
Cost-effectiveness analysis (CEA)	Analyses the costs of two or more similar initiatives in comparison to their effects by using a context-specific measure
Cost utility analysis (CUA)	Analyses the costs of two or more initiatives in comparison to their effects, where the measure of effectiveness is in quality-adjusted life years; identifies 'value for money' across initiatives with different target outcomes
Quality-adjusted life year (QALY)	A composite measure of health-related quality of life and mortality. One QALY denotes a full year with perfect health; fractions of a QALY denote a year with imperfect health
Incremental cost-effectiveness ratio (ICER)	The ratio of additional costs to additional outcomes associated with a new intervention in comparison to a comparator
Cost-effectiveness threshold	Refers to the maximum amount a decision-maker is prepared to pay for an additional unit of health effect; typically defined as a monetary amount per QALY
Net costs	The accumulation of all costs and savings related to an activity (i.e. the sum of costs related to the intervention, future cost savings, and avoided costs)
Net health effects	The accumulation of all health effects related to an activity (i.e. the sum of health effects over time)

Sources: Drummond et al., 2015; York Health Economics Consortium, 2016.

References

Drummond, M., Sculpher, M.J., Claxton, K., Stoddart, G.L., and Torrance, G.W. (2015). *Methods for the Economic Evaluation of Health Care Programmes*. Oxford: Oxford University Press.
York Health Economics Consortium. https://yhec.co.uk

Cost and quality improvement

The reduction of undesirable variation in healthcare is not a costless activity. Where possible, a QI initiative should aim to improve quality and decrease costs, that is, to provide better 'value for money' (see ⇒ Chapters 2 and 13).

Cost of poor-quality healthcare

Poor-quality healthcare imposes unnecessary burdens and costs on patients, health systems, and societies.

- It is estimated that 1 in 10 patients experience an adverse event while receiving hospital care (Connolly et al., 2021).
- Healthcare experiences the 60:30:10 ratio challenge—that is, 60% of healthcare complies to evidence-based guidelines, 30% is waste or low value, and 10% is harm (Braithwaite et al., 2020).

Costs accrue to both healthcare systems and society (Box 7.1).

> **Box 7.1 Examples of costs associated with poor-quality care**
>
> - *Healthcare cost*: treatment of safety failures from adverse events, estimated to cost 15% of hospital budgets (Slawomirski et al., 2017)
> - *Societal cost*: work absences from adverse event-related sickness and disability

Cost of high-quality healthcare

QI activities aim to improve patient and staff experiences and to achieve better health outcomes. However, delivery of high-quality healthcare can be costly, often due to the use of more expensive technologies and medications, as well as higher-skilled staff.

'Value for money' of quality improvement initiatives

To appraise the 'value for money' of a QI initiative, one needs to assess whether the QI initiative is better and cheaper than current practice. This requires an assessment of costs and outcomes. Two possibilities occur:

1. Initiatives that are clearly superior in both costs and health outcomes are called '*dominant*' initiatives. These offer 'value for money' by providing a clear gain in outcome and saving in costs. An example is provided in Box 7.2;

> **Box 7.2 Example of a QI initiative to reduce prescribing errors**
>
> A QI initiative employing an electronic patient record aimed at reducing medication errors may improve health outcomes and save costs. The electronic system may be less prone to human error and facilitate automated checking of contraindicated medications, leading to reduced adverse drug effects.
>
> The electronic system may also be faster to use, requiring less labour inputs, and so be less costly. Such an initiative that demonstrates health improvements and cost savings relative to paper-based records would therefore be 'dominant' over the status quo.

2. Initiatives that are inferior to the status quo are called 'dominated initiatives' or 'non-dominant over the status quo' (e.g. where the initiative improves outcomes and increases costs or reduces desired outcomes and decreases costs).

Many healthcare interventions are non-dominant, as it is often not possible to achieve health improvements without increasing costs (Drummond et al., 2015). These initiatives require further assessment by using a cost-effectiveness (CEA) or cost utility analysis (CUA) to determine if it is justifiable to adopt a more costly service (Box 7.3).

Box 7.3 Example of a more costly QI initiative to reduce falls

A QI initiative to reduce falls may use more expensive change strategies (e.g. more costly drugs, low-rise beds, better case management, weekly audit meetings) which may be more effective than the status quo.

There is a trade-off between increased effect (improved outcomes) and additional cost. The QI initiative is therefore denoted as 'non-dominant'. To determine the effects relative to costs requires a cost-effectiveness analysis. To identify 'value for money' among initiatives targeting different outcomes, a cost utility analysis is required.

References

Braithwaite, J., Glasziou, P., and Westbrook, J. (2020). The three numbers you need to know about healthcare: the 60–30–10 challenge. *BMC Medicine*, 18(1), p. 102. doi: 10.1186/s12916-020-01563-4.

Connolly, W., Rafter, N., Conroy, R.M., Stuart, C., Hickey, A., and Williams, D.J. (2021). The Irish National Adverse Event Study-2 (INAES-2): longitudinal trends in adverse event rates in the Irish healthcare system. *BMJ Quality and Safety*, 30(7), pp. 547–58. doi: 10.1136/bmjqs-2020-011122.

Drummond, M., Sculpher, M.J., Claxton, K., Stoddart, G.L., and Torrance, G.W. (2015). *Methods for the Economic Evaluation of Health Care Programmes.* Oxford: Oxford University Press.

Slawomirski, L., Auraaen, A., and Klazinga, N. (2017). *The economics of patient safety: strengthening a value-based approach to reducing patient harm at national level.* OECD Health Working Papers, No. 96. Paris: OECD Publishing.

Health economic evaluation designs for QI

The field of health economics offers evaluation designs of varying complexity to estimate the costs and cost-effectiveness of a QI initiative.

Activities of health economic evaluation

The activities required to establish costs and cost-effectiveness are outlined in Figure 7.1.

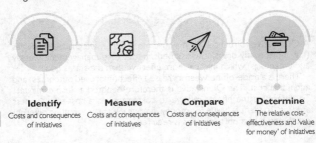

Identify
Costs and consequences of initiatives

Measure
Costs and consequences of initiatives

Compare
Costs and consequences of initiatives

Determine
The relative cost-effectiveness and 'value for money' of initiatives

Figure 7.1 Activities of health economic evaluation.

When deciding on the design of the health economic evaluation, it is important to consider the timing of the assessment and the health economic perspective to be adopted.

Timing of a health economic assessment

Health economic assessments can be conducted before (*ex ante*) an initiative is selected for implementation or after (*ex post*) an initiative has been implemented (Table 7.2).

- *Before*-assessments are required when there is a need to influence the resource allocation for a QI initiative in real time. For example, these may be included in the write-up of a business case for an initiative.
- *After*-assessments are used to account for resources used and to appraise actual costs and outcomes of the initiative.

These assessments help decision-makers to understand the costs and cost-effectiveness of a QI initiative.

Table 7.2 Timing of health economic assessment

Before (ex ante)	• Estimates anticipated costs and outcomes of a future QI initiative in comparison to alternatives
	• Uses expected values to assess which QI initiatives offer the best potential for improved outcomes and more effective resource utilization
After (ex post)	• Conducted when the QI initiative has been implemented and data on actual costs and outcomes are available
	• Provides a better foundation for decisions related to future iterations of a QI initiative, including the potential for spread or scale-up and wider dissemination

Adopting a health economic perspective

A health economic perspective or viewpoint needs to be adopted to decide whose costs and outcomes are to be included in the analysis (Drummond et al., 2015).

- The perspective may be that of the patient, the healthcare system, the government, or society as a whole.
- It is important to apply the perspective consistently.
- Most guidelines for CEA recommend which perspective to adopt. For example, the National Institute for Health and Care Excellence (NICE, 2022) in England and Wales recommends a healthcare perspective, whereas the Dutch Zorginstituut Nederland (2016) recommends a societal perspective.

Partial health economic evaluations

A partial health economic evaluation examines the basic costs and/or outcomes of a QI initiative. A cost description is an important first step in any design and is a useful cost-identifying exercise in its own right. An additional step to compare the costs identified to the costs of other similar initiatives (cost analysis) helps to identify where cost savings may be achieved.

There are three types of partial evaluation, as indicated in Table 7.3.

Table 7.3 Types of partial health economic evaluation

Cost descriptions without comparisons to status quo or alternatives	
Cost description	Outlines the costs and resource use of a QI initiative. No health or process outcomes are described
Cost outcome description	Describes the costs and outcomes of a single QI initiative. Does not examine the relationship between costs and outcomes
Partial evaluation with comparisons to status quo or alternatives	
Cost analysis	Outlines the costs and resource use of a QI initiative in comparison to one or more alternatives. The alternative may be the status quo (i.e. continuing care as normal). No outcomes are considered or are assumed identical

Drummond et al., 2015.

Cost outcome descriptions are useful for QI initiatives with no baseline data on the status quo and where comparisons of improvement using pre- and post-data is not possible. An example is when an organization introduces QI initiatives to target issues not normally measured as part of routine care or performance monitoring. These initiatives will require prospective data collection to form a baseline (see ⊙ Chapter 13).

Partial evaluations that do not include any comparison of an initiative to the status quo or any other comparator cannot be used to determine cost-effectiveness and 'value for money'.

Table 7.4 summarizes key characteristics of partial evaluations.

Table 7.4 Key characteristics of partial evaluations

Technical definition	• Examines either costs or outcomes only, or both • Except for cost analysis, a comparator is not used
Purpose	• Informs stakeholders about the basic costs and/or outcomes of the QI initiative • Identifies opportunities for cost savings • Provides cost and outcome categories prior to a full evaluation
Limitations	• Does not examine the relationship between costs and outcomes or utilize a comparator initiative, and therefore does not estimate or establish cost-effectiveness • The lack of assessment of the relationship between costs and outcomes means partial evaluations are not suitable for informing investment decisions

Drummond et al., 2015; Turner et al., 2021.

Full health economic evaluations

A full health economic evaluation examines the cost and outcomes of a QI initiative in comparison to current practice.

• The relationship between costs and outcomes is examined, as well as whether the initiative has had an impact on costs and quality.
• A full health economic evaluation may examine cost-effectiveness to provide an assessment of 'value for money'.

Concepts used in a CEA are shown in Box 7.4.

Box 7.4 Concepts used in a cost-effectiveness analysis

The *incremental cost-effectiveness ratio* (*ICER*) represents the trade-off between costs and health effects in initiatives that are non-dominant over the status quo (e.g. higher costs and better quality). It is calculated as a ratio between the difference in costs and the difference in the selected measure (e.g. events avoided or quality-adjusted life year (QALY)).

$$ICER = \frac{\text{Incremental cost}}{\text{Incremental effect}}$$

The ICER can be interpreted as the cost required to gain one additional unit of effect.

The *cost-effectiveness* (*CE*) *threshold* is usually determined based on social preferences, not by clinicians or patients. The CE threshold refers to the maximum amount a decision-maker will pay for an additional unit of effect. A cost-effective initiative is an initiative where the ICER is below the CE threshold. The CE threshold is typically defined in cost per QALY, as opposed to other health outcomes.

Health Improvement and Quality Authority, 2020; York Health Economics Consortium, 2016.

There are three types of full evaluation and they differ in how they measure outcomes (such as process changes or health effects) (Drummond et al., 2015). These are indicated in Table 7.5.

Table 7.5 Types of full economic evaluations

Cost-effectiveness analysis (CEA)	• CEA uses a context-specific measure of QI effectiveness (e.g. falls avoided) related to the cost, in comparison to alternatives
	• Effects are conveyed in natural units (e.g. falls avoided) and are not monetized
	• For QI initiatives identified as 'non-dominant' (i.e. 'both outcome and cost increasing' or 'both outcome and cost decreasing'), calculation of the ICER (e.g. cost per fall avoided) is required to estimate the cost-effectiveness of the initiative
	• ICERs defined in terms of non-QALY health outcomes do not permit comparisons to CE thresholds
Cost utility analysis (CUA)	• CUA expresses health outcomes as QALYs across different QI initiatives (e.g. QIs to reduce falls, pressure ulcers, and sepsis) and uses this common outcome to compare the cost-effectiveness of these initiatives
	• Uses the QALY as the outcome measure, and calculates the ICER and compares it to a CE threshold
	• CE thresholds vary between countries and are often not explicitly stated. The United Kingdom uses an explicit cost-effectiveness threshold range of £20 000–30 000/QALY (National Institute for Health and Care Excellence, 2022)
Cost–benefit analysis (CBA)	• CBA applies a monetary value to the resources consumed and the health consequences from an initiative in comparison to resources and health consequences from use of alternatives
	• This generates a comparison of the assessed value with the actual costs
	• It is not commonly applied in health economics and is not typically a recommended approach

Application of cost-effectiveness analysis to quality improvement

CEA is the primary method recommended for the measurement of cost-effectiveness of QI initiatives and alternative interventions targeting the same health outcome (e.g. falls avoided).
• Based on the CEA, if a particular QI initiative has been identified as more cost-effective, where possible, a CUA is useful as a follow-up step to fully determine the 'value for money', in comparison to initiatives targeting other outcomes (e.g. sepsis, deaths).

- A CUA is able to determine if an initiative offers sufficient 'value for money', as it compares the cost per QALY to the CE threshold. This is a proxy for the opportunity cost of other healthcare interventions (i.e. what the funding could be spent on instead).
- Comparison to the CE threshold permits indirect comparison of the intervention to opportunity costs elsewhere in the health system.

Table 7.6 summarizes the key characteristics of full evaluations, including how they may be best used in QI initiatives and their limitations.

Table 7.6 Key characteristics of full evaluations

Technical definition	Compares relative cost-effectiveness across initiatives by identifying 'health effects per cost' or 'cost per health effects' among alternatives
	Using QALYs and the CE threshold, a CUA compares the 'value for money' of a QI initiative among alternative courses of action
	Comparison of cost–benefit is less frequently used
QI purpose	Produces data about cost-effectiveness and 'value for money' to influence investment decisions
Limitations	For a CUA, generating QALY estimates from QI initiatives can be onerous

Process outcomes in cost-effectiveness analysis

Health economic evaluation typically seeks to assess outcomes in terms of health improvements.

- In some circumstances, QI initiatives might be able to demonstrate improvements in aspects of healthcare processes, although they might not be able to capture data on health improvements.
- In cases where process improvements are linked with unambiguous health improvements, these process improvements may be considered a reasonable proxy for (unobserved) health improvements.
- A pragmatic approach to CEA in such circumstances is to consider whether a QI initiative can achieve 'dominance' (superiority in both costs and health outcomes) in terms of cost per process outcome.

An example of a process-based outcome is the waiting time to see a clinician on admission to an emergency department. As a reduction in delay in receiving medical care might be linked with better outcomes, an initiative that achieves shorter waiting times could reasonably be assumed to be improving health outcomes.

How to use the cost-effectiveness plane

When one applies CEA or CUA, the anticipated or established outcomes of an economic analysis can be illustrated in a cost-effectiveness plane. This is represented in a quadrant diagram, as shown in Figure 7.2.

- The cost-effectiveness plane depicts the incremental costs and outcomes of an initiative relative to an alternative initiative or to maintaining the status quo, which is referred to as 'the origin' or the graph's centre point O in Figure 7.2.
  - The incremental effects are shown on the horizontal axis, with beneficial effects (positive outcomes) being those to the right of the origin.
  - The incremental costs of the initiative are shown on the vertical axis, with the portion below the origin representing cost savings (negative costs).
  - In the case of a CUA, the amount a decision-maker will pay for improvement (the CE threshold) is indicated by a diagonal line. The threshold may be made explicit by health economic advisory bodies such as NICE.
- Initiatives in the south-east (SE) quadrant have 'better effects and less costly initiatives' and are attractive to funders and do not require further analysis.
- Initiatives in the north-west (NW) quadrant with 'worse effects and more costly initiatives' are dominated by the status quo and are unattractive to funders and do not require further analysis.
- Initiatives in the north-east (NE) quadrant with 'better effects and more costly initiatives' and in the south-west (SW) quadrant with 'worse effects and less costly initiatives' require an ICER assessment to decide whether the QI project is cost-effective.

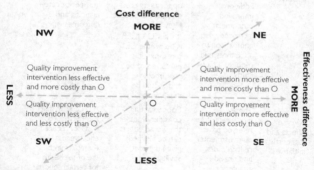

Figure 7.2 The cost-effectiveness plane.
Adapted from Drummond et al., 2015.

Examples of decision-making based on analysis using the cost-effectiveness plane are presented in Table 7.7.

Table 7.7 Decision-making using the cost-effectiveness plane

Quadrant	Interpretation	Recommended decision	Example
SE 'Better effects and less costly initiatives'	These initiatives dominate the status quo, as they improve both cost and health outcomes and are clearly favourable	Implement the QI initiative	A care bundle which decreases the risk of surgical site infections without increasing the workload of hospital staff
NW 'Worse effects and more costly initiatives'	These initiatives are dominated by the status quo, as they are worse in both costs and health outcomes and are not cost-effective	Do not implement or stop the QI initiative	A novel care pathway that allocates additional staff time to patients with a defined health condition, but was shown to worsen health outcomes from QI evaluation
NE 'Better effects and more costly initiatives'	Adoption of these initiatives requires further consideration of the trade-off between additional improved outcome at increased cost; comparison to a CE threshold requires a CUA study	Prior to acting, consider whether the higher costs can be paid, given budgetary constraints and the opportunity costs of using the budget elsewhere. If the CUA ICER is below the CE threshold, it is perceived to be cost-effective and should be implemented	An enhanced system of multidisciplinary team meetings which consumes additional staff time but results in superior care planning and outcomes
SW 'Worse effects and less costly initiatives'	These initiatives (often referred to as disinvestments) reduce costs and provide an inferior standard of care	Prior to acting, consider whether the worse effects can be justified, given the cost savings	Any decision that accepts reduced costs for reduced effectiveness. An example may be use of telehealth for certain cohorts. Telehealth may lower patient experience; yet implementation might be justified by patient and provider cost savings, compared to in-person consultations

Signposting

York Health Economics Consortium (2016). *Cost-effectiveness threshold*. Available at: 🔗 https://yhec.co.uk/glossary/cost-effectiveness-threshold/ (accessed 10 September 2023).

York Health Economics Consortium (2016). *Incremental cost-effectiveness ratio (ICER)*. Available at: 🔗 https://yhec.co.uk/glossary/incremental-cost-effectiveness-ratio-icer/ (accessed 10 September 2023).

York Health Economics Consortium (2016). *Unit costs*. Available at: 🔗 https://yhec.co.uk/glossary/unit-costs/ (accessed 10 September 2023).

Further reading

Crealey, G. and O'Neill, C. (2021). *A review of economic evaluation methodologies for the assessment of arts and creativity interventions for improving health and wellbeing in older adults. Institute of Public Health in Ireland.* Available at: 🔗 https://publichealth.ie/wp-content/uploads/2021/09/Arts-and-creativity-economic-report-final.pdf (accessed 10 September 2023).

Hoomans, T. and Severens, J.L. (2014). Economic evaluation of implementation strategies in health care. *Implementation Science*, 9, p. 168. doi: 10.1186/s13012-014-0168-y.

References

Drummond, M., Sculpher, M.J., Claxton, K., Stoddart, G.L., and Torrance, G.W. (2015). *Methods for the Economic Evaluation of Health Care Programmes.* Oxford: Oxford University Press.

Health Information and Quality Authority (2020). *Guidelines for the economic evaluation of health technologies in Ireland 2020.* Available at: 🔗 https://www.hiqa.ie/reports-and-publications/health-technology-assessment/guidelines-economic-evaluation-health (accessed 10 September 2023).

National Institute for Health and Care Excellence (2022). *NICE health technology evaluations: the manual.* Available at: 🔗 https://www.nice.org.uk/process/pmg36/chapter/introduction-to-health-technology-evaluation (accessed 10 September 2023).

Turner, H.C., Archer, R.A., Downey, L.E., *et al.* (2021). An introduction to the main types of economic evaluations used for informing priority setting and resource allocation in healthcare: key features, uses, and limitations. *Frontiers in Public Health*, 9, p. 722927. doi: 10.3389/fpubh.2021.722927.

Zorginstituut Nederland (2016). *Guideline for economic evaluations in healthcare.* Available at: 🔗 https://english.zorginstituutnederland.nl/publications/reports/2016/06/16/guideline-for-economic-evaluations-in-healthcare (10 September 2023).

Health economics in a quality improvement initiative

A health economic assessment of a QI initiative may include:
- Cost descriptions;
- Cost analysis;
- Cost outcome descriptions;
- CEA;
- CUA.

Table 7.8 describes the cost categories relevant to QI initiatives. Societal costs should only be included if this is part of the health economic perspective being adopted for the initiative.

Table 7.8 Cost categories for quality improvement initiatives

QI development costs	Costs of planning a QI initiative (e.g. stakeholder consultation exercises, gathering non-routine data to establish the opportunity for improvement, securing funding and managerial support)
QI implementation costs	Costs of doing the improvement using PDSA or Lean, for example, and documentation of the effects and costs
Intervention costs	Costs of establishing the QI change ideas (e.g. guidelines, staff training, information for patients)
Healthcare costs	Costs of care (e.g. staff time, consumables, facilities) Cost savings (negative costs): the lower quantity of resource use and costs (i.e. the value of resource use) for a given use which results in capacity savings that can be used elsewhere Avoided costs: avoided resource use and costs due to avoided future complications and incidents Nets costs: overall cost of implementation minus avoided costs
Societal costs	Overall costs incurred by society, not only including health system and broader government costs, but also costs for patients and members of the public, including out-of-pocket expenses (e.g. pharmacy and travel costs), productivity losses (e.g. time out of work), and informal care cost

Example of a cost description

Cost assessment involves the identification, quantification, and valuation of the costs of a QI initiative over a specified time period. To describe the costs of a QI initiative, follow the steps outlined in Table 7.9.

Table 7.9 Steps in conducting a cost description

1. **Identify the relevant resources**	Develop a gross list of resource items that are important to quantify and decide how best to quantify them
2. **Determine the quantities of resource use (q)**	In before-assessments, quantities are estimated based on experience, literature, or expert views. After-assessments are based on records of actual resource use, indicated by the initiative data collection
3. **Establish the unit cost or prices (p)**	Unit costs may vary, depending on the quantity of resource use involved, and may only be determined when the quantity to be used is decided. An estimate for the unit cost should be used
4. **Calculate the overall cost**	Multiply the quantities of resource use (q) by their unit costs (p)

For example, the cost description for a QI project aiming to reduce falls in an inpatient ward within 6 months is shown in Table 7.10. The evaluation is conducted from the healthcare perspective. Specifically, Table 7.10 describes the unit cost (p), quantities (q), and total cost for each resource in the QI initiative.

Table 7.10 Average cost per patient of a QI initiative aimed at reducing falls on an inpatient ward

Cost category	Quantity (q)	Unit cost, £ (p)	Total cost, £ (= q × p)
Pre-implementation QI costs			
Consultation meeting with patients and families	Two consultations	1-hour staff nurse facilitation per consultation Hourly rate: 19	38
Establishment of baseline falls rate over 6 months	One audit	5-hour audit by staff nurse Hourly rate: 19	95
QI implementation costs			
Staff nurse documentation of patient compliance to guideline and falls rate	1 hour per day, 7 days per week	Hourly rate: 19	133 per week

(Continued)

Table 7.10 (Contd.)

Cost category	Quantity (q)	Unit cost, £ (p)	Total cost, £ (= q × p)
Intervention costs			
Non-slip socks (one-off costs on ward)	10 patients require 7 pairs each (70 pairs required in total)	19 per pair	1330
Healthcare costs			
Laundry costs	Two loads per week	5 per load	10 per week
Cleaner time	2 hours per week	11 per hour	22 per week

Example of a cost analysis

The cost description in Table 7.10 can be extended to a cost analysis by contrasting the provided costs with the costs of an alternative falls prevention strategy occurring during the same time frame. To make the cost comparison of several interventions easier, the costs in Table 7.10 can be further aggregated into one-off costs that occur before or during implementation of the QI initiative, and running costs, as presented in Table 7.11.

Table 7.11 Summary of additional costs per 10 patients

Cost type	Costs (£)
Pre-implementation costs per 10 patients	133
Implementation costs (one-off)	1330
Implementation/running costs per 10 patients	165 per week 4290 (26 weeks)
Total costs of implementation	5753

Example of a cost outcome description

In Table 7.12, data on the outcome measure (number of falls) and the associated costs are shown to demonstrate a cost outcome description.

Without a comparative option, the usefulness of the analysis in Table 7.12 is limited. Taken together, the analyses presented in Tables 7.10 (cost description), 7.11 (cost analysis), and 7.12 (cost outcome description) provide the cost of the QI initiative. Nonetheless, the evidence for change in targeted outcomes and consequential savings and avoided costs is missing.

A full economic evaluation is required and can be conducted once sufficient baseline data become available. The next section provides an alternative scenario where baseline data are available, making a full economic evaluation possible.

Table 7.12 Cost outcome description of a QI project aimed at reducing falls on an inpatient ward

Number of falls over 6 months before the QI initiative	No baseline data available, but noted as a common problem on the ward
Number of falls over 6 months with the QI initiative	Four, which seemed lower than the preceding 6 months, but no data to support the claim
Cost of falls incurred	Six added bed days per injured patient, approximately £6000 per patient = £24000
Total costs of QI implementation	£5753

Example of a cost-effectiveness analysis

When comparative data are available, it is possible to identify whether a QI initiative is 'dominant over/dominated by' the status quo or 'non-dominant'. If 'non-dominance' is identified, the additional step of the ICER is calculated.

- Table 7.13 describes a QI initiative to reduce falls, in which the assessment indicates 'better effects (fewer falls), less costly' (dominance) over the status quo.
- Table 7.14 describes an alternative trajectory of the QI initiative, whereby the assessment indicates 'better effects (fewer falls), more costly' (non-dominance) over the status quo.

Note that the descriptive analyses in Tables 7.11 and 7.12 include £133 pre-implementation costs. These would usually be excluded from a CEA, as they are not required for the ongoing spread or scale-up of the QI initiative. So the cost of the QI initiative is £5620, rather than £5753.

The analysis in Table 7.13 suggests cost-effectiveness (better than status quo or alternatives, i.e. dominance) as the intervention both improves effects (falls are reduced) and there is a net cost saving of £30380. The

Table 7.13 Cost-effectiveness analysis of a QI initiative to reduce falls on an inpatient ward

Number of falls over 6 months before the QI initiative	10
Number of falls with the QI initiative	4
Number of falls avoided with the QI initiative	6
Costs avoided	Six avoided bed days per injured patient, approximately £6000 per patient = £36000
Cost of QI implementation	£5620
Net costs saved	£30380

Table 7.14 Calculating an ICER for a QI initiative to reduce falls using pager and bed rails

Patient outcomes before the QI initiative	10 falls
Cost before the QI initiative	£60 000 (10 falls at £6000 per fall)
Patient outcomes during the QI initiative	4 falls (i.e. cost of £24 000)
Cost of the QI initiative	£42 500 = 10 × (£350 + £3900)
Cost during the QI initiative	£66 500 (4 falls £24 000 + cost of QI £42 500)
Cost-effectiveness ratio	$$\frac{£66500 - £60000}{4-10} = \frac{£6500}{-6}$$ £1083 cost increase per patient fall avoided

analysis provides confidence to decision-makers that the QI reduced overall costs and improved health (avoided falls).

To illustrate a more costly initiative with better outcomes on the same ward, with same number of patients, a more expensive change idea to reduce falls includes: a pendant pager call bell with alarm at £350 per patient and the purchase of floor level adjustable low beds at £3900 per patient = £42 500 across 10 patients.

On initial assessment of cost and outcomes, this initiative was assessed to be *health improved but net costs increased* (i.e. non-dominant). In this situation, a cost-effectiveness ratio is calculated to determine the exact nature of the relationship between cost and outcome in comparison to the status quo (Table 7.14).

The result in Table 7.14 confirms that this QI initiative reduced falls (a health improvement) but increased costs. While we can determine the cost-effectiveness ratio achieved here is £1083 increase in cost per patient fall avoided, to fully determine whether the initiative is 'value for money', we need outcomes quantified in terms of QALYs gained to perform a comparison against a CE threshold.

Example of a cost utility analysis

A CUA measures health effects in QALYs. These are measured on a scale of 0 to 1 where 1 is full health and 0 would be death. Every incremental point below 1 represents increasing morbidity and a decreasing quality of life. A QALY is assessed by using standardized formulae related to the specific illness.

- In the above example, a gain in QALYs would arise from the falls that have been avoided.
- Assuming that the six avoided falls would have resulted in harm, an affected person would have experienced a reduction in their

health-related quality of life (e.g. less mobility, more pain, and potentially earlier death).

• These consequences can be quantified using QALYs. On a quality of life scale from 0 to 1, each patient may have hypothetically lost an average of 0.2 QALYs over the following year.

• By preventing these falls, the QI initiative may have achieved 6×0.2 QALYs = 1.2 QALYs.

• This implies that the ICER of the QI initiative is £6500/1.2 QALYs = £5417 per QALY.

• With a threshold value of £30 000/QALY set by NICE, the cost-effectiveness ratio would indicate that the QI initiative is cost-effective and represents good 'value for money'.

Top tips

Use the principles of health economics to determine which QI initiatives are cost-effective and provide 'value for money'. This is an important part of any QI process. Follow the steps below:

1. Determine who the decision-makers are and which criteria they use for determining cost-effectiveness.
2. Consider the utility of a partial health economic evaluation.
   a. Is an analysis without comparison to an alternative strategy useful in your context?
   b. This may be useful to determining the baseline costs and health outcomes of the status quo.
3. A full economic evaluation, including a comparison to at least one or more alternatives, is necessary to meaningfully inform decisions.
4. If conducting a full economic evaluation:
   a. Make the health economic perspective clear (e.g. the healthcare system, patient, or society);
   b. Consider if a CEA using context-specific metrics will be sufficient to guide a decision;
   c. If planning a CUA, consider where QALY weights for the relevant health outcomes can be sourced.

Signposting

Healthcare Improvement Scotland (2020). *Economic evaluation in quality improvement: a starter guide.* Available at: ✆ https://ihub.scot/media/7453/a-starter-guide-to-economic-evaluation.pdf (accessed 10 September 2023).

Summary

- Health economic evaluation offers decision support related to effectiveness in resource utilization.
- Cost analysis aims to report on the use of resources and express the cost of providing healthcare in monetary terms.
- Cost outcome analyses aim to report outcomes and relevant costs of single QI initiatives.
- Full health economic evaluations examine the relationship between the costs and outcomes of a QI initiative in comparison to the status quo or alternative initiatives (e.g. adverse events avoided per cost and in comparison to alternative QI initiatives).
- The ratio between incremental cost and incremental outcomes indicates the cost-effectiveness of a new initiative in comparison to an alternative programme.

Further reading

Arefian, H., Vogel, M., Kwetkat, A., and Hartmann, M. (2016). Economic evaluation of interventions for prevention of hospital acquired infections: a systematic review. *PLoS One*, 11(1), p. e0146381. doi: 10.1371/journal.pone.0146381.

De La Perrelle, L., Radisic, G., Cations, M., Kaambwa, B., Barbery, G., and Laver, K. (2020). Costs and economic evaluations of quality improvement collaboratives in healthcare: a systematic review. *BMC Health Services Research*, 20(1), p. 155. doi: 10.1186/s12913-020-4981-5.

Glied, S. and Smith, P.C., eds. (2013). *The Oxford Handbook of Health Economics*. Oxford: Oxford University Press.

Nuckols, T. K., Keeler, E., Morton, S. C., Anderson, L., Doyle, B., Booth, M., Shanman, R., Grein, J., & Shekelle, P. (2016). Economic evaluation of quality improvement interventions for bloodstream infections related to central catheters: a systematic review. *JAMA Internal Medicine*, 176(12), pp. 1843–54. doi.org/10.1001/jamainternmed.2016.6610

Nuckols, T.K., Keeler, E., Morton, S., *et al.* (2017). Economic evaluation of quality improvement interventions designed to prevent hospital readmission: a systematic review and meta-analysis. *JAMA Internal Medicine*, 177(7), pp. 975–85. doi: 10.1001/jamainternmed.2017.1136.

Solid, C.A. (2021). *Return on Investment for Healthcare Quality Improvement*. Cham: Springer Nature.

Thompson, C., Pulleyblank, R., Parrott, S., and Essex, H. (2016). The cost-effectiveness of quality improvement projects: a conceptual framework, checklist and online tool for considering the costs and consequences of implementation-based quality improvement. *Journal of Evaluation in Clinical Practice*, 22(1), pp. 26–30. doi: 10.1111/jep.12421.

Co-producing health and person-centred care

Key points

- Person-centred care is at the core of all that we do in healthcare.
- The concept has evolved from patient-centred to person-centred, which indicates that patients as people have a wider context than their illness.
- Asking '*What matters to you?*' opens the door to meaningful interactions between the patient and the clinician.
- Understanding the *lived experience* of people who receive care facilitates the provision of person-centred care.
- Co-production allows for the sharing of power in a respectful and equal way.
- Shared decision-making allows people to be in control of their health.
- People should always be part of the improvement team to bring knowledge, challenge, and accountability.

Introduction

The conventional understanding of healthcare is that healthcare is a 'product' that we as professionals 'sell' to our patients, the customers (Foster and Batalden, 2021). Yet healthcare is simultaneously both technical and relational, so it is more than providing care (Ballatt et al. 2020).

- In ◌ Chapter 1, the concepts of Quality 1.0 and Quality 2.0 were introduced as approaches to enable quality through improvements in the 'product', as well as standardization of the delivery process.
- As a result, we have witnessed tremendous advances in the technical aspects of healthcare, such as safety and effectiveness, and the relational aspect has often been neglected.
- In other words, the people behind the patient and the professional provider of care have been ignored, often resulting in poor experience for both.

In this chapter, we will explore how you can include patients as people in your improvement project and in your clinical work. Although we will not be focusing on person-centred care (PCC) in clinical practice, the philosophy of the approach in improvement work can translate into your day-to-day clinical practice.

There are many definitions of PCC. An all-encompassing one is in Box 8.1.

Box 8.1 Definition of person-centred care

'"Person-centered care" means that individuals' values and preferences are elicited, and once expressed, guide all aspects of their health care, supporting their realistic health and life goals. Person-centered care is achieved through a dynamic relationship among individuals, others. who are important to them, and all relevant providers. This collaboration informs decision-making to the extent that the individual desires.'

Goodwin, 2015.

Defining the problem or challenge

As noted in ◌ Chapter 1, over the past century, healthcare has achieved considerable success with increased life expectancy and tackling major diseases.

- One could argue most of the gain has been due to public health measures such as immunization, clean water, nutrition, and improving social conditions.
- Disease management and the impact of the changing nature of healthcare on PCC can be understood through the concept of industrialization, which is characterized by innovation and change powered by technological solutions.
- Industrialization can also result in depersonalization and alienation, as processes are standardized and automated.
- This is manifested by patient dissatisfaction with the service and experience and by clinician or healthcare worker burnout.

Prior to the medical advances of the twentieth century, healthcare was more personal, often with a direct relationship between the healer and the person seeking care within the community.
- The healthcare professional had a limited range of interventions.
- Care was provided more closely to the home of the person requiring care and often within the community, surrounded by their kin.

The care that we provide now is:
- Less personal and more technical than before;
- Designed around the management of disease rather than around the holistic management of a person with a disease;
- Subspecialized, with the division of labour, the introduction of technology, and a decreased emphasis on generalization;
- Medicalized at every point, with the benefit of cure for many conditions (e.g. infectious diseases, cancer, cardiac conditions), with a resultant increasing life expectancy.

On an individual level, a person is divided into either a disease or an organ entity, and is not seen in a holistic way.
- Physical health is separated from mental well-being.
- Natural experiences, like childbirth and often death, are made into medical processes.

On a meso- and macro-level, healthcare is organized in large industrial complexes, which we call hospitals, isolated from the community in which the person lives.
- Technical improvements in healthcare, as well as increasing burden of long-term conditions, have resulted in rising healthcare costs, with diminishing value (Elwyn et al., 2020).
- The system rewards subspecialties and downgrades the generalists.
- Success has created the challenges of an ageing population and multiple comorbidities, for which the new industrial system has not been prepared.
- As healthcare enters the next industrial revolution of digitalization, the next challenge for PCC will develop unless the paradigm is changed.
- Finally, as has happened with industrialization in other industries, patients and healthcare workers experience alienation and often despair, which, for healthcare workers, we call burnout.

Why is person-centred care important to people receiving care?

PCC is central to all that we do and is a key component of developing high-quality healthcare. From a quality improvement (QI) perspective, PCC is essential for:
- Respecting a person's rights, including autonomy, so as to support informed consent, truth-telling, and confidentiality;
- Improving health gain in terms of patient behaviour, recovery, and outcomes;
- Improving organizational performance by the use of patient-provided information, including experience and outcome measures;
- Achieving the triple aim of improving the experience of care, improving the health of populations, and reducing per capita costs of healthcare (Berwick et al., 2008).

In Box 8.2 and Box 8.3 examples of good and poor person centred care are described.

After losing his 27-year-old daughter due to an adverse event at the Hospital Israelita Albert Einstein, in 2015, Francisco Cruz Lima, an engineer aged 60, decided to fight to promote changes in the procedures and behaviour of the hospital's professionals. The report on the adverse event led to the Patient Safety Program, named Júlia Lima in her honour. A foundation of the Program is the Patient Council, which is based on the concepts of person-centred care and patient experience. The key is promoting healthcare provider empathy, communication, and positive attitude. The Council was established to show the institutional commitment to person-centred care, continuous improvement, and transparency in patient safety processes. New members who have been a patient or a caregiver having suffered an adverse event or a near miss join each year. They must be willing to have mature and often difficult conversations to help professionals and the institution to improve its processes. Members are voluntary and sign a contract. Meetings are held quarterly, with a leader from the institution serving as a liaison to facilitate and guide the discussions and learning. Members have the opportunity to discuss and participate in new projects, process mapping in event investigations, and participate in focus groups, among other activities.

With permission of Albert Einstein Hospital – São Paulo, Brazil.

The principle that patients need to come first is widely held. To achieve this, organizations may create a patient and family association (PFA) to create a path to co-production and patient engagement. However, in the 'real-world' of day-to-day operations, staff may believe that the existence of the PFA means they are person-centred. A centralized committee in an office does not translate to person-centred care. Person-centred care is not a forum or a committee for completing superficial tasks, such as reviewing patient brochures or food menus, or involving them in meaningless conversations or helping with complaints and grievances. Rather it is a mindset and culture of treating patients as partners and as people who can co-produce solutions. An active approach can help the institution in a horizontal and reciprocal way. Without this change in thinking, great ideas, organizational energy, better value, better experience for all patients, families, and workforce, and goodwill from the volunteers may be lost.

Why is person-centred care important to the clinician?

PCC requires us to move from a 'product'-dominant logic (i.e. health as a commodity) to a 'service'-dominant logic where we provide a service that must add value to health, and not only to cure disease.

The perception of the professional as the expert and the patient as a passive recipient of care will be replaced by an equal partnership between the service provider and the person we call a patient. Such collaborative care ensures that the needs of all people are met and is broadly referred to as 'person-centred care'.

Further reading

Berwick, D.M. (2009). What 'patient-centered' should mean: confessions of an extremist. *Health Affairs*, 28(Supplement 1), pp. w555–65. doi: 10.1377/hlthaff.28.4.w555.

Coulter, A. and Oldham, J. (2016). Person-centred care: what is it and how do we get there? *Future Hospital Journal*, 3(2), pp. 114–16. doi: 10.7861/futurehosp.3-2-114.

Groene, O. (2011). Patient centredness and quality improvement efforts in hospitals: rationale, measurement, implementation. *International Journal for Quality in Health Care*, 23(5), pp. 531–7. doi: 10.1093/intqhc/mzr058.

References

Ballatt, J., Campling, P., and Maloney, C. (2020). *Intelligent Kindness: Rehabilitating the Welfare State*. Cambridge: RCPsych Publications.

Berwick, D.M., Nolan, T.W., and Whittington, J. (2008). The triple aim: care, health, and cost. *Health Affairs (Project Hope)*, 27(3), pp. 759–69. doi: 10.1377/hlthaff.27.3.759.

Elwyn, G., Nelson, E., Hager, A., and Price, A. (2020). Coproduction: when users define quality. *BMJ Quality and Safety*, 29(9), p. 711–16. doi: 10.1136/bmjqs-2019-009830.

Foster, T. and Batalden, P. (2021). New ways of working: health professional development for effective coproduction. *International Journal for Quality in Health Care*, 33(Supplement 2), pp. ii6–7. doi: 10.1093/intqhc/mzab055.

Goodwin, C. (2015). Person-centered care: a definition and essential elements. *Journal of the American Geriatrics Society*, 64(1), pp. 15–18. doi: 10.1111/jgs.13866.

Background to person-centred care

Evolution of person-centred care

Although the concept of patient-centred care surfaced about 30 years ago and seemed to be a simple concept, healthcare providers have found it difficult to implement. The term patient-centred has evolved to person-centred in recognition that patients are people who happen to be patients for part of their lives.

Levels of person-centred care

PCC has become internationally recognized over the past 20 years as a dimension of the broader concept of high-quality healthcare, especially following the publication of *Crossing the Quality Chasm* (Institute of Medicine, 2001). The report outlined four levels that define quality from the perspective of the patient and their family (Table 8.1).

Table 8.1 Levels of person-centred care

Experience	How an individual experiences the care received. The experience must be candid, and support and encourage the participation and/or activation of the patient and their families or caregivers
Clinical microsystem p. 269	Refers to the service, department, section, process, or programme designed to deliver care (i.e. where frontline teams work). At this level, patients and families should actively participate in the design of the service and how it is delivered
Organizational	Refers to the organization considered as a whole. At this level, patients and families should participate in all the key committees across the organization to ensure the patient's voice is being considered in the strategy
Environmental	At the regulatory level, the perspectives of patients and their families should inform healthcare policies at every level—local, regional, national, and international. People as patients would be able to help these agencies in setting the expectations at all other levels and align reimbursement and incentives to result in person-focused care. People and their families would be involved in healthcare decision-making at every level, allowing people, especially women, rather than the state, to manage their own bodies

Dimensions of person-centred care

Six dimensions for PCC were proposed in *Crossing the Quality Chasm* (Institute of Medicine, 2001) (Box 8.4).

These domains are the foundation of PCC delivery and the measurement of how it is achieved.

Box 8.4 Institute of Medicine's domains of person-centred care

* Respect for patients' values, preferences, and expressed needs
* Coordination and integration of care
* Provision of information, communication, and education
* Ensuring physical comfort
* Providing emotional support, and relieving fear and anxiety
* Involvement of family and friends

Crossing the Quality Chasm, Institute of Medicine, 2001

How does this impact our role?

While considering a broader perspective of healthcare participation through the lens of patients, how people receive care has become a central point of the work of PCC. The challenge was summarized by Conway as follows: *'When you have 9000 things going on, you don't want to sit down and figure out how to partner with your patients. The paternalistic model of care is the way we have organized ourselves, simply to get the work done'* (Conway, 2009).

As the view of what constitutes person (patient)-centred care broadened, the role of patient advocates underwent a simultaneous transition in many organizations, from a reactive complaint management role into a more proactive change agent and advocacy role. This required giving people agency and using many of the techniques that will be described in ⊃ Chapters 10 and 11.

The following sections will provide some ways in which clinical practice and improvement projects can be person-centred.

Further reading

Berwick, D.M. (2009). What 'patient-centered' should mean: confessions of an extremist. *Health Affairs*, 28(Supplement 1), pp. w555–65. doi: 10.1377/hlthaff.28.4.w555.

References

Conway, J. (2009). Quoted in: *Delivering great care: engaging patients and families as partners*. Available at: ℘ http://www.ihi.org/resources/Pages/ImprovementStories/DeliveringGreatCareEngagingPatientsandFamiliesasPartners.aspx (accessed 10 September 2023).

Institute of Medicine (US) Committee on Quality of Health Care in America (2001). *Crossing the Quality Chasm: A New Health System for the 21st Century*. Washington, DC: National Academies Press.

What is person-centred care?

Why is person-centred care important?

Over the last 20 years, healthcare has witnessed profound changes in the relationship between people and how care is delivered by the healthcare workforce and how it is perceived by patients and their families. A first step to take is to know what PCC is from the viewpoint of the people receiving care, and why it is important to them.

- PCC is a concept that affects our thought processes and the way in which everyday responsibilities are performed by medical staff and carers.
- It is more than an action, but rather a philosophical approach and a state of mind to the way in which care is delivered.
- PCC is completely centred around the person who is receiving care.
- The term is constantly changing and developing as the needs of patients evolve.

The Institute of Medicine defined patient-centred care as: '*Providing care that is respectful of, and responsive to, individual patient preferences, needs and values, and ensuring that patient values guide all clinical decisions*' (Institute of Medicine, 2001).

- This approach requires a true partnership between individuals and their healthcare providers.
- It might sound a quite simple approach, but in the real world, it is still a challenging way of working for most healthcare organizations and clinical teams.
- As noted in ⊃ Chapter 1, the Institute of Medicine included patient-centred care as one of six domains of quality, though in reality, PCC surrounds every domain of care.
- A chasm exists between the kind of care that patients receive and the kind of care they should have and what they want to have.
- A fundamental change in the system of care is required to deliver PCC.

Collins (2014) defines PCC as comprising four principles (Figure 8.1):
- Care that is personalized to the individual person;

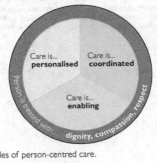

Figure 8.1 Principles of person-centred care.
Reproduced with permission of The Health Foundation.

- Care that is coordinated around the patient as a person;
- Care that enables the patient to take control of his/her health;
- Care whereby the person is treated with dignity, compassion, and respect.

To achieve this level of PCC, the concept of shared decision-making (SDM) proposed by Barry and Edgman-Levitan (2012) is essential. They highlighted that the most important attribute of patient-centred care is active engagement of patients when healthcare decisions are made—that is, when they arrive at a crossroads of medical options and the diverging paths may have different and important consequences to patients and their families.

How is person-centred care beneficial?

The path to changing the way in which one views PCC starts with the individual, which is why patient-directed care should stand at the core of all that we do and should be an integral part of every improvement project.
PCC has many benefits for patients as people:

- Patients will feel more motivated when following a plan in which they have actively participated and that is focused on their specific needs;
- PCC helps patients work towards their goals and reach important milestones;
- Patients' emotional, personal, and social needs will be considered and delivered;
- PCC encourages activation and independence, and provides patients and their families with more responsibility, which can be a self-motivating factor;
- PCC creates a better environment in care as patients feel comfortable;
- The quality of care is improved, which may have so many beneficial consequences such as improved and rapid recovery, with resultant cost reduction;
- PCC can improve patients' long-term interest in their health if they are involved in decision-making on the recovery process, which is truly beneficial if they have more responsibility over their own health.

All these benefits mentioned above create more cost-effective and time-efficient services, as care quality is improved and patients are more cooperative with their personalized plans.

How does asking 'what matters to you' make a difference?

The concept of including the lived experience and the preferences of the person (whom we call the 'patient') in all decision-making is simple, yet only recent in healthcare. Other industries aim to understand what the consumer would want, so that the product developed and delivered meets the individual needs of the consumer. Perhaps, because one does not choose to be ill and the knowledge has been held by the health profession in the past, the concept of delivering *what really matters* to people has only just emerged.

- An essential component of the person-centred philosophy of SDM (Barry and Edgman-Levitan, 2012) is asking a person '*What really matters to you?*', instead of the traditional '*What is the matter or wrong with you?*', which superficially seems to be a simple change. However, it brings in a complex change in the relationship between the provider of care and the receiver of care.

- By asking the question, the provider of care—be it a doctor, nurse, physiotherapist, dentist, or any other professional—has opened the door to a set of values that we discussed in ➲ Chapter 1 in the multidimensional model:
  - *Respect* for the views of the person being asked;
  - Treating the patient as a *person* who has views and a life outside the construct of the illness, sick role, or consultation paradigm;
  - Incorporating caring and *kindness* as part of the interaction;
  - Committing to providing what the patient, as a member of a wider *kinship*, really wants;
  - *Sharing decisions* on what needs to be done and how it can be achieved.
- The question '*What matters to you?*' opens up a space for the patient as a person to express their values, ideas, desires, and wants. It invites both the patient as a person and the healthcare professional as a person to frame the next stage of the interaction, now not only between patient and clinician, but also between two people.
- The question recognizes the humanity of both individuals and changes the dynamics of the interactions.
- This is the complexity of the intervention as we, as caregivers, need to change the way in which we think—from only finding out what is wrong (diagnosis) based on the symptoms that a person has of an illness to adding the finding out of what the person really wants.
- The patient also has to be liberated from the sick role and the cultural norm of powerlessness in the face of illness as an adversity.

In an improvement project, it is important to assess whether the aim of the project and the outcomes will produce what matters to the people affected by the project, be it patients or providers of care.

In Box 8.5 the concept of *What matters to you?* is illustrated.

Box 8.5 What Matters to You?

Every year, there is a *What Matters to You?* day run by the international organization What Matters To You? (What Matters To You, n.d.).

Many stories are available, and some examples include:

- A child in a hospital who wants people to knock on the door and introduce themselves if they come into her room;
- A lady with dementia who wants to know how her pet is doing every day;
- A lady with cancer who wants to live as long as she can to attend her daughter's wedding;
- A child who wants to be able to play normally with her friends even while on treatment.

What is the lived experience of people?

To provide PCC, we need to understand the experience of both the person receiving care, called the patient, and the person delivering care, called the doctor, nurse, therapist, etc. Wolf et al. (2014, 2021) examined personal experience and postulated that we need to talk about the lived human experience, rather than about person experience alone, if we really want to develop PCC.

- The human experience is defined by looking at all interactions across the total continuum of care, without boundaries on the person's journey.
- The breadth of experience is important, especially with a person who has a long-term condition.
- Human experience will be influenced by the culture of each organization or clinical team encountered, and how PCC is defined and delivered.
- As it is human experience, we look at the experience of staff and patients as humans, rather than at their previously defined role in their interactions.

The human experience concept is shown in Figure 8.2.

What is a quality improvement designed by the lived experience?

As one decides on what to improve and how this may impact the people in the process, one needs to ensure the following:

- The proposed improvement will improve the lived experience of those delivering care—that is, the new process should make it easier to achieve the desired outcomes, and not more difficult to deliver.
- The lived experience of the patient is improved—that is, they receive the care that they want to receive in the way that meets what matters to them.
- Methods such as experience-based co-design use the lived experience of everyone in the process to co-design the new process (see ⊙ Chapter 14).
- To assess the delivery of a person-centred experience, the Donabedian framework is used and the following questions are asked:
  - What *structures* need to be in place (e.g. organization culture);
  - Whether the *processes* of care are person-centred;
  - Whether the *outcomes* achieved are desirable for person-centredness (Santana et al., 2017).
- In clinical day-to-day care, using methods such as SDM will help ensure co-production of a positive lived experience for all.

Signposting

What Matters to You? Available at: ⌨ https://wmty.world (accessed 10 September 2023).

Further reading

Gaille, M. (2019). 'Patient's lived experience'. *Medicine, Health Care and Philosophy*, 22(3), pp. 339–42. doi: 10.1007/s11019-019-09896-5.

Hirpa, M., Woreta, T., Addis, H., and Kebede, S. (2020). What matters to patients? A timely question for value-based care. *PLoS One*, 15(7), p. e0227845. doi: 10.1371/journal.pone.0227845.

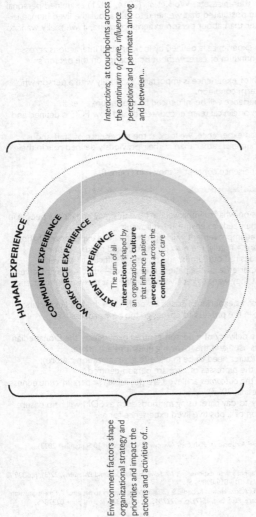

Interactions, at touchpoints across the *continuum of care*, *influence* perceptions and permeate among and between...

HUMAN EXPERIENCE

COMMUNITY EXPERIENCE

WORKFORCE EXPERIENCE

PATIENT EXPERIENCE

The sum of all *interactions* shaped by an organization's **culture** that influence patient **perceptions** across the **continuum** of care

...patients, family members and care partners, the healthcare workforce, and the communities that healthcare organizations serve.

Environment factors shape organizational strategy and priorities and impact the actions and activities of...

Figure 8.2 An integrated view of human experience in healthcare.
Reproduced with permission of the Beryl Institute (Wolf et al. 2021).

Kebede, S. (2016). Ask patients 'What matters to you?' rather than 'What's the matter?' *BMJ*, 354, p. i4045. doi: 10.1136/bmj.i4045.

Montori, V.M. (2020). *Why We Revolt: A Patient Revolution for Careful and Kind Care.* Rochester, MN: Mayo Clinic Press.

Olsen, C.F., Debesay, J., Bergland, A., Bye, A., and Langaas, A.G. (2020). What matters when asking, 'what matters to you?' — perceptions and experiences of health care providers on involving older people in transitional care. *BMC Health Services Research*, 20(1), p. 317. doi: 10.1186/s12913-020-05150-4.

Trzeciak, S., Booker, C., and Mazzarelli, A. (2019). *Compassionomics: The Revolutionary Scientific Evidence that Caring Makes a Difference.* Pensacola, FL: Studer Group.

References

Barry, M.J. and Edgman-Levitan, S. (2012). Shared decision making — the pinnacle of patient-centered care. *New England Journal of Medicine*, 366(9), pp. 780–1. doi: 10.1056/nejmp1109283.

Collins, A. (2014). *Measuring what really matters: a thought paper.* London: The Health Foundation. Available at: https://www.health.org.uk/sites/default/files/MeasuringWhatReallyMatters.pdf (accessed 10 September 2023).

Santana, M.J., Manalili, K., Jolley, R.J., Zelinsky, S., Quan, H., and Lu, M. (2017). How to practice person-centred care: a conceptual framework. *Health Expectations*, 21(2), pp. 429–40. doi: 10.1111/hex.12640.

What Matters to You? (n.d.). Available at: https://wmty.world (accessed 10 September 2023).

Wolf, J.A., Niederhauser, V., Marshburn, D., and LaVela, S.L. (2014). Defining patient experience. *Patient Experience Journal*, 1(1), 7–19. doi: 10.35680/2372-0247.1004.

Wolf, J.A., Niederhauser, V., Marshburn, D., and LaVela, S.L. (2021). Reexamining 'defining patient experience': the human experience in healthcare. *Patient Experience Journal*, 8(1), pp. 16–29. doi: 10.35680/2372-0247.1594. Available at: https://pxjournal.org/journal/vol8/iss1/4/.

Co-production of health

(See → Chapters 1, 2, 10, 14, and 16.)

What is co-production?

The concepts of co-production area core theme of the philosophy of quality improvement in the book.

* In → Chapter 1 in the discussion of the quality improvement journey it is stated that the next stage for quality improvement will be Quality 3.0 where people actively take part in designing and co-producing for health not only for management of disease.
* In → Chapter 2 the concept of co-production with people receiving care is introduced.
* In → Chapter 11 how to design a QI project with staff is discussed.
* The method of experience-based co-design is discussed in → Chapter 14.
* Application of co-production in a QI project is discussed in → Chapter 17.

Co-production in healthcare has been defined as '*The interdependent work of users and professionals to design, create, develop, deliver, assess and improve the relationships and actions that contribute to the health of individuals and populations*' (Batalden et al., 2015) This goal is one that has been developed in other services and is complex in delivery. Four key principles of co-production have been identified in social care and these can be transferred to the healthcare setting as shown in Table 8.2.

Table 8.2 Principles of co-production in social care

Equality	All people within the process have assets that they bring to co-production on an equal basis. The focus is on solutions rather than on problems
Diversity	Co-production should reflect the diversity of the population within the process or service, and no one should be excluded (see → Chapter 5). Attention must be paid to include: <ul><li>People from the black and minority ethnic communities</li><li>The lesbian, gay, bisexual, and transgender communities</li><li>People who communicate differently</li><li>People with dementia</li><li>Older people who need a high level of support</li><li>People who are not affiliated to any organized group or 'community'</li></ul>
Accessibility	Accessibility is about ensuring that everyone has the same opportunity to take part in an activity fully, in the way that suits them best
Reciprocity	It is important to ensure that people receive something back for putting something in and to build on people's desire to feel needed and valued. The idea has been linked with 'mutuality', and all parties involved have responsibilities and expectations

Adapted from Co-Production in Social Care – What is it and how to do it, 2022.

- Co-production requires sharing of power, whereby power held by professionals is ceded and there is an equal partnership between healthcare providers and planners and people receiving care.
- These equal partnerships are often difficult to achieve, as it is a challenge to the current culture and design of healthcare systems.

The co-production ladder

The co-production ladder can assist you in determining where a clinical service or an improvement process is in terms of co-production and sharing of power (Figure 8.3).

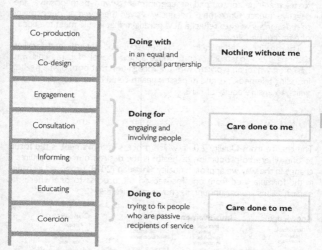

Figure 8.3 The co-production ladder.

Adapted with permission from Thinklocalactpersonal.org.uk (2019). *Think Local Act Personal*. [online] Available at: ℘ https://www.thinklocalactpersonal.org.uk/. Accessed (10 September 2023).

- Most clinical practice starts at the bottom of the ladder, and to move up the ladder, one needs to engage the patient with SDM and self-management strategies.
- Often healthcare improvement projects or service design have consulted patient groups, rather than include them in designing the solution.

In Box 8.6 an example of coproduction during the COVID pandemic is described.

Box 8.6 Example of co-production

In quality improvement, co-production of solutions requires involvement of all stakeholders in a project from the very start. Often we identify a problem and then develop solutions without involving all of the people in the process (i.e. patients and healthcare workers). An example is the redesign of services in the post-coronavirus disease 2019 (COVID-19) period.

Before the COVID-19 pandemic, in many clinics, there were long waiting times and often people could not have their problem solved without visiting a hospital clinic. During the pandemic, there was a move to telemedicine for outpatient appointments, with both positive and negative impact. Once the pandemic was over, there was an opportunity to redesign services to reflect a new paradigm that would meet the needs of different people.

The quality redesign team contacted staff and patients and families to bring them together to co-produce a new model of care. This was based on what had worked, with the recognition that both digital health, including telemedicine, and in-person health could be harnessed, without waits, to ensure equity of care.

Why is co-production in projects on quality and safety important?

The change from Quality 2.0, in which process improvement is the focus, to one where co-production of health is the desired outcome requires a change in the way we approach quality. Batalden (2018) proposed a change in the formula used from one focused on the process to one where the person's aims are paramount, as shown in Figure 8.4.

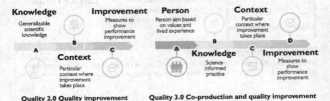

Figure 8.4 From process improvement to co-production of health.
Based on Batalden, 2018.

To achieve this transformation in the way needed to improve care requires the human experience, combining the lived experience of both patients and clinicians with scientific knowledge and how the system works to co-produce solutions.

An improvement project including people as equal partners and sharing decision-making will make a real difference to the project. Co-production could also have cost benefits, as services may be used more efficiently.

Co-production and learning systems

A foundation of co-production is that knowledge is not the prerogative of one group, and in healthcare, that is usually the professional.
- Batalden (2018) proposed that co-production involves joint working between service users and professionals to create, design, produce, deliver, and assess the relationships and interactions that will result in health of individuals and populations.
- To achieve this, we need to create a learning environment, and these could also occur in learning health systems (Gremyr et al., 2021).
- In a learning environment, there will be shared systems and users of the service will own the quality and will define what really matters (Elwyn et al., 2020).
- In the clinical environment, co-production is evident in SDM where patients and professionals assess, design, decide, and deliver care together and learn together in a micro-learning system (see ⮕ Involving people in clinical care—shared decision-making, p. 178).

As one approaches an improvement project, creating a learning system builds the milieu for collaborative change.

Barriers and facilitators to co-production

Barriers to effective and successful co-production include (Batalden et al., 2015; Holland-Hart et al., 2018; Palumbo and Manna, 2017):
- Lack of awareness of what co-production is or what it means;
- A healthcare culture that is founded on a top–down approach and is resistant to change;
- Power differentials between clinicians and patients;
- Poorly designed systems that make it difficult for staff to interact meaningfully with people receiving care;
- Difficulty for staff to communicate in a timely and effective way;
- Inadequate communication among key participants;
- Time constraints to making changes;
- Lack of motivation for change by clinicians and policy;
- Preconceptions of what patients can do;
- Diversity of populations, so that not all are included;
- Tension between the need to decrease variation and the need to be person-centred with co-production;
- Perceived financial constraints;
- Health literacy of people receiving care.

To address these barriers, one needs to:
- Prepare both patients and clinical teams for a new way of thinking;
- Develop a culture of empowerment and sharing of power;
- Partner with community organizations when designing projects or service improvements;
- Ensure there is diverse membership in a co-production team.

How to measure co-production on quality and safety

As with all improvement, unless one can measure, one will not know if there has been improvement. For co-production, one can measure the process and outcomes from the perspectives of the patient, providers, and organization (Marsilio et al., 2021). In Table 8.3, a range of measures are listed to demonstrate the breadth of measures that are required (Marsilio et al., 2021).

Table 8.3 Measures to assess co-production

Focus	Measure
Organization	Cultural changes
	Cost efficiency of the programme
	Trust among different participants
	Loyalty
	Behavioural intentions of consumers to use or recommend the service
	Innovation and adaptability/flexibility of co-production
Person/ professional	Job satisfaction levels
	Staff well-being and burnout
	Work engagement and turnover
	Motivation at work
	Behavioural changes
	Trust in professionals/relationship strength
Person/patient	**Experience and outcomes**
	• Health status and outcomes
	• Satisfaction with the process
	• Patient-reported experience and outcomes
	Clinical
	• Activation as a patient
	• Empowerment to make decisions
	• Self-management of health conditions
	• Self-efficacy
	• Self-esteem
	• Self-confidence
	• Eustress
	• Burden of disease
	Behaviour
	• Learning
	• Changes in behaviour/attitude
	• Relationship with other strengths
	• Issue awareness
	• Individual cost savings

Signposting

Batalden, P. (2022). *The power of coproduction* (podcasts). Available at: ℘ https://ju.se/center/icohn/podcasts/the-power-of-coproduction.html (accessed 10 September 2023).

Batalden, P., Nelson, E., and Foster, T., eds. (2021). *International Journal for Quality in Health Care*, 33(Supplement 2) https://academic.oup.com/intqhc/issue/33/Supplement_2 (accessed 10 September 2023).

Coalition for Personalised Care. Available at: ℘ https://www.coalitionforpersonalisedcare.org.uk (accessed 10 September 2023).

Co-Production Collective. Available at: ℘ https://www.coproductioncollective.co.uk/ (accessed 10 September 2023).

International Coproduction Health Network (ICoHN). Available at: ℘ https://ju.se/center/icohn.html (accessed 10 September 2023).

Further reading

Robert, G., Locock, L., Williams, O., Cornwell, J., Donetto, S., and Goodrich, J. (2022). *Co-Producing and Co-Designing* (Elements of Improving Quality and Safety in Healthcare series). Cambridge: Cambridge University Press.

References

Batalden, M., Batalden, P., Margolis, P., et al. (2015). Coproduction of healthcare service. *BMJ Quality and Safety*, 25(7), pp. 509–17. doi: 10.1136/bmjqs-2015-004315.

Batalden, P. (2018). Getting more health from healthcare: quality improvement must acknowledge patient coproduction—an essay by Paul Batalden. *BMJ*, 362, p. k3617. doi: 10.1136/bmj.k3617.

Elwyn, G., Nelson, E., Hager, A., and Price, A. (2020). Coproduction: when users define quality. *BMJ Quality and Safety*, 29(9), pp. 711–16. doi: 10.1136/bmjqs-2019-009830.

Gremyr, A., Andersson Gäre, B., Thor, J., Elwyn, G., Batalden, P., and Andersson, A.-C. (2021). The role of co-production in learning health systems. *International Journal for Quality in Health Care*, 33(Supplement 2), pp. ii26–32. doi: 10.1093/intqhc/mzab072.

Holland-Hart, D.M., Addis, S.M., Edwards, A., Kenkre, J.E., and Wood, F. (2018). Coproduction and health: public and clinicians' perceptions of the barriers and facilitators. *Health Expectations*, 22(1), pp. 93–101. doi: 10.1111/hex.12834.

Marsilio, M., Fusco, F., Gheduzzi, E., and Guglielmetti, C. (2021). Co-production performance evaluation in healthcare. A systematic review of methods, tools and metrics. *International Journal of Environmental Research and Public Health*, 18(7), p. 3336. doi: 10.3390/ijerph18073336.

Palumbo, R. and Manna, R. (2017). What if things go wrong in co-producing health services? Exploring the implementation problems of health care co-production. *Policy and Society*, 37(3), pp. 368–85. doi: 10.1080/14494035.2018.1411872.

Social Care Institute for Excellence (2022). *Co-production in social care: what it is and how to do it: at a glance*. Available at: ℘ https://www.scie.org.uk/publications/guides/guide51/at-a-glance/ (accessed 10 September 2023).

Involving people in clinical care—shared decision-making

What is empowerment and shared decision-making?

Barry and Edgman-Levitan (2012) stated that the '*most important attribute of patient-centered care is the active engagement of patients when fateful health care decisions must be made — when an individual patient arrives at a crossroads of medical options, where the diverging paths have different and important consequences with lasting implication.*'

However, the construct of healthcare with the traditional hierarchical paradigm has prevented the widespread introduction of SDM. The National Institute for Health and Care Excellence (NICE, 2021) defines SDM as '*a collaborative process that involves a person and their healthcare professional working together to reach a joint decision about care*'.

SDM can take place:
- In the acute care setting where the decision is made on treatment (e.g. to take a medication or not);
- In chronic care where advance planning of how long-term treatment can be delivered is shared;
- In all settings choosing what tests to do and which treatment options are most suitable (Choosing Wisely, available at: ℘ https://www.cho osingwisely.org, accessed 10 September 2023)).

SDM requires weighing up of the risks of each option and the consequences of each decision in an unbiased way, so that a fair representation of each option is discussed and a joint decision is made.
- This implies that there is sharing of power as people are enabled to decide, based on the evidence and their own values and beliefs. This can include declining to be treated.
- The transfer of agency (see ➲ Chapter 10) is a central part of the SDM process.

How to facilitate empowerment and shared decision of care

Elwyn et al. (2012) proposed a three-step model to implement SDM (Figure 8.5):
- *Choice talk*: introducing choice to the person;
- *Option talk*: describing options, often by integrating the use of patient decision support. Programmes such as Choosing Wisely (available at: ℘ https://www.choosingwisely.org, accessed 10 September 2023) can provide the option choices available;
- *Decision talk*: helping patients to explore preferences and make decisions.

Within the process of SDM, goal setting, which is an integral part of self-management, would be the next step to add once a decision has been made (Elwyn and Vermunt, 2019). Goal setting will be part of any improvement project. Use of Teach-back (available at: ℘ http://www.teachbacktraining. org/home, accessed 10 September 2023) can assist in ensuring that the decisions and options have been understood.

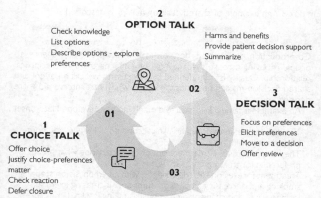

Figure 8.5 Model for clinical shared decision-making.
Based on Elwyn et al., 2012.

SDM incorporates the elements of co-production (Elwyn et al., 2020) where the people receiving care are in control of their health by:

- *Co-assessing* the current status of the problem with the clinician;
- *Co-deciding* what to do, as per their own goals and values;
- *Co-designing* what the treatment or management plan will be;
- *Co-delivering* the agreed interventions, so that they are jointly owned.

These principles are integral to improvement projects where patients can be part of the improvement team within a learning health system.

How does one measure successful shared decision-making?

If SDM is part of an improvement project, one can measure success at several levels (Elwyn et al., 2015):

- Impact on the patient in terms of involvement in the process of care, patient-reported measures, experience, and clinical outcomes;
- Impact on the clinical staff in the way they interact with one another as a group or on an individual level, joy in work, general well-being, and belief systems;
- Impact on the organization in terms of culture and cost benefits;
- Healthcare system level where SDM can be a key part of integrated care and the redesign of how policy is developed and delivered.

In Box 8.7 an example of shared decision making is described.

Box 8.7 Example of shared decision-making

Co-production and shared decision-making involve giving agency to people receiving care, so that they can be equal partners in a reciprocal relationship. Quality is then defined by the person we call a patient and shared decision-making becomes the way in which care interventions are decided upon.

An example is James, a 45-year-old man who has developed late-onset diabetes.

- The diabetes team *co-assess* his clinical condition, lifestyle, and home environment with him.
- They then discuss the treatment options and *co-decide* what his preference for treatment would be.
- Treatment focuses on lifestyle changes, with an emphasis on stopping smoking and decreasing alcohol consumption, increasing exercise, losing weight, and changing diet, as well as taking insulin. James *co-designs* the treatment programme with his family, as well as with the treatment team, so that he feels he owns the solution, with clear treatment goals that he has set himself.
- James and his family then discuss how he can ensure that this is successful and they *co-deliver* the treatment in partnership with the diabetes team nurse. At the same time, they discuss ways in which James can then *self-manage* diabetes within the family setting and become self-sufficient in his diabetes management.

Signposting

Choosing Wisely. *Promoting conversations between providers and patients.* Available at: ℘ https://www.choosingwisely.org (accessed 10 September 2023).

General Medical Council (2020). *Decision making and consent.* Available at: ℘ https://www.gmc-uk.org/ethical-guidance/ethical-guidance-for-doctors/decision-making-and-consent (accessed 10 September 2023).

National Institute for Health and Care Excellence (2021). *Shared decision making.* Available at: ℘ https://www.nice.org.uk/guidance/ng197 (accessed 10 September 2023).

Teach-back. Available at: ℘ http://www.teachbacktraining.org/home (accessed 10 September 2023).

Further reading

Carmona, C., Crutwell, J., Burnham, M., and Polak, L. (2021). Shared decision-making: summary of NICE guidance. *BMJ*, 373, p. n1430. doi: 10.1136/bmj.n1430.

Elwyn, G., Edwards, A., Wensing, M., Hibbs, R., Wilkinson, C., and Grol, R. (2001). Shared decision making observed in clinical practice: visual displays of communication sequence and patterns. *Journal of Evaluation in Clinical Practice*, 7(2), pp. 211–21. doi: 10.1046/j.1365-2753.2001.00286.x.

References

Barry, M.J. and Edgman-Levitan, S. (2012). Shared decision making: pinnacle of patient-centered care. *New England Journal of Medicine*, 366(9), pp. 780–1. doi: 10.1056/nejmp1109283.

Elwyn, G., Frosch, D., Thomson, R., et al. (2012). Shared decision making: a model for clinical practice. *Journal of General Internal Medicine*, 27(10), pp. 1361–7. doi: 10.1007/s11606-012-2077-6.

Elwyn, G., Frosch, D.L., and Kobrin, S. (2015). Implementing shared decision-making: consider all the consequences. *Implementation Science*, 11, p. 114. doi: 10.1186/s13012-016-0480-9.

Elwyn, G., Nelson, E., Hager, A., and Price, A. (2020). Coproduction: when users define quality. *BMJ Quality and Safety*, 29(9), pp. 711–16. doi: 10.1136/bmjqs-2019-009830.

Elwyn, G. and Vermunt, N.P.C.A. (2019). Goal-based shared decision-making: developing an integrated model. *Journal of Patient Experience*, 7(5), pp. 688–96. doi: 10.1177/2374373519878604.

National Institute for Health and Care Excellence (2021). *Shared decision making*. Available at: ✄ https://www.nice.org.uk/guidance/ng197 (accessed 17 August 2023).

Involving people in a project

What is people involvement in projects?

Involvement of people receiving care and their families in improvement projects is an important part of being person-centred. The purpose of involvement is:

- To be able to address *what really matters* to people by including them from the start and seeing the issues through their lens;
- To improve the challenges of their lived experience of their disease and of their experience of the way they receive care.

Why is people involvement in projects important?

All improvement aims to change something, be it processes, outcomes, or experience, to be better for people.

- People who are patients bring different dimensions when looking at a problem and often may have solutions that professionals do not see.
- To add value the people in the process, either the patient or staff member, need to be active participants in defining the programme and what needs to be changed.

Types of involvement

Often funders or government agencies will ask for a patient to be part of an improvement initiative. This can result in tokenism and disillusion and failure in active participation, unless clear principles are followed (Fereday and Rezel, 2019). People involvement (as patients) has different levels, from passive to more active roles:

- Focus groups to obtain a group understanding of what the problems are in the process, based on the lived experience of the patients;
- Consultation which is more passive and is about finding out what people think, rather than having them actively involved;
- Collaboration where the patient is more active, but the service providers are still in control;
- Active and equal membership in the improvement team;
- Part of a process of experience-based co-design (see ⊃ Chapter 14);
- Active co-production at every stage of the improvement process, in which there is an equal partnership and the patient may lead the programme of change.

Principles of patient involvement

Underlying these approaches are several principles and values that, if adopted, will increase the success of patient participation in change (Figure 8.6).

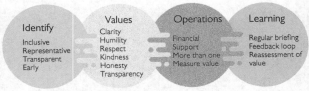

Identify
Inclusive
Representative
Transparent
Early

Values
Clarity
Humility
Respect
Kindness
Honesty
Transparency

Operations
Financial
Support
More than one
Measure value

Learning
Regular briefing
Feedback loop
Reassessment of
value

Figure 8.6 Principles for patient participation.
Based on Fereday, S., Rezel, K. (2019) Patient and public involvement in quality improvement. Healthcare Quality Improvement Partnership (HQIP).

- The reason for person involvement must be made clear and be constantly reviewed to assess whether the purpose is constant.
- People need to be asked early on in the process to ensure that the design of the project is enhanced.
- The person representing the patient group needs to be able to provide a comprehensive approach. This may be difficult to achieve in a heterogeneous population.
- When asking for a person to be involved, inclusivity is essential, especially if one has the perspective of equity as a key outcome.
- All actions must be transparent, as this will enhance engagement.
- The value of patient involvement must be assessed.
- There must be regular bidirectional feedback to ensure the value of patient participation.
- Support for patients as participants needs to be considered (e.g. travel costs, other subsistence requirements such as childcare).

Challenges in involving people in projects

It is not as easy as it may appear to co-produce and to involve people in projects, as there are many challenges that have to be addressed. In Table 8.4, possible challenges and solutions are provided to guide patient participation in a project.

Table 8.4 Challenges and potential solutions for patients in quality improvement

Challenge	Potential solutions
Rationale	Clarify the rationale for the role, and define the scope of the role
	Think through why patient involvement in the project is required—if this is not done, patient representation can be tokenistic
	Define the role to be played, so it is not ambiguous
Potential scope of the role	*Knowledge broker*
	As a provider of knowledge of the lived experience of how the service is delivered or of the illness itself
	Influencer
	As an influencer to direct discussion and to influence decisions made and how the project is developed and implemented
	Expertise
	Specific expertise as an advocate or in any other area
	This can be patient-facing developing material for patients or staff-facing with training and education
	Be flexible in the role to be played
Who should be invited?	This depends on the purpose and role of patient participation, the quality gap to be addressed, and the improvement methodology
	Focus on equity to ensure that disadvantaged groups can be part of the process

(Continued)

Table 8.4 *(Contd.)*

Challenge	Potential solutions
How to advertise for people to be part of the process?	Depending on the scope, this can be formal or informal; if there is a Patient Council, then they can assist in recruitment
How to ensure diversity and equity is addressed? (See ⊙ Chapter 5)	Consider who will be affected by any service improvement to decide on how to have active participation Partner with community organizations and actively seek out representatives from communities that may be disadvantaged Provide support for those who need financial, pastoral, or technical support
Are patient advocates or patients the best option?	Patients and patient advocates provide a unique perspective; through their personal lived experience though they may need to be able to apply this more generally. Ensure patients have the qualities and ability to be able to contribute to the activity in a meaningful and rewarding way
Are patient representatives paid or reimbursed for costs?	In general, most are voluntary, with all expenses covered to enable participation (e.g. travel, childcare)
How to manage expectations, especially if one cannot deliver all that is requested?	Be transparent at all times and realistic as to what can be achieved; do not promise something that cannot be delivered Clear roles and responsibilities for patients will assist in management of expectations
How to change the power dynamics that may exist as one moves to equal participatory co-production?	Ensure early involvement, preferably at the planning stage Actively promote and facilitate a non-hierarchical structure Provide training for staff and constantly monitor the power dimensions Value every opinion; engender trust and respect, and always be humble
Inclusivity and communication	Consider how to include people disadvantaged by illness, ethnicity, location, language, etc. Establish effective communication channels through social media, and patient stories

Based on Armstrong *et al.*, 2013, Bergerum *et al.*, 2019, and Bergerum *et al.*, 2020.

Each of these challenges can be resolved by using the techniques of co-production and require a culture of respect, kindness, and transparency. Understanding the power paradigm is essential, given the hierarchical nature of healthcare. The power differential is at every level, from clinical consultation where SDM is not routine to the micro-, meso-, and macrosystem levels where healthcare is still organized in a paternalistic way (Ocloo et al., 2020). To make progress, we need to:

- Acknowledge the power dynamics;
- Assess who has power and who has not;
- Design systems that allow for the power to be shared and address the prevailing power;
- Facilitate agency for those who have no power, be it patients or staff members (see ⮕ Chapter 10).

Signposting

Fereday, S. and Rezel, K. (2019). *Patient and public involvement in quality improvement.* Healthcare Quality Improvement Partnership. Available at: 🔗 https://www.hqip.org.uk/resource/a-guide-to-patient-and-public-involvement-in-quality-improvement/#.YncMlS8RpN0 (accessed 10 September 2023).

Further reading

Alidina, S., Martelli, P.F., Singer, S.J., and Aveling, E.-L. (2019). Optimizing patient partnership in primary care improvement. *Health Care Management Review*, 46(2), pp. 123–34. doi: 10.1097/hmr.0000000000000250.

Bombard, Y., Baker, G.R., Orlando, E., et al. (2018). Engaging patients to improve quality of care: a systematic review. *Implementation Science*, 13(1), pp. 1–22. doi: 10.1186/s13012-018-0784-z.

Todd, S., Coupland, C., and Randall, R. (2020). Patient and public involvement facilitators: could they be the key to the NHS quality improvement agenda? *Health Expectations*, 23(2), pp. 461–72. doi: 10.1111/hex.13023.

Wiig, S., Storm, M., Aase, K., et al. (2013). Investigating the use of patient involvement and patient experience in quality improvement in Norway: rhetoric or reality? *BMC Health Services Research*, 13(1), p. 206. doi: 10.1186/1472-6963-13-206.

References

Armstrong, N., Herbert, G., Aveling, E.-L., Dixon-Woods, M., and Martin, G. (2013). Optimizing patient involvement in quality improvement. *Health Expectations*, 16(3), pp. e36–47. doi: 10.1111/hex.12039.

Bergerum, C., Engström, A.K., Thor, J., and Wolmesjö, M. (2020). Patient involvement in quality improvement—a 'tug of war' or a dialogue in a learning process to improve healthcare? *BMC Health Services Research*, 20(1), p. 1115. doi: 10.1186/s12913-020-05970-4.

Bergerum, C., Thor, J., Josefsson, K., and Wolmesjö, M. (2019). How might patient involvement in healthcare quality improvement efforts work—a realist literature review. *Health Expectations*, 22(5), pp. 952–64. doi: 10.1111/hex.12900.

Fereday, S. and Rezel, K. (2019). *Patient and public involvement in quality improvement.* Healthcare Quality Improvement Partnership. Available at: 🔗 https://www.hqip.org.uk/resource/a-guide-to-patient-and-public-involvement-in-quality-improvement/#.YncMlS8RpN0 (accessed 10 September 2023).

Ocloo, J., Goodrich, J., Tanaka, H., Birchall-Searle, J., Dawson, D., and Farr, M. (2020). The importance of power, context and agency in improving patient experience through a patient and family centred care approach. *Health Research Policy and Systems*, 18(1), p. 10. doi: 10.1186/s12961-019-0487-1.

Top tips

- Always see patients as people who have a wider experience than the illness they have.
- Ask 'What matters to you?' and be prepared to open the door to a meaningful interaction.
- Ask 'What matters to me?' as a caregiver, as this will help to define the values of care.
- Discover the lived experience of the person, so that care can be improved.
- Embrace co-production as the way to work with people at every level.
- At a clinical level, adopt SDM within daily clinical practice.
- Ask who should be involved in an improvement project, and have respectful and transparent interactions with the patient member of the team.

Summary

PCC is both a philosophical approach to healthcare as well as a method to deliver care that really matters to people.

The foundation of PCC is based on understanding and embracing the *lived experience* of people delivering and receiving care. To achieve PCC, the culture and design of care will need to change.

Co-production of health as Quality 3.0 offers the people called healthcare professionals to partner in an equal and transparent way with the people called patients to deliver co-designed and co-produced solutions to the challenge of healthcare within complex systems.

The outcome is respectful, coordinated care that enables people to reach their potential with dignity in an integrated and coordinated model of care. To achieve relevant outcomes in our quality improvement projects, we need to involve the people in the process at every stage of the improvement process.

Person-centred care resources

Several websites provide information on the philosophy, theory, and practice of person-centred care.

Beryl Institute https://www.theberylinstitute.org/

Institute for Patient and Family Centred Care https://www.ipfcc.org/

International Consortium for Healthcare Outcome Measures https://www.ichom.org/

International Alliance of Patients' Organizations: (IAPO) https:// www.iapo.org.uk/

Picker Institute https://www.picker.org/

Planetree International https://www.planetree.org/

Point of Care Foundation https://www.pointofcarefoundation.org.uk

World Patient Alliance https://www.worldpatientsalliance.org

Summary

Person-centred care resources

Standards in healthcare

(Quality 1.0)

Key points
- Standards provide regulation and enhance operation across a wide variety of sectors.
- Standards are developed by individuals and groups with expertise in their field in collaboration with key stakeholders.
- Standards are implemented by organizations.
- Standards in healthcare ensure safe, high-quality care for patients.
- There are different ways to measure standards, which include guidelines, external evaluation, regulation, accreditation, certification, and inspection.
- Adherence to standards may be regulated by regulatory bodies or implemented privately within organizations and then utilized for processes such as accreditation and certification.
- Inspection assesses whether standards are met or not, and plays an important role in external evaluation.
- Clinical guidelines and pathways provide internal standards for clinical teams.

The need for standards in healthcare

Why are standards important?

Every day, as we go about our daily activities, we interact with processes and systems that are subject to standards. Standards help processes to reach a certain level of quality and ensure safety. For example:

- Food hygiene standards ensure that restaurants are safe for their customers;
- Fire standards ensure that buildings people visit are safe;
- Air regulatory standards ensure that people can fly safely.

Standards provide regulation and enhance operations across a wide variety of sectors. When systems and processes fail, it is often due to the absence of standards.

Every country has its own bodies for standards in different sectors. The International Organization for Standardization (ISO) oversees over 166 national standards bodies and publishes standards across a wide variety of areas.

What is the concept of standards in healthcare?

In → Chapter 1, the concept of *Quality 1.0* was introduced.

- Ernest Codman, a surgeon in Boston, was the pioneer in developing standards in healthcare in the early part of the twentieth century, when he developed the concept of the 'end results system'.
- Clinicians and hospitals could follow their patients and receive feedback to ensure that the desired outcomes were realized and to facilitate continual improvement. This concept of external evaluation was initially rejected by Codman's institution.
- Nowadays clinical guidelines, certification, accreditation, inspection, and external evaluation are critically important components for ensuring the quality of healthcare (Figure 9.1).

In this chapter, an understanding of the process for developing standards is provided, as measurements against standards are a crucial first step in the quality improvement journey.

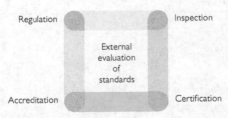

Figure 9.1 Types of standards used in healthcare.

What is the role of a healthcare professional?

It is important for all who work in healthcare to understand their role in maintaining standards and how to take part in an external evaluation, either by the regulator or by the accreditation body. This will enable safe-quality care to be provided to those who require it.

Standards can help to:
- Assess and improve the quality of a health service;
- Determine what type of care should be offered and identify gaps in the current systems;
- Improve health and safety in the workplace;
- Identify best practices, leading to reliable and higher-quality health services for patients and service users.

How do standards fit in with quality improvement?

The Juran Trilogy, discussed in ⮑ Chapter 3, calls for quality planning, control, and improvement.
- This is the quality management system, and standards are at its core as part of quality control.
- Standards in healthcare set expectations and assist healthcare professionals in providing consistency in care and identifying the minimum standards.
- When faced with challenging or unfamiliar scenarios, standards can help guide frontline staff and provide clarity around clinical roles and responsibilities, progression, and training, and help alleviate any undue stress.
- Using improvement methodologies allows healthcare professionals to continually improve processes to ensure that standards are consistently met.

Further reading

Codman, E.A. (2009). The classic: the registry of bone sarcomas as an example of the end-result idea in hospital organization. 1924. *Clinical Orthopaedics and Related Research*, 467(11), pp. 2766–70. doi: 10.1007/s11999-009-1048-7.

Dagi, T.F. and Dagi, L.R. (2019). Commentary: Ernest Codman and the impact of quality improvement in neurosurgery: a century since the idea of the 'end result'. *Neurosurgery*, 84(2), pp. E120–1. doi: 10.1093/neuros/nyy526.

Different approaches to standards

How to define standards

There are different ways to measure standards. Table 9.1 provides the definitions for each of these. These are complementary and support each other.

Table 9.1 Definitions of approaches to standards

	Description	Common examples
Standards	Standards set out a framework upon which a system operates	NICE sets out standards (e.g. end-of-life care standard)
Guidelines and clinical pathways	Guidelines support organizations and their staff in decision-making and promote best practice Clinical pathways are standardized, evidence-based multidisciplinary management plans, with an inbuilt evaluation of implementation	Royal College of Obstetricians and Gynaecologists (RCOG) (e.g. maternal collapse in pregnancy and the puerperium guideline)
External evaluation	Evaluates performance against a defined set of standards, using external evaluators. It occurs in accreditation, regulation, inspection, and certification	Evaluation of the registrar training programme by the Royal College of Physicians (RCP)
Regulation	Carried out by an independent body and ensures that standards set out by commissioners are achieved by organizations and individuals working within them	Care Quality Commission (CQC) inspects and rates NHS and independent (private) hospitals
Accreditation	A self-assessment and external peer review process used by health and social care organizations to accurately assess their level of performance in relation to established standards and to implement ways to continuously improve the health or social care system	International Society for Quality in Health Care (ISQua) Joint Commission International Accreditation Canada CHKS
Certification	Processes whereby an organization is reviewed by governmental/non-governmental evaluators and performance is assessed and accredited based on set standards. Certification assesses and awards additional qualifications beyond minimum requirements	European Society of Human Reproduction and Embryology (ESHRE) certification programmes in reproductive medicine, for nurses, midwives, and clinical embryologists

Table 9.1   *(Contd.)*

	Description	Common examples
Inspection	Inspection is performed by an external organization on site and ensures that clinical practice adheres to paper-based reporting within the organization	Health Improvement Scotland to identify good practice and to address areas for improvement

NICE, National Institute for Health and Care Excellence.

Signposting

Accreditation Canada. Available at: ℘ https://accreditation.ca (accessed 10 September 2023).

Care Quality Commission (CQC). Available at: ℘ https://www.cqc.org.uk (accessed 10 September 2023).

CHKS. Available at: ℘ https://www.chks.co.uk (accessed 10 September 2023).

European Society of Human Reproduction and Embryology (ESHRE). Available at: ℘ https://www.eshre.eu (accessed 10 September 2023).

Healthcare Improvement Scotland. Available at: ℘ https://www.healthcareimprovementscotland.org (accessed 10 September 2023).

Improving Quality in Physiological Services Accreditation (IQIPS). Available at: ℘ https://www.ukas.com/accreditation/standards/iqips/ (accessed 10 September 2023).

International Organization for Standardization (ISO). Available at: ℘ https://www.iso.org (accessed 10 September 2023).

International Society for Quality in Health Care (ISQua). Available at: ℘ https://isqua.org (accessed 10 September 2023).

Joint Commission International. Available at: ℘ https://www.jointcommissioninternational.org (accessed 10 September 2023).

National Institute for Health and Care Excellence (NICE). Available at: ℘ https://www.nice.org.uk (accessed 10 September 2023).

Royal College of Obstetricians and Gynaecologists (RCOG). Available at: ℘ https://www.rcog.org.uk (accessed 10 September 2023).

Royal College of Physicians (RCP). Available at: ℘ https://www.rcplondon.ac.uk (accessed 10 September 2023).

United Kingdom Accreditation Service (UKAS). Available at: ℘ https://www.ukas.com (accessed 10 September 2023).

The Quality Standard for Imaging (QSI). Available at: ℘ https://www.rcr.ac.uk/clinical-radiology/service-delivery/quality-standard-imaging-qsi (accessed 10 September 2023).

Standards development

How are standards developed?

Standards are developed by individuals and groups with expertise in their field in collaboration with key stakeholders.

- Standards are applicable to all areas of healthcare, including organizations, individual departments, healthcare professionals, service users, consumables, and equipment.
- The standard development process has several stages, as listed in Box 9.1.

Box 9.1 Standards development

1. Identify the topic and the purpose of the standard.
2. Form a standards development committee, including experts, service providers, and service users.
3. Undertake a comprehensive literature review to assess the available best evidence for the standard.
4. Develop a draft standard by consensus—a Delphi approach can be used.
5. Publish the draft standard for consultation.
6. Review feedback and amend, and then agree on a final version.
7. Publish and implement the standard.
8. Measure the impact of the standard on the identified topic it addresses.
9. Revise the standard as required following the above process.

The developed standards should be:

- Relevant (i.e. measure what is important for quality for the patients and providers);
- Based on the latest evidence for the item being assessed;
- Achievable in that implementation of the standard will lead to quality of care being improved;
- Measurable so that the current state and improvement over time can be demonstrated.

Greenfield (2012) reviewed standard development and concluded that there is a lack of robust empirical evidence examining the development, writing, implementation, and impact of healthcare accreditation standards.

In the past, patients or patient organizations have not been included in standard development. It is now recommended that standards are co-produced with the people delivering care, as well as with those receiving care.

How are standards implemented?

- Following development, standards are intended to be implemented by organizations.
- Adherence to the standards may be regulated by regulatory bodies or implemented within organizations and then be the basis for external evaluation by accreditation and certification.

Signposting

The organizations listed below develop standards.

International

International Organization for Standardization (ISO). Available at: ✍ https://www.iso.org (accessed 10 September 2023).

International Society for Quality in Health Care External Evaluation Association (ISQuaEEA). Available at: ✍ https://ieea.ch (accessed 10 September 2023).

Australia

Australian Council on Healthcare Standards (ACHS). Available at: ✍ https://www.achsi.org (accessed 10 September 2023).

Canada

Accreditation Canada. Available at: ✍ https://accreditation.ca (accessed 10 September 2023).

Jordan

Health Care Accreditation Council (HCAC). Available at: ✍ https://hcac.jo/en-us/ (accessed 10 September 2023).

South Africa

Council for Health Service Accreditation of Southern Africa (COHSASA). Available at: ✍ https://cohsasa.co.za (accessed 10 September 2023).

United Kingdom

CHKS. Available at: ✍ https://www.chks.co.uk (accessed 10 September 2023).

United States

Joint Commission International. Available at: ✍ https://www.jointcommissioninternational.org (accessed 10 September 2023).

Further reading

Braithwaite, J., Vincent, C., Nicklin, W., and Amalberti, R. (2018). Coping with more people with more illness. Part 2: new generation of standards for enabling healthcare system transformation and sustainability. *International Journal for Quality in Health Care*, 31(2), pp. 159–63. doi: 10.1093/intqhc/mzy236.

Greenfield, D., Civil, M., Donnison, A., Hogden, A., Hinchcliff, R., Westbrook, J., and Braithwaite, J. (2014). A mechanism for revising accreditation standards: a study of the process, resources required and evaluation outcomes. *BMC Health Services Research*, 14, p. 571. doi: 10.1186/s12913-014-0571-8.

Hammond, W.E., Jaffe, C., and Kush, R.D. (2009). Healthcare standards development. The value of nurturing collaboration. *Journal of AHIMA*, 80(7), pp. 44–52.

Hinchcliff, R., Greenfield, D., Westbrook, J.I., Pawsey, M., Mumford, V., and Braithwaite, J. (2013). Stakeholder perspectives on implementing accreditation programs: a qualitative study of enabling factors. *BMC Health Services Research*, 13, p. 437. doi: 10.1186/1472-6963-13-437.

Shaw, C.D. (2015). How can healthcare standards be standardised? *BMJ Quality and Safety*, 24(10), pp. 615–19. doi: 10.1136/bmjqs-2015-003955.

Reference

Greenfield, D., Pawsey, M., Hinchcliff, R., Moldovan, M., and Braithwaite, J. (2012). The standard of healthcare accreditation standards: a review of empirical research underpinning their development and impact. *BMC Health Services Research*, 12, p. 329. doi: 10.1186/1472-6963-12-329.

External evaluation

How does external evaluation work?

Inspection has an important role in external evaluation.
- Inspection aims to assess whether standards are met or not.
- Inspection addresses 'decoupling', which is the discrepancy between clinical practice and paper-based reporting within organizations.
- Inspection is initiated and performed by an external organization.

The aim of inspection is to:
- Ensure adherence to standards and guidelines;
- Provide certification and accreditation;
- Promote high-quality, evidence-based healthcare.

Following an inspection, an organization is expected to acknowledge non-conformities and take accountability for implementing necessary changes. The evidence for inspection is variable, as there have been few published studies. Now there is a growing body of anecdotal evidence to suggest that external regulation which includes inspection identifies good, as well as poor, practice and enables improvement initiatives to be implemented.

An inspection framework has three actions, as shown in Table 9.2 (Hood, 1999).

Table 9.2 Inspection framework

Setting direction	Action taken at a systems level such as creation of legislation or national guidelines
Detection	Actions directed towards an individual organization to ensure adherence to standards of care
Enforcement	Actions taken at an organizational level to implement changes following detection of non-conformities

What is the role of the inspector or surveyor?

An external regulator, inspector, or surveyor:
- Assesses and inspects performance against an agreed standard;
- Gathers information from routine data, patient outcomes, and interviews with staff and patients;
- Identifies variation from the standard;
- Investigates non-conformance to standards and the reasons for deviation from standards;
- Recommends a framework to prevent serious failures;
- Recommends action to address issues that have been found;
- Identifies potential quality improvement to meet standards;
- Reports the findings to the organization, the regulatory body, and the public.

Further reading

Flodgren, G., Gonçalves-Bradley, D.C., and Pomey, M.-P. (2016). External inspection of compliance with standards for improved healthcare outcomes. *Cochrane Database of Systematic Reviews*, 12(12), CD008992. doi: 10.1002/14651858.cd008992.pub3.

Graf, B. and Richards, M. (2014). Inspection as a driver for quality improvement. *Future Hospital Journal*, 1(2), pp. 76–9. doi: 10.7861/futurehosp.14.020.

Schaefer, C. and Wiig, S. (2017). Strategy and practise of external inspection in healthcare services: a Norwegian comparative case study. *Safety in Health*, 3, p. 3. doi: 10.1186/s40886-017-0054-9.

Weenink, J.-W., Wallenburg, I., Leistikow, I., and Bal, R.A. (2021). Publication of inspection frameworks: a qualitative study exploring the impact on quality improvement and regulation in three healthcare settings. *BMJ Quality and Safety*, 30(10), pp. 804–11. doi: 10.1136/bmjqs-2020-011337.

Reference

Hood, C. (1999). *Regulation Inside Government: Waste Watchers, Quality Police, and Sleaze-Busters*. Oxford: Oxford University Press.

Types of inspection or evaluation

Inspection can be undertaken in several ways, each of which is described below.

External regulation

External regulation is carried out by an independent body and ensures that standards set out by healthcare commissioners are achieved by organizations and individuals working within them.

- Regulators can be established by the Department of Health (DoH) to regulate public and private health sectors.
- There are different models in that some are arm's-length bodies, either separate from the DoH or they could be part of it.
- The regulator can include the quality improvement organization or be totally separate. Hospital inspection is part of the licensing of health service providers.

External regulation plays a critical role in ensuring that there are minimum standards of care to ensure the public receives safe and high-quality care.

Factors that may prevent an organization from meeting minimum standards include time, resources, and finances, which can result in shortcomings in care (Dixon, 2005).

In Box 9.2 different types of regulation is explained.

> **Box 9.2 Examples of regulators**
>
> *England*
> The Care Quality Commission (CQC; available at: ℘ https://www.cqc.org.uk, accessed 10 September 2023) regulates all health and social care services. The role of the CQC includes: registering care providers; monitoring, inspecting, and rating services; acting where required to ensure safety for service users; and providing and publishing independent views. The output of an external evaluation is the award of a recognized status to an organization and is valid for a defined period of time.
>
> *Scotland*
> Healthcare Improvement Scotland (available at: ℘ https://www.healthcareimprovementscotland.org, accessed 10 September 2023) regulates care to ensure that healthcare services meet the required standards of care, good practice is identified, and areas for improvement are addressed. Inspectors undertake announced and unannounced inspections of healthcare services. These involve a physical inspection of the clinical areas and discussions with staff.
>
> *Wales*
> Healthcare Inspectorate Wales (HIW, available at: ℘ https://bcuhb.nhs.wales, accessed 10 September 2023) is the independent inspectorate and regulator of all healthcare in Wales. Its purpose is to provide independent and objective assurance on the quality, safety, and effectiveness of healthcare services, making recommendations to healthcare organizations to promote improvements.

Northern Ireland

The Regulation and Quality Improvement Authority (RQIA, available at: 🔖 https://www.rqia.org.uk, accessed 10 September 2023) is the independent body responsible for monitoring and inspecting the availability and quality of health and social care services in Northern Ireland, and encouraging improvements in the quality of those services.

Ireland

The Health Information and Quality Authority (available at: 🔖 https://www.hiqa.ie, accessed 10 September 2023) is an independent authority that regulates and inspects health organizations. The aim is to drive high-quality and safe care for people using health and social care services.

Accreditation and certification

Accreditation and certification entail the review of an organization by external evaluators.

- Performance is assessed against an agreed set of standards.
- Accreditation and certification are often used interchangeably and are closely linked, though they have different steps (Table 9.3).
- Accreditation has played a central role in healthcare for over 100 years and is now evident in over 70 countries. It is an established process to ensure safe and high-quality patient-centred care.
- Although accreditation in healthcare continues to expand, research to support its effectiveness has been limited.
- Accreditation can promote change and professional development.
- Some studies suggest that the process of accreditation can have negative effects on healthcare organizations by distracting and rechannelling energy and investment away from primary clinical goals.
- Many countries employ an accrediting body to act as its assessor of the quality of healthcare as part of the regulatory process.

Table 9.3 Differences between accreditation and certification

Accreditation	Assesses the compliance of organizations to recognized standard/scheme
	Non-governmental evaluator
	Inspector employed by an accreditation body
	Requires on-site evaluation, though after the COVID-19 pandemic, remote evaluation has been introduced
	Often a voluntary process for organizations
Certification	Audit on conformity to recognized standard or scheme
	Governmental or non-governmental evaluator
	Inspector employed by organizations/individuals
	Audits organizations, individuals, or products

Accreditation is either voluntary, in which a hospital or hospital group includes accreditation as part of an ongoing quality programme. Alternatively, accreditation may be used by a department of health as part of their quality assurance programme, as demonstrated in the case study in Box 9.3.

A service line can be certified by a professional body to ensure the service meets international standards, as demonstrated in the case study on stroke services in Box 9.4, or national certification as shown in Box 9.5.

Box 9.3 Case study: accreditation on a national level

The Faroe Islands have three hospitals, none of which had ever received accreditation. A study was designed to assess seven clinical conditions at these facilities before and after accreditation.

The Danish Institute for Accreditation in Healthcare carried out the initial assessments for accreditation.

- All standards being assessed were modified in line with local Faroe legislation.
- The seven clinical conditions were assessed by using process performance measures before and after accreditation.
- The outcome of the study demonstrated that the likelihood of patients receiving full recommended care was significantly higher following accreditation.
- This finding highlights the fact that those improvements implemented in processes in preparation for accreditation can have a positive impact on clinical care.

Bergholt, M.D., Falstie-Jensen, A.M., Hibbert, P., *et al.* (2021). The association between first-time accreditation and the delivery of recommended care: a before and after study in the Faroe Islands. *BMC Health Services Research*, 21(1), p. 917. doi:10.1186/s12913-021-06952-w.

Box 9.4 Example of certification of a clinical service

The European Stroke Organisation (ESO) aims to improve care and reduce the number of deaths due to stroke. The organization provides certification with external evaluation to measure the capabilities of stroke centres in Europe based on the ESO's stroke recommendations.

Specific aims are to:

- Reduce variation in clinical processes by standardizing processes with clinical pathways and guidelines;
- Improve clinical outcomes with improved processes (e.g. ensuring door-to-decision time is within 30 minutes);
- Provide a benchmark for the quality of stroke management, so that stroke centres can measure how well they do in meeting high standards;
- Facilitate the development of clinical teams and expertise in stroke management;
- Enhance a culture of excellence across the organization;
- Strengthen public confidence in the quality of the care delivered.

European Stroke Organisation (n.d.). *Stroke Unit and Stroke Centre Certification*. Available at: https://eso-stroke.org/projects/stroke-unit-and-stroke-centre-certification/ (accessed 10 September 2023).

Ringelstein, E.B., Chamorro, A., Kaste, M., *et al.* (2013). European Stroke Organisation recommendations to establish a stroke unit and stroke center. *Stroke*, 44(3), pp. 828–40. doi: 10.1161/strokeaha.112.670430.

Box 9.5 Case study: evaluation of a service line by a Royal College of Physicians case study

Dr Biggs was informed by the hospital Chief Executive Officer that following feedback from trainees, an external evaluator from the Royal College of Physicians would evaluate the gastroenterology training programme at their tertiary referral hospital. The gastroenterology service was well regarded nationally for its clinical service as a tertiary referral national service. The training programme received an extremely poor external evaluation with a number of critical recommendations:

* It was poorly structured, with no defined learning objectives or curriculum;
* There was no process in place for evaluation or mentorship of the trainees;
* There were no additional educational activities for trainees, and the pass rate of their trainees for the membership examination was dismal;
* Feedback from trainees suggested that they were unsupported and overworked, and felt on completion of the programme that they would not be able to function independently.

The evaluation demonstrated the value of the assessment, and an action plan was implemented to improve the learning and training experience.

Further reading

Carrasco-Peralta, J.A., Herrera-Usagre, M., Reyes-Alcázar, V., and Torres-Olivera, A. (2019). Healthcare accreditation as trigger of organisational change: the view of professionals. *Journal of Healthcare Quality Research*, 34(2), pp. 59–65. doi: 10.1016/j.jhqr.2018.09.007.

Greenfield, D., Iqbal, U., O'Connor, E., Conlan, N., and Wilson, H. (2021). An appraisal of healthcare accreditation agencies and programs: similarities, differences, challenges and opportunities. *International Journal for Quality in Health Care*, 33(4), p. mzab150. doi: 10.1093/intqhc/mzab150.

Greenfield, D., Lawrence, S.A., Kellner, A., Townsend, K., and Wilkinson, A. (2019). Health service accreditation stimulating change in clinical care and human resource management processes: a study of 311 Australian hospitals. *Health Policy*, 123(7), pp. 661–5. doi: 10.1016/j.healthpol.2019.04.006.

Hovlid, E., Braut, G.S., Hannisdal, E., *et al.* (2020). Mediators of change in healthcare organisations subject to external assessment: a systematic review with narrative synthesis. *BMJ Open*, 10(8), p. e038850. doi: 10.1136/bmjopen-2020-038850.

Hovlid, E., Høifødt, H., Smedbråten, B., and Braut, G.S. (2015). A retrospective review of how nonconformities are expressed and finalized in external inspections of health-care facilities. *BMC Health Services Research*, 15, p. 405. doi: 10.1186/s12913-015-1068-9.

Hussein, M., Pavlova, M., Ghalwash, M., and Groot, W. (2021). The impact of hospital accreditation on the quality of healthcare: a systematic literature review. *BMC Health Services Research*, 21(1), p. 1057. doi: 10.1186/s12913-021-07097-6.

Jha, A.K. (2018). Accreditation, quality, and making hospital care better. *JAMA*, 320(23), p. 2410. doi: 10.1001/jama.2018.18810.

Lam, M.B., Figueroa, J.F., Feyman, Y., Reimold, K.E., Orav, E.J., and Jha, A.K. (2018). Association between patient outcomes and accreditation in US hospitals: observational study. *BMJ*, 363, p. k4011. doi: 10.1136/bmj.k4011.

Rooney, A.L. and van Ostenberg, P.R. (1999). *Licensure, accreditation, and certification: approaches to health services quality*. Bethesda MD: USAID, Quality Assurance Project.

Swiers, R. (n.d.). *Assessing the value of accreditation to health systems and organisations*. Available at: https://ahha.asn.au/system/files/docs/publications/evidence_brief_no.18_assessing_the_value_of_accreditation.pdf (accessed 10 September 2023).

World Health Organization (2022). *Health care accreditation and quality of care: exploring the role of accreditation and external evaluation of health care facilities and organizations*. Available at: 𝒮 https://www.who.int/publications/i/item/9789240055230 (accessed 10 September 2023).

Reference

Dixon, J. (2005). *Regulating health care: the way forward*. London: The King's Fund.

Learning in the external evaluation

Learning from external evaluation

For an external evaluation to be of any value, it should be embedded in a learning healthcare system which aims to continually improve its processes to achieve desired outcomes, as set by the organization's strategic vision.

- Although many healthcare organizations aim to improve quality and safety of care, many are unsuccessful when it comes to measuring outcomes.
- To improve from the findings of the external evaluation process, an organization should aspire to be a learning health system (see Chapter 12).
- Learning health systems are 'systems in which science, informatics, incentives, and culture are aligned for continuous improvement and innovation, with best practices seamlessly embedded in the delivery process. Patients and families are active participants in all elements, and new knowledge captured as an integral by-product of the delivery experience' (Institute of Medicine, 2007).
- Learning health systems can provide actionable knowledge, which enable improvements in patient outcomes and experience.

In a learning health system, translation of knowledge—that is, what needs to be done—into tangible action to achieve the outcomes is complex. Graham et al. (2006) proposed that the knowledge to action cycle comprises two key components:

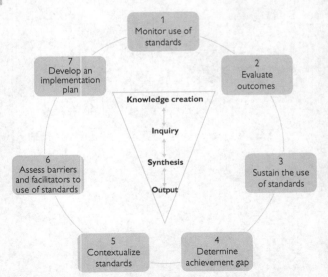

Figure 9.2 The knowledge to action cycle adapted to the accreditation process.
Based on Graham et al., 2006 and Mitchell, J.I., Graham, I.D., Nicklin, W., 2020.

- Knowledge creation (e.g. creation of the latest evidence to achieve quality care);
- Knowledge action or application cycle (i.e. application of the knowledge to real-time implementation).

If one applies this logic to the external evaluation process, one can see that the challenge is in consistent implementation of the standard to achieve the desired outcomes. Therefore, learning from the process of external evaluation is fundamental to its success. This cycle can be applied to the accreditation process, as outlined in Figure 9.2.

Standards can only be successful if all involved in reaching the standard use them as a learning opportunity—that is, learning about what is required for achievement of good outcomes, learning about the challenge of implementation, and learning how to continually improve.

References

Graham, I.D., Logan, J., Harrison, M.B., et al. (2006). Lost in knowledge translation: time for a map? *Journal of Continuing Education in the Health Professions*, 26(1), pp. 13–24. doi: 10.1002/chp.47.

Institute of Medicine (US) Roundtable on Evidence-Based Medicine; Olsen, L., Aisner, D., and McGinnis, J.M., eds. (2007). *The Learning Healthcare System: Workshop Summary*. Washington, DC: National Academies Press.

Mitchell, J.I., Graham, I.D., and Nicklin, W. (2020). The unrecognized power of health services accreditation: more than external evaluation. *International Journal for Quality in Health Care*, 32(7), pp. 445–55. doi: 10.1093/intqhc/mzaa063.

Internal clinical standards

Clinical guidelines

Guidelines are established based on the most up-to-date research and evidence (Table 9.4).

- They require continuous review and evaluation, and allow for certification and accreditation.
- Guidelines support organizations and their staff in decision-making and promote best practice. An evaluation framework is shown in Figure 9.3

Table 9.4 Research evidence use and guideline development

Guideline appraisal	Regular review, best in real time. Both internal and external reviews
	A checklist should be used (e.g. AGREE—a reporting checklist to assist guideline developers)
	The checklist should be adapted to be specific to the guideline
Scheduling of updates	Routine monitoring to establish whether updates are required
	Routine review of newly published research to update guidelines on a continuous basis
	Independent external periodic review of guidelines
	Consider the establishment of a guideline panel to ensure regular review and updates of guideline
Evaluation of recommendations and impact of guidelines	Provide advice regarding impact assessment and practical support
	Randomized evaluations
Responsibility for ensuring that important uncertainties are addressed by future research	Develop a process to keep up-to-date with the literature and national recommendations

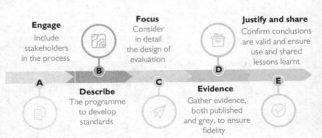

Engage
Include stakeholders in the process

Focus
Consider in detail the design of evaluation

Justify and share
Confirm conclusions are valid and ensure use and shared lessons learnt

A — B — C — D — E

Describe
The programme to develop standards

Evidence
Gather evidence, both published and grey, to ensure fidelity

Figure 9.3 Guideline evaluation framework.

Guideline committees play an important role and should identify areas where uncertainties exist that require further research to establish evidence.

Clinical care pathways

Clinical care pathways play an important role in improving patient outcomes. They act as tools to drive evidence-based healthcare. The definition of a clinical care pathway is given in Box 9.6.

> ### Box 9.6 European Pathway Association definition
>
> A care pathway is a complex intervention for the mutual decision-making and organization of care processes for a well-defined group of patients during a well-defined period. Defining characteristics of care pathways include:
> - An explicit statement of the goals and key elements of care, based on evidence, best practice, and patients' expectations and their characteristics;
> - Facilitation of communication among team members and with patients and families;
> - Coordination of the care process by coordinating the roles and sequencing the activities of the multidisciplinary care team, patients, and their relatives;
> - Documentation, monitoring, and evaluation of variances and outcomes;
> - Identification of appropriate resources.
>
> From European Pathway Association. *About care pathways: E-P-A definition of care pathway.* Available at: https://e-p-a.org/care-pathways/ (accessed 10 September 2023).
>
> Vanhaecht, K., De Witte, K., and Sermeus, W. (2007). *The Impact of Clinical Pathways on the Organisation of Care Processes.* PhD dissertation. KU Leuven: Katholieke Universiteit Leuven.

Rotter *et al.* (2019) summarized the purpose of clinical pathways as follows:
- Translate guidelines into local practice and context;
- Specify the specific steps in treatment or care, often with a time frame within which the action is to be taken;
- Standardize care for a clinical problem or a part of the treatment episode.

Studies have shown that implementation of clinical pathways can lead to a reduction in length of hospital stay, cost, and rate of complications, and improved clinical documentation.

In many European countries, clinical pathways are regarded as a way to ensure that people receive the evidence-based care they need when they require it.

The challenge remains in implementation, and patient involvement can assist in ensuring the pathways are followed. Careful assessment of adherence is required and real-time assessment of implementation is generally built into the pathways.

Signposting

AGREE. *AGREE reporting checklist*. Available at: 🔗 https://www.agreetrust.org/resource-centre/agree-reporting-checklist/ (accessed 10 September 2023).

Centers for Disease Control and Prevention. *Program evaluation*. Available at: 🔗 https://www.cdc.gov/evaluation/ (accessed 10 September 2023).

European Pathway Association. Available at: 🔗 https://e-p-a.org (accessed 10 September 2023).

National Institute for Health and Care Excellence (NICE). Available at: 🔗 https://www.nice.org.uk (accessed 10 September 2023).

Further reading

Oxman, A.D., Schünemann, H.J., and Fretheim, A. (2006). Improving the use of research evidence in guideline development: 14. Reporting guidelines. *Health Research Policy and Systems*, 4, p. 26. doi: 10.1186/1478-4505-4-26.

Vanhaecht, K., De Witte, K., Panella, M., and Sermeus, W. (2009). Do pathways lead to better organized care processes? *Journal of Evaluation in Clinical Practice*, 15(5), pp. 782–8. doi: 10.1111/j.1365-2753.2008.01068.x.

Reference

Rotter, T., de Jong, R.B., Lacko, S.E., *et al*. (2019). Clinical pathways as a quality strategy. In: Busse, R., Klazinga, N., Panteli, D., *et al*., eds. *Improving Healthcare Quality in Europe: Characteristics, Effectiveness and Implementation of Different Strategies* (Health Policy Series, No. 53.). Copenhagen: European Observatory on Health Systems and Policies; p. 12.

Top tips

Summary

Top tips

- Appreciate the importance of setting standards to ensure quality and safety in healthcare.
- Recognize the role in maintaining standards within an organization.
- Identify gaps within an organization and actively contribute to the development of standards to address these deficiencies.
- Consider all key aspects involved in the measurement of standards.
- Actively encourage and participate in external evaluation.

Summary

- Every day we interact with processes and systems that are subject to standards. Standards help processes to reach a certain level of quality and ensure safety.
- Standards can help to:
  - Assess and improve the quality of health service;
  - Determine what type of care should be offered and identify gaps in the current systems;
  - Improve health and safety in the workplace;
  - Identify best practices, leading to reliable and higher-quality health services for patients and service users.
- By incorporating improvement methodologies, standards can allow healthcare professionals to continually improve processes, to ensure that standards are consistently met.
- Inspection has an important role in external evaluation. The aim of inspection is to:
  - Ensure adherence to standards and guidelines;
  - Provide certification and accreditation;
  - Promote high-quality, evidence-based healthcare.
- Inspection can be undertaken in several ways:
  - External regulation;
  - Accreditation;
  - Certification.
- Clinical guidelines and clinical pathways are key components of internal clinical standards.
- These evaluation systems are critically important to ensure the provision of safe and high-quality healthcare.

Chapter 10

The Lens of Psychology

Key points

- The beliefs and attitudes of people influence their actions and therefore are of vital importance in any quality improvement project.
- Working with people involved in a process—both patients and providers of care—is the foundation for quality.
- There are several methods you can use to build the *will* for change, and this will ensure the success of the project.

Introduction

In this chapter, we aim to provide practical ways in which you can build and develop an improvement culture within a team and harness the power of the most important improvement element—the team and its people. Improvement requires more than the technical or 'hard' skills. Success is dependent on winning over peoples' hearts and minds, often termed 'soft' skills. In Figure 10.1, this is conceptualized.

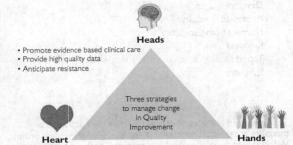

Heads
• Promote evidence based clinical care
• Provide high quality data
• Anticipate resistance

Three strategies
to manage change
in Quality
Improvement

Heart
• Invoke values of altruism and humanism
• Appeal to emotion
• Understand root cause of resistance
• Coproduce

Hands
• Use rigorous QI methodology
• Identify champions
• Gather critical mass of supporters

Figure 10.1 Engaging the hearts and mind for change.
Reproduced with permission from Shaikh, U., Lachman, P (2021).

What is the psychology of improvement?

Psychology of improvement is the adaptive, human side of change. Deming, one of the leaders in improvement science, defines psychology as the way in which people think and feel, what motivates them, what demotivates them, and how they behave, including when they encounter change (Deming, 1986). Understanding psychology is one of the four lenses of Deming's System of Profound Knowledge.

In this chapter, we will provide some of the theory, and in ⊃ Chapter 11, we will propose several steps that you can take to ensure you can engage the people who are involved in the change process.

Why is it important?

In healthcare, there is often a significant delay between what we know and what we do in practice. Connecting with how people think and behave—their psychology—is essential to effect real and lasting change. Sinek (2011) proposed the theory of the Golden Circle and postulated that for change to be successful, there are three phases:

• *WHY* the change is required—this is where the purpose is defined and is about winning the hearts and minds, the psychology of change;

- *HOW*—the technical skill required to achieve the desired purpose—the desired outcome;
- *WHAT*—the outcome that is required.

Unless we have people on board, the change and improvement will not be successful or sustained. Quality improvement may be self-limiting, unless we take into account socio-behavioural factors such as emotional experience of the people in the system when implementing change. System dynamics and working with management and organizational models are essential if change is to be sustainable (Mandel and Cady, 2022).

References

Deming, W.E. (1986). *Out of the Crisis*. Cambridge, MA: MIT Center for Advanced Engineering Study.

Mandel, K.E. and Cady, S.H. (2022). Quality improvement as a primary approach to change in healthcare: a precarious, self-limiting choice? *BMJ Quality and Safety*, 31(12), pp. 860–6. doi: https://doi.org/10.1136/bmjqs-2021-014447.

Shaikh, U. and Lachman, P. (2021). Using the head, heart, and hands to manage change in clinical quality improvement in the time of COVID-19. *IJQHC Communications*, 1(1), p. Iyab012. doi: 10.1093/ijcoms/Iyab012.

Sinek, S. (2011). *Start With Why: How Great Leaders Inspire Everyone To Take Action*. London: Penguin.

The hierarchy of needs

What is the quality issue?

When one starts an improvement project, one needs to understand the psychological basis for action and what motivates people to perform well. Maslow (1943) proposed the theory of a *hierarchy of human needs* to explain human behaviour.

- Maslow postulated that humans have various levels of requirements, ranging from survival and security to love and integration, and from self-esteem to self-actualization.
- We are obliged to satisfy our fundamental needs before we can focus on those needs that are less pressing.
- For that reason, a person who is hungry must address their need for food sooner than their need for safety, love, or belonging.

Why is this important for quality of health and healthcare?

Application of Maslow's hierarchy helps healthcare professionals to deliver comprehensive care of the total person, not only for survival (i.e. physical health), but also towards restitution of pre-illness function of mind, body, and spirit (i.e. holistic care).

What is the theory?

Maslow's paradigm has five levels of needs that must be attained to foster healthy well-being for an individual (Figure 10.2).

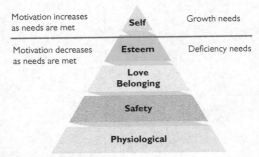

Figure 10.2 Maslow's hierarchy of needs.
♪ https://www.simplypsychology.org/maslow.html.

- The lower two levels of the hierarchy concentrate on physiological insufficiencies and correlate with safety issues, such as security and stability, which play an imperative role in the immediate survival of an individual.
- The three higher levels address psychological needs that take into account the feelings of belonging or love, self-esteem, and self-actualization (i.e. creativity or self-realization of potential).
- For a healthcare worker on the frontline, the theory can be applied as follows:
  - All doctors and nurses need their basic physical needs of food, nutrition, sleep, etc. met, so they can function safely;

- The above alone is not sufficient to build a safe and effective team to deliver quality care;
- One needs a sense of belonging and self-esteem in order to be in a psychologically safe space to work.

How does one use the theory to improve clinical care?

By applying Maslow's theory, we can analyse and understand the care pathways within different clinical settings.

Intensive care unit

- Once basic and physiological needs are met, patients and their families can progress to matters concerning psychological and complex-ordered needs.
- Survivorship *physically* is no longer a far-sighted goal.
- Considerable brain function, happiness, and physical capabilities of the patient should all be considered, so that important needs can be addressed and combined into care in the intensive care unit.

Palliative care

Zalenski and Raspa (2006) applied Maslow's paradigm to hospice care. They were able to treat distressing symptoms such as pain, dyspnoea, and physical and emotional fears, as well as provide acceptance and respect in the face of a terminal illness.

Other clinical areas

Maslow's paradigm has been applied in the management of patient care and survivorship in diverse areas such as emergency medicine, falls prevention, haemodialysis, cognitive rehabilitation, and management of traumatic brain injury and severe intellectual disability. In Box 10.1 the application of Maslow's theory is demonstrated.

Box 10.1 Case study to illustrate the application of Maslow's theory

Maslow's hierarchy of needs can be used as a framework for revolutionizing the culture of primary and secondary care. One can create interdisciplinary teams of providers to apprehend, prioritize, and address higher-ordered prerequisites associated with patient survivorship.

The interdisciplinary teams of physicians, nurses, physiotherapists, and social workers can connect with the patient and their family to discuss the ever-changing culture of holistic care and what this means to and for the patient. For example, after discharge from the intensive care unit, a person may be incapacitated and unable to complete straightforward physical activities, and may have fragmentary pain and discomfort for a protracted period.

A discussion with the person and their families to assist them in understanding the natural life post-discharge from the intensive care unit would enable them to understand potential cognitive, psychological, and physical disorders which may seem unrelated to the hospitalization or illness.

Based on: Jackson, J.C., Santoro, M.J., Ely, T.M., Boehm, L., Kiehl, A.L., Anderson, L.S. and Ely, E.W. (2014). Improving patient care through the prism of psychology: application of Maslow's hierarchy to sedation, delirium, and early mobility in the intensive care unit. *Journal of Critical Care*, [online] 29(3), pp. 438–44. doi: 10.1016/j.jcrc.2014.01.009.

References

Jackson, J.C., Santoro, M.J., Ely, T.M., et al. (2014). Improving patient care through the prism of psychology: application of Maslow's hierarchy to sedation, delirium, and early mobility in the intensive care unit. *Journal of Critical Care*, 29(3), pp. 438–44. doi: 10.1016/j.jcrc.2014.01.009.

Maslow, A. (1943). A theory of human motivation. *Psychological Review*, 50(4), pp. 370–98.

Zalenski, R.J. and Raspa, R. (2006). Maslow's hierarchy of needs: a framework for achieving human potential in hospice. *Journal of Palliative Medicine*, 9(5), pp. 1120–7. doi: 10.1089/jpm.2006.9.1120.

Intrinsic and extrinsic motivation

Intrinsic and extrinsic motivation

What is the quality issue?

When people perform their work or other activities, they do so for different reasons. If we understand why a person does something, then we can use that motivation as a key to unlock the improvement process.

- Intrinsic motivation is doing something for the personal satisfaction that engaging in that activity provides. This could include a sense of fulfilment gained by providing care to a person to help them feel better or more comfortable.
- Extrinsic motivation is doing something because it leads to a separate outcome such as a reward, recognition, or avoidance of punishment.

Why is this important for quality of health and healthcare?

- To create the environment needed for improvement, we need to move away from systems driven by fear and extrinsic motivation towards those driven by intrinsic motivation.
- Intrinsic motivation helps to generate creativity, engagement, adaptive learning, and achievement—all of which help to advance and sustain improvement. In improvement work, we want individuals to intrinsically decide to improve care.

What is the theory?

Improvers need to understand *what matters* to other people to unleash their intrinsic motivation.

- Each member of the improvement team must be asked *what matters* to them, so that everyone affected by the change can voice why the change is or is not valuable to them.
- Understanding which aspects of the change are valuable to different people allows leaders not to judge this source of motivation, but to enable people to access it repeatedly to promote and sustain the improvement.

How does one use the theory to improve care?

There are many methods of unleashing intrinsic motivation, including designing motivational tasks to carry out improvement efforts, incorporating play into improvement design, and celebration as a ritual to create community within the improvement team (see ⮊ Learning from Excellence, p. 226).

Another approach is the use of public narrative, as described by Ganz (2011). This includes three elements, as indicated in Box 10.2.

> ### Box 10.2 Ganz's public narrative
>
> 1. *Self*: personal stories to connect with the emotions of our values to enable mindful action
> 2. *Us*: collective stories to connect with the emotions of the values shared by the whole team participating in the action
> 3. *Now*: stories that provide a narrative for how the challenges we face in the here and now can be responded to with hope, followed by mindful action, rather than by fearful reaction

This framework helps teams to communicate the motivations that are behind their improvement efforts such as dignity and respect or love and kindness. The three elements interact with each other, as demonstrated in Figure 10.3.

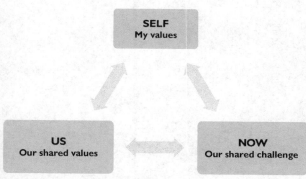

Figure 10.3 Developing shared values.
Adapted from Ganz (2011).

Improvement leaders need to create the space for these stories to be shared, allowing the entire team to be reminded of why we care. This, in turn, motivates others to make intentional choices to adopt and sustain improvement efforts. In Box 10.3 an example of intrinsic motivation is given.

Box 10.3 Case study on intrinsic motivation

Dr Michael Rose, an anaesthetist at McLeod Regional Medical Center in South Carolina, recognized the importance of unleashing intrinsic motivation in his team for adoption of the surgical safety checklist. Despite efforts to raise awareness, train, incentivize, and mandate the use of the checklist, adoption rates were around 30%.

Dr Rose invited the team to open meetings where they shared stories of 'self'—what motivated them to do the work they do, to pursue their profession, and to care for patients. Through these stories, the staff connected to one another and to their intrinsic motivations around patient care. Dr Rose then highlighted how their improvement work around the surgical safety checklist brought them all closer to achieving what drew them to medicine in the first place—to care for people, safely.

The results followed, with a sustained 100% utilization of the checklist and a resulting 35% decrease in patient mortality. Creating space for these conversations allowed the team to connect to their shared humanity, unleashing individuals, the team, and the organization to improve and change together.

Based on: Hilton, K., Anderson, A. (2018). *IHI Psychology of Change Framework to Advance and Sustain Improvement*. Boston, Massachusetts: Institute for Healthcare Improvement; 2018 (available at: ℘ ihi.org).

Reference

Ganz, M. (2011). Public narrative, collective action, and power. In: Odugbemi, S. and Taeku, L., eds. *Accountability through Public Opinion: From Inertia to Public Action*. Washington, DC: The World Bank; pp. 273–89.

Developing agency

What is the quality issue?

Ownership of an improvement project and the ability to generate ideas and solutions at the point of work is an important concept for improvers.

Often trainees and other healthcare workers feel powerless to effect change. Agency is essential if you are going to facilitate improvement. '*Agency is the ability to choose to act with purpose. It can be described as feeling that we are in the driving seat when it comes to our actions*' (Moore, 2016).

Why is this important for quality of health and healthcare?

For members of the healthcare team to be in a position to effect change, they need to feel they have the agency—both the power and the courage— to do so. The people best placed to make improvements within our system often do not have the agency to make changes that would improve the problems they see.

- They may have heavy workloads which prevent them from taking the time to change the way in which things are done in their unit.
- They may have had previous experiences of punitive measures taken when others deviated from standard practices, and therefore be unwilling to take the personal risk involved in initiating change.

As leaders in the healthcare setting, it is important to activate the agency of team members—to make sure they have both the power and the courage to choose to act to improve the quality of patient care.

What is the theory?

Power is often thought of as a position or a title, or sometimes as a personality trait or quality. But this is not the case, and it is important for the team to understand this in order for them to achieve a sense of agency in their work.

- Power is relational—it is about building numerous interdependent relationships, which, in turn, can be leveraged to achieve an aim It is the *ability* to act with purpose.
- Courage stems from knowing ourselves and being in relationship with what is happening around us. It is having the emotional resources to be able to choose to act, even in the face of difficulty or uncertainty. It is the *emotional* resource to choose to act in the face of difficulty or uncertainty

The combination of this power and courage—*people's agency*—can be considered at a number of different levels:

- *Self*: an individual's agency to make their own choices;
- *Interpersonal*: the collective agency of people acting together within the healthcare team;
- *System*: an institution or organization's structures, processes, and conditions which support the exercise of agency.

How does one use the theory to improve care?

A number of elements need to be considered in order to activate the agency of the healthcare team.

These include:
- Unleashing people's intrinsic motivation to galvanize their commitment to act;
- Co-designing and co-producing change—the people most affected by the change will have the most interest in designing and committing to change in ways that are meaningful to them;
- Distributing power so that each team member can contribute their unique skills and attributes to produce change;
- Creating a culture of improvement where action is the norm—demonstrating people as being courageous and exercising their power—making future action all the more achievable.

In Box 10.4 a case study on agency is demonstrated.

Box 10.4 Case study: agency in action

Tricia is a registrar on the medical ward. She notices that the house officers with whom she is working do not feel that they are part of the team and feel powerless to make decisions (i.e. they are always told what to do and cannot decide how they do the tasks).

She has recently read about the importance of team members being able to feel that they belong and have some power in their decision-making. She decides to start an improvement project to ensure that, despite the type of work being undertaken, the house officers would feel that they can make decisions on some aspects of their work.

The intervention is simple. Every morning she asks them '*How do you feel?*' and '*What matters to you today?*'. Then, as the daily tasks are decided, she asks them how they would like to complete the tasks and empowers them to design the work processes for the day. She has given them a degree of *agency*, and the morale of the team improves, measured by a daily morale meter.

Reference

Moore, J.W. (2016). What is the sense of agency and why does it matter? *Frontiers in Psychology*, 7. doi: 10.3389/fpsyg.2016.01272.

Further reading

Heimans, J. and Timms, H. (2014). Understanding 'new power'. *Harvard Business Review*. Available at: https://hbr.org/2014/12/understanding-new-power (accessed 10 September 2023).

Heimans, J. and Timms, H. (2018). *New Power: How Power Works in Our Hyperconnected World—and How To Make It Work for You*. Toronto, ON: Vintage Canada.

Mannion, R., Exworthy, M., Wiig, S., and Braithwaite, J. (2023). The power of autonomy and resilience in healthcare delivery. *BMJ*, 382, p. e073331. doi: 10.1136/bmj-2022-073331.

Ocloo, J., Goodrich, J., Tanaka, H., Birchall-Searle, J., Dawson, D., and Farr, M. (2020). The importance of power, context and agency in improving patient experience through a patient and family centred care approach. *Health Research Policy and Systems*, 18(1), p. 10. doi: 10.1186/s12961-019-0487-1.

Appreciative inquiry

What is the quality issue?

Healthcare is a complex endeavour, and processes and outcomes continually need to be improved to achieve optimum outcomes. Clinical teams work hard and try to deliver care, often under trying circumstances and with limited resources.

Traditionally, improvement projects start with finding out what is not working well and then applying theory and method to improve. In appreciative inquiry, we find out what is working well and then build on this to develop the improved system. An *appreciative inquiry* approach can engender and facilitate agency. It looks for the best in people and in teams to discover what makes them effective in all their activities (Cooperrider and Whitney, 2005).

Why is this important for quality of health and healthcare?

Team morale is an important factor to consider, as one develops an improvement project or processes to improve care. The development of individual and team resilience engineering (RE) and psychological safety is an essential part of a safe working environment. *Appreciative inquiry* is an effective method to build on strengths, rather than focusing on what is not working well.

Appreciative inquiry differs from problem-solving in that it:
- Looks to the future, rather than concentrating on what has not worked in the past;
- Promotes generative thinking rather than critical analysis;
- Allows solutions to emerge, rather than planning them in advance;
- Is co-produced with people rather than directed at them;
- Focuses on positive deviance (i.e. what is working well) rather than on negative deviance (i.e. what is not working);
- Is based on the positive relationships among people rather than on the negative tensions that may exist.

How does one use the theory to improve care?

Five key steps are taken to implement *appreciative inquiry*, as indicated in Figure 10.4.

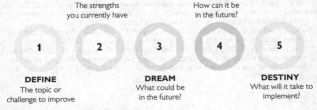

DISCOVER
The strengths
you currently have

DESIGN
How can it be
in the future?

1 **2** **3** **4** **5**

DEFINE
The topic or
challenge to improve

DREAM
What could be
in the future?

DESTINY
What will it take to
implement?

Figure 10.4 Appreciative inquiry.

- *Define the topic*: the team comes together to jointly decide on the process in the system to work on. The focus is not on problem-solving, but rather on enhancing good practice.
- *Discover the strengths*: explore where there is good work happening (i.e. the positive)—who and what is working well, and what the strengths in the team are. What of ourselves are we bringing to work?
- *Dream of what could be*: paint a positive picture for the future—what the future can look like, what outcomes we can achieve with 'blue sky' thinking.
- *Design*: what the future *process* can look like and how we will achieve this—that is, what can we emulate and build on to reach the goals we have set?
- *Destiny*: how we will get to the outcomes and future state—that is, what do we need to do to achieve the dream? This focuses on generating solutions by using positive motivation and energy.

The basis is about building relationships and moving from a transactional approach to one that is value-based. In this process, people feel valued and are able to deliver more than what is asked. The approach is also part of the Learning from Excellence Safety II approach (i.e. learning from the positive, rather than from the negative).

Further reading

Cooperrider, D. (2012). *What is appreciative inquiry?* Available at: 🔗 https://www.davidcooperrider.com/ai-process/ (accessed 10 September 2023).

Cooperrider, D.L. and McQuaid, M. (2012). The positive arc of systemic strengths: how appreciative inquiry and sustainable designing can bring out the best in human systems. *Journal of Corporate Citizenship*, 2012(46), pp. 71–102. doi: 10.9774/gleaf.4700.2012.su.00006.

Sandars, J. and Murdoch-Eaton, D. (2017). Appreciative inquiry in medical education. *Medical Teacher*, 39(2), pp. 123–7. doi: 10.1080/0142159x.2017.1245852.

Reference

Cooperrider, D.L. and Whitney, D. (2005). *Appreciative Inquiry: A Positive Revolution in Change*. San Francisco, CA: Berrett-Khoeler Publishers.

Learning from Excellence

What is the quality issue?

In healthcare, we approach patient safety by learning from what goes wrong and trying to minimize these scenarios. In doing this, we neglect to learn from the wealth of experience gained from when things go right, which is most of the time. By looking at what works well and why it has been successful, we can celebrate, build community, and unleash intrinsic motivation within teams.

Resilience Engineering (RE) is based on insights from complexity science, and quality results from clinicians' ability to adapt safely to difficult situations such as a surge in patient numbers, missing equipment, or difficult and unforeseen physiological problems. Progress in applying these insights to improve quality has been slow, despite the theoretical developments.

Why is this important for quality of health and healthcare?

The Learning from Excellence approach enables the study of a system's ability to adapt and succeed under varying conditions. This is essential in a system that is ever-changing and increasing in complexity.

What is the theory?

- RE is an approach to how work is accomplished in complex adaptive systems such as healthcare.
- It explicitly argues that organizations can adapt to pressures to make the system work and maintain good outcomes in spite of problems and challenges.
- Healthcare workers are therefore seen as the key to creating safety, rather than being cast as the weak link in the system, prone to error and responsible for adverse outcomes.
- RE argues that it is the variability in the healthcare environment that drives the need for adaptation. For example, surges in patient numbers, multiple patients deteriorating at the same time, lack of equipment, and inappropriate staffing are all common variations in the conditions of work that require adaptation by workers.
- This way of thinking is different to the assumptions underpinning most quality improvement efforts that attempt to constrain human behaviour by specifying via protocols what actions should be taken, based on past problems identified through incident reporting and audits or identification of waste through Lean principles.
- These ideas appeal to clinicians and safety researchers, because they reflect the reality of the messy clinical world in which conditions cannot always be anticipated and solutions sometimes need to be improvised.
- However, they need further interpretation and elaboration to move from a description of how work is achieved to how it can inform quality improvement.
- Human performance in healthcare almost always goes right, not because staff strictly follow a set of predefined rules and behaviours, but because they are constantly making adjustments needed under varying conditions of work.
- These adjustments are vital to maintain an acceptable level of performance in a system that is increasing in complexity.

- Actively looking for, seeking to understand, and celebrating what goes right in each system can be an investment not only in safety, but also in productivity, as well as improving resilience and boosting staff morale. This is the feel-good factor of achievement.

How does one use the theory to improve care?

- A 'Learning from Excellence' initiative involves asking people, staff, and patients to report excellence when they see it.
- A system similar to an adverse event reporting system can be used to capture the reports.
- A champion within the team can help to propel the initiative forward—that is, someone who has received an excellence report is more likely to look for excellence in their colleagues, as well as continue to display the behaviour/action which led to the initial report.
- Analysis of the reports can then be used to understand moments of excellence from which a wider team or audience can learn, as well as ensuring that time, resources, and environments are available for current examples of excellence to continue.
- Once teams are familiar with the Learning from Excellence process, specific areas of care or behaviours can be targeted to effect improvement.

In Box 10.5 a Case study on Learning from Excellence is described.

Box 10.5 Case study on Learning from Excellence

The team at Birmingham Children's Hospital paediatric intensive care unit hypothesized that antimicrobial stewardship could be enhanced through positive feedback for certain behaviours of healthcare professionals.

They ran a Learning from Excellence initiative over 6 months, during which positive feedback for behaviours which had been identified to facilitate antimicrobial stewardship was given. Selected reports were also followed with appreciative inquiry interviews to reinforce positive feedback.

In comparison to a comparable period the year before, there was a 6.5% decrease of antimicrobial consumption. Broad-spectrum antibiotic consumption falling by 17.6%.

Based on: Jones, A. S., Isaac, R. E., Price, K. L., & Plunkett, A. C (2019). Impact of Positive Feedback on Antimicrobial Stewardship in a Pediatric Intensive Care Unit: A Quality Improvement Project. Pediatric quality & safety, 4(5), e206. https://doi.org/10.1097/pq9.00000 00000000206.

Signposting

Learning from Excellence. Available at: ℘ https://learningfromexcellence.com (accessed 10 September 2003).

References

Baxter, R. and Lawton, R. (2022). The Positive Deviance Approach (Elements of Improving Quality and Safety in Healthcare series). Cambridge: Cambridge University Press.

Kelly, N., Blake, S., and Plunkett, A. (2016). Learning from excellence in healthcare: a new approach to incident reporting. Archives of Disease in Childhood, 101(9), pp. 788–91. doi: 10.1136/archdischild-2015-310021.

Kindness

Kindness is so vital to our practice of healthcare that it cannot be separated from our clinical work. This work, whether as an individual, a team, or an organization, is both technical and relational at the same time, and it is crucial not to disregard the importance of the relational element or to see it as a mere question of 'being nice'. Kindness is an integral part of the multidimensional quality improvement model discussed in ⮑ Chapter 1.

Kindness is both:

- an obligation to our *kin* born of understanding of our connectedness; and
- the natural expression of our attitudes and feelings arising from this connectedness.

Kindness is a binding, creative, and problem-solving force that inspires and directs the attention and efforts of people and organizations towards building relationships with those they care for. It is not a 'nice' side issue in the project of competitive progress; rather it is the *glue* of cooperation required for such progress to be of most benefit to most people (Campling et al., 2020).

The importance of kindness is simple—it is an essential component of any part of healthcare practice if excellence is to be achieved. In the same way that the sports psychologist is recognized as being equally as important as the coach in elite sporting endeavours, how we relate to each other and to our patients cannot be underestimated by the healthcare team.

> 'The quality of practice, its efficiency, the safety of the patient, and the outcomes of the work depend at least as much on the relational, psychological dimensions of practice as on the "evidence base", the system design, the technical skills or the equipment and facilities available.'
>
> John Ballat

Kindness not only impacts the healthcare experience for the patient, but also benefits the experience of the healthcare provider at the same time. As Phillips and Taylor (2010) described: 'Real kindness changes people in the doing of it ... it mingles our needs and desires with the needs and desires of others, in a way that so-called self-interest never can.'

Kindness is a word that can need rescuing, as in the modern culture of competitive individualism, it has been sentimentalized and marginalized, rather than representing a core moral value of being in solidarity with human needs (Phillips and Taylor, 2010).

Campling et al. (2020) advocated that we look upon kindness in healthcare as 'intelligent kindness'. The adjective 'intelligent' signals to us that it is possible to think about the conditions needed for kindness in a sophisticated way, and that clinical, managerial, leadership, and organizational skills and systems can be leveraged to promote compassionate care.

The concept of 'intelligent kindness' is an essential part of quality of care and is integral to a quality improvement project. When one engages with people either at work or in a project, apply the following principles:

- *Develop kinship*: working together to recognize and bear in mind kinship (i.e. being 'of a kind' and 'in it together'), depending on one another for survival, well-being, and success—in our relationships with one another and with those with whom we work to heal or treat or involve in the project;
- *Value the awareness of kinship*: understanding and valuing the way in which such an awareness, and consequent attitude to others, can build productive and effective relationships and direct your attention, responsiveness, decisions, and actions in our work as people, as colleagues, and as skilled clinicians;
- *Focus on kindness*: understanding and working with the factors that promote or work against such a stance, or approach, in individuals, groups, organizations, and communities;
- *Promote kindness*: recognizing and promoting what is involved in integrating this perspective into training and continuing education, clinical practice, professional supervision, and service design, development, and management.

A virtuous cycle of kindness

When kinship is recognized and kindness is practised, multiple further benefits can ensue in a 'virtuous cycle', which, in turn, reinforces the sense of kinship itself.

- A virtuous circle is an economic concept introduced by Adam Smith, which describes how the growth of capital stimulates more comsumption, which, in turn, will increase economic growth.
- More recently, it has been attributed to Jeff Bezos from Amazon, who postulated that more customers would result in more choice of products, which would result in more customers, etc. (i.e. each step in the virtuous cycle generates a positive outcome).
- This concept has been adopted in '*intelligent kindness*', and an adapted cycle is shown in Figure 10.5.

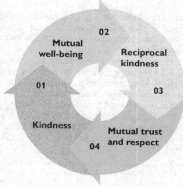

Figure 10.5 Example of a virtuous cycle.

In healthcare, this concept is important in the attainment of well-being of all healthcare providers and patients. In the planning and designing of healthcare and its systems, we should continually aim to develop a virtuous cycle of well-being, and avoid that which works against it.

How does one use the theory to improve care?

All improvement work needs to consider both the relational and kinship dimension of our work, together with the technical knowledge, skills, care pathways, and system design where necessary.

- Both systems are essential, and both depend on each other.
- They need to be considered honestly, with genuine understanding and appropriate importance consistently given to the relational side, while recognizing the challenges that applying this perspective may pose.
- Offering 'resilience training' or lunchtime yoga to overworked staff with unhealthy working conditions who are unable to take lunch breaks simply will not do.

These two systems are inadequate alone and cannot be considered in isolation. A role and task system could become factory-like or robotic if designed without attention to the relational, whereas a relational system without appropriate science or structure may be comfortable and well-meaning, but ultimately be ineffective and inefficient.

Attention to the relational optimizes the application of the technical, and vice versa

All levels of each system also need to be considered due to their inevitable effect on one another. For example, building relationships between teams, while neglecting those within them, would have little positive effect. In Box 10.6 an example on the impact of compassion pm stress is described in a case study.

Box 10.6 Case study on impact of compassion of clincal outcome

A team in the emergency department of a busy urban hospital hypothesized that patient perception of healthcare provider compassion was associated with the subsequent development of post-traumatic stress disorder (PTSD) symptoms.

They performed a prospective cohort study of patients presenting with a life-threatening emergency requiring life-sustaining treatment in the emergency department. They measured patient perception of healthcare provider compassion in the emergency department, and (blinded to these results) assessed PTSD symptoms 1 month post-discharge.

After adjusting for potential confounders, they found that patients who perceived their healthcare providers to have greater compassion were less likely to develop PTSD symptoms (odds ratio 0.93, 95% confidence interval 0.89–0.98) 1 month post-discharge.

Moss, J., Roberts, M.B., Shea, L., Jones, C.W., Kilgannon, H., Edmondson, D.E., Trzeciak, S. and Roberts, B.W (2019). Healthcare provider compassion is associated with lower PTSD symptoms among patients with life-threatening medical emergencies: a prospective cohort study. Intensive Care Medicine, [online] 45(6), pp.815–822. doi:10.1007/s00134-019-05601-5.

Signposting

Gathering of Kindness. Available at: https://www.gatheringofkindness.org (accessed 10 September 2003).

Further reading

Allwood, D., Koka, S., Armbruster, R., and Montori, V. (2022). Leadership for careful and kind care. *BMJ Leader*, 6(2), pp. 125–9. doi: 10.1136/leader-2021-000451.

Ballatt, J., Campling, P., and Maloney, C. (2020). Intelligent kindness. *IPPR Progressive Review*, 27(1), pp. 75–83. doi: 10.1111/newe.12187.

Campling, P. (2015). Reforming the culture of healthcare: the case for intelligent kindness. *BJPsych Bulletin*, 39(1), pp. 1–5. doi: 10.1192/pb.bp.114.047449.

Klaber, R.E. and Bailey, S. (2019). Kindness: an underrated currency. *BMJ*, 367, p. l6099. doi: 10.1136/bmj.l6099.

Lachman, P., Batalden, P., and Vanhaecht, K. (2020). A multidimensional quality model: an opportunity for patients, their kin, healthcare providers and professionals in the new COVID-19 period. *F1000Research*, 9, p. 1140. doi: 10.12688/f1000research.26368.1.

Louiset, M., Allwood, D., Bailey, S., Klaber, R., and Bisognano, M. (2023). Let's reconnect healthcare with its mission and purpose by bringing humanity to the point of care. *BMJ Leader*, leader-2023-000747. Advance online publication. Available from: https://doi.org/10.1136/leader-2023-000747.

Montori, V.M. (2020). *Why We Revolt: A Patient Revolution for Careful and Kind Care*. Rochester, MN: Mayo Clinic Press.

Montori, V.M. and Allwood, D. (2022). Careful, kind care is our compass out of the pandemic fog. *BMJ*, 379, p. e073444. doi: 10.1136/bmj-2022-073444.

Trzeciak, S., Booker, C., and Mazzarelli, A. (2019). *Compassionomics: The Revolutionary Scientific Evidence that Caring Makes a Difference*. Pensacola, FL: Studer Group.

References

Campling, P., Ballatt, J., and Maloney, C. (2020). *Intelligent Kindness*. Cambridge: Cambridge University Press.

Phillips, A. and Taylor, B. (2010). *On Kindness*. London: Penguin Books.

Top tips

In an improvement programme, remember to be:

- Humble at all times;
- Respectful of the work people are doing;
- Encouraging and empowering, so that people feel valued;
- Kind—kindness will produce kindness in return, as well as success in what you ask of people.

As you develop the *will* for people to be part of the programme:

- Make the case for change, so that it matters to the people involved;
- Always provide a vision for change;
- Be open and transparent at all times;
- Build agency and use appreciative inquiry to find out what really matters in the lived experience of all.

Summary

- Quality improvement is a complex endeavour involving changing the way in which people interact with one another and their environment.
- Of the four Lenses of Profound Knowledge, the psychology of change will determine whether your improvement project will succeed or not.
- The methods provided in this chapter are complementary, and one needs to know when to use them in each context.
- Ultimately, people will only change if the new way has benefits. This is the foundation of all change.

How to make change happen

Key points

- Leadership for quality and safety is an essential factor in developing change.
- A safe culture will encourage people to embrace change.
- Creating a common purpose will ensure there is a vision for change.
- Co-designing change will engender ownership of the process.
- Equity is an essential component of change.
- Taking time to build the right quality team will help a project succeed.
- Maintaining gains needs to ensure change fatigue is addressed.
- All change needs to include sharing of the learning gained.

How to challenge hierarchies and power

What is the quality issue?

Much of what we do in healthcare is related to power and how it is distributed or managed. Hierarchies exist and these have power differentials. Power is not a title, position, personal quality, or trait.

- Power is relational and is produced by several interdependent relationships that can be leveraged to achieve a specific aim. Building these relationships over time builds power with those people and, in turn, can assert power over those who initially were resistant to change.
- Distributing power means that many people within a system, across numerous boundaries and levels, work together interdependently to create the conditions to achieve a shared goal. While their positional authority may be different, their contributions are all necessary for success.

Why is this important for quality of health and healthcare?

Challenge to the traditional hierarchies is important, as it can:

- Activate people's agency (i.e. by distributing power to make decisions);
- Achieve bigger goals by splitting larger objectives into numerous smaller projects;
- Help to scale up improvements in different contexts.

What is the theory?

Four actions are recommended to change the power dynamic (Figure 11.1):

1. Creating a shared purpose.

Defining the collective work of the group, rather than that of an individual, suggests that all partners are equal in this effort. This can also help

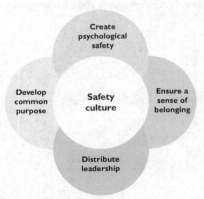

Figure 11.1 Developing a safe improvement culture.

Adapted from Psychology of Change Framework, Boston, Massachusetts, The Institute for Healthcare Improvement (IHI), 2018.

overcome previously negative intergroup relationships by creating a mutually shared positive purpose (see microsystems in ➔ Chapters 12 and 17).

2. Distributed leadership structure.

A visual can help people see themselves as sharing power with one another, emphasizing that everyone's share of the work is based on their unique skills and that each part is necessary to achieve the shared purpose.

- Those with positional authority need to actively distribute power to those without.
- For others, recognize and appreciate when someone in a position of authority practises these behaviours—thank them and show appreciation publicly. You will motivate them and others to behave in this way again.

3. Create psychological safety (see ➔ Chapter 10).

Establishing psychological safety within the improvement team requires taking steps to create a climate where people feel safe to speak up with ideas, questions, or concerns.

- Psychological safety has been shown to be the most important element in what makes effective teams. Within healthcare itself, teams with higher levels of psychological safety have been shown to make fewer mistakes and therefore to have better patient safety outcomes.
- Psychologically safe teams have greater staff job satisfaction and a reduction in staff turnover.
- Recognizing shared purpose in our work, acting with curiosity, showing vulnerability, and responding productively when team members speak up are ways in which you can create psychological safety within the team.

4. Engender a sense of belonging.

Teams are stronger when every member feels that they belong to the team and share the purpose of the team. A sense of belonging will be facilitated if the first three actions are achieved. With this, the team and team members will be better placed to deliver the desired outcomes.

Further reading

Bevan, H. and Henriks, G. (2021a). Creating tomorrow today: seven simple rules for leaders Blog one. *BMJ Leader*, 1 February 2021. Available at: https://blogs.bmj.com/bmjleader/2021/02/01/creating-tomorrow-today-seven-simple-rules-for-leaders-by-helen-bevan-and-goran-henriks/ (accessed 10 September 2023).

Bevan, H. and Henriks, G. (2021b). Creating tomorrow today: seven simple rules for leaders. Blog two: Define our shared purpose. *BMJ Leader*, 16 February 2021. Available at: https://blogs.bmj.com/bmjleader/2021/02/16/creating-tomorrow-today-seven-simple-rules-for-leaders-blog-two-define-our-shared-purpose-by-helen-bevan-and-goran-henriks/ (accessed 10 September 2023).

Bevan, H. and Henriks, G. (2021c). Creating tomorrow today: seven simple rules for leaders. Blog 3: Root our transformation efforts in a sense of belonging. *BMJ Leader*, 24 March 2021. Available at: https://blogs.bmj.com/bmjleader/2021/03/24/creating-tomorrow-today-seven-simple-rules-for-leaders-blog-three-root-our-transformation-efforts-in-a-sense-of-belonging-by-helen-bevan-and-goran-henriks/ (accessed 10 September 2023).

Bevan, H. and Henriks, G. (2021d). Creating tomorrow today: seven simple rules for leaders. Blog 4: Predict and prevent: start at an earlier stage ('upstream') in the intervention or care processes. *BMJ Leader*, 24 December 2021. Available at: https://blogs.bmj.com/bmjleader/2021/12/24/creating-tomorrow-today-seven-simple-rules-for-leaders-blog-four-predict-and-prevent-start-at-an-earlier-stage-upstream-in-the-intervention-or-care-processes-by-helen-bevan/ (accessed 10 September 2023).

Bevan, H. and Henriks G. (2021e). Creating tomorrow today: seven simple rules for leaders. Blog five: Support people to build their agency at every level of the system. *BMJ Leader*, 16 June 2022. Available at: https://blogs.bmj.com/bmjleader/2022/06/16/creating-tomorrow-today-seven-simple-rules-for-leaders-blog-four-support-people-to-build-their-agency-at-every-level-of-the-system-by-helen-bevan-and-goran-henriks/ (accessed 10 September 2023).

Edmondson, A. (1999). Psychological safety and learning behavior in work teams. *Administrative Science Quarterly*, 44(2), pp. 350–83. doi: 10.2307/2666999.

Heimans, J. and Timms, H. (2018). *New Power: How Power Works in Our Hyperconnected World—and How To Make It Work for You*. Toronto, ON: Vintage Canada.

Hilton, K. and Anderson, A. (2018). *IHI psychology of change framework to advance and sustain improvement*. IHI White Paper. Boston, MA: Institute for Healthcare Improvement. Available at: https://www.ihi.org (accessed 10 September 2023).

How to co-design and co-produce change

(See ➔ Chapters 2, 8, and 14.)

What is the quality issue?

For an improvement intervention to be effective, it must be meaningful to the people most affected by the change. They will have the greatest interest in designing improvements that are important to themselves and have a unique insight into what is workable and realistic, which is an essential element of sustainable improvement.

The concept of 'all teach, all learn' encapsulates the principle that everyone who touches, or is involved in, improvement at every level has something to contribute. Identifying and engaging all these stakeholders are the essential first step in people-driven change, rather than starting by focusing on the process itself and ideas of how to improve it.

What is the theory?

There are five properties of changes that make them favourable to being adopted (Rogers, 2003), as shown in Box 11.1.

This acknowledges that, because improvement involves people, it cannot simply operate from an evidence-based standpoint. The proposed change must be workable for both the people implementing the change as well as those affected by it. Involving all stakeholders from the outset is essential for this to be achieved.

Another important concept that helps us as improvers is the concept of 'humble enquiry', which is the 'fine art of drawing someone out, of asking questions to which you do not know the answer, of building a relationship based on curiosity and interest in the other person' (Schein, 2013). This is vital in building those authentic relationships with which teams can co-produce change successfully.

Box 11.1 Rogers' properties of change

- Responsiveness to the need of those involved
- Compatibility with the local context
- Simplicity (i.e. easy to implement)
- Trialability—can be tried and tested
- Observability—the benefit can be seen

How does one use the theory to improve care?

Four actions are required:

- Identifying the key stakeholders in a proposed change;
- Taking the time to see the whole system from the perspective of each stakeholder before building a strategy for change. This includes seeing problems through the lens of the staff member, and importantly through the lens of the patient how the problem impacts them;
- Identifying how each stakeholder connects with others;
- Viewing everyone as having an equal status as a 'partner' in the improvement effort.

In doing this, be conscious of your own biases and how these will affect tests of change and how you design change. To really co-design and co-produce change, we must inquire, listen, see, and commit to one another, creating authentic relationships with those involved.

When crafting an aim statement, ensure that you can identify *who* is involved and *why* the change is being made.

References

Rogers, E.M. (2003). *Diffusion of Innovations*, 5th edition. New York, NY: Free Press.

Schein, E.H. and Schein, P.A. (2021). *Humble Inquiry: The Gentle Art of Asking Instead of Telling*. Oakland, CA: Berrett-Koehler Publishers.

How to engage stakeholders to ensure equity

What is the quality issue?

Healthcare workers and the people receiving care come from diverse backgrounds. In improvement work, we need to acknowledge this in the planning and implementation of our improvement projects.

- The challenge of incorporating diversity into the quality improvement process is one that has only recently been accepted as an essential approach to take.
- As discussed in ⮕ Chapter 5, health inequalities are determined by several interrelated factors. These include ethnicity and gender; the exclusion of specific groups, including people who are homeless; socio-economic factors, including levels of income and dispossession; and geography.
- The impact of health inequalities requires us to address underlying structural issues, such as prejudice and racism, which propel the social determinants of health.
- This can be difficult within clinical teams but is a challenge that we need to take.
- A multidisciplinary approach is required, including equity at the core, together with patient-centred outcomes.
- We also need to look at how this impacts clinical teams themselves.

In Box 11.2 actions required to decrease inequity are listed.

Box 11.2 Inequity in the National Health Service (NHS)

A report by the NHS England Race and Health Observatory calls for the following action to be taken:

- Enforcing guidelines on ethnic monitoring data;
- Producing better NHS statistics;
- Investing in interpreter services;
- Working to build trust with ethnic minority groups and key community organizations;
- Investing in research to understand the impact of racism on healthcare.

These five actions can all translate into how we conduct quality improvement projects and include assessment of equity in every project.

Khapada et al. (2022).

Why is this important for quality of health and healthcare?

Within every improvement programme, there is the opportunity to address equity, even if the issue may appear to be beyond the remit of a particular project.

- Quality improvement methods can preserve or aggravate health inequities across subpopulations.
- The approach is to ask the question at the start: 'Is what we plan to do going to improve any inequities the target population is experiencing?'

How does one use the theory to improve care?

Five steps can help you to address the equity challenge (see ➲ Chapter 5):
1. *Engage better* by including a wider range of participants in improvement processes to ensure you capture the lived experience of all;
2. *Measure* and use data better by stratifying to detect inequity;
3. *Design better* by tackling barriers identified through your stakeholders representing disadvantaged groups;
4. *Improve better* by moving beyond the established scope of quality improvement by tackling gaps in the health system structure, such as human resources, systems, health financing, and governance associated with disparities, including social determinants health;
5. *Learn better* with a learning system (see ➲ Chapter 12).

Reference

Kapadia, D., Zhang, J., Salway, S., et al. (2022). *Ethnic inequalities in healthcare: a rapid evidence review.* Available at: ⏧ https://www.nhsrho.org/wp-content/uploads/2022/02/RHO-Rapid-Review-Final-Report_v.7.pdf (accessed 10 September 2023).

How to connect to organizational mission, vision, and values

What is the quality issue?

To achieve sustainable change, you need to consider the mission, vision, and values of your organization.

- A shared common purpose where individuals at every level of the organization feel a collective desire to make processes and outcomes better every day, in a valiant and continuous approach.
- A successful quality improvement project should connect to the wider mission and goals of the organization. This is essential if the project is to be sustained in the longer term.
- Quality is not one person's or one team's role. Seek wider buy-in from across your organization, and support from the quality director and/or quality and safety team who can facilitate and help you to improve and achieve excellence.

Why is this important for quality of health and healthcare?

- It will be easier to achieve buy-in across the wider healthcare and management team for projects with aims aligning with an organization's missions and visions.
- It is important for the longer-term sustainability of a project that its aims reflect the goals of the organization as a whole.
- It is important to align with visions/goals, so as not to inadvertently create conflict within or between teams.

What is the theory?

As discussed in ⊃ Chapter 10, Developing agency, p. 222 and ⊃ Appreciative inquiry, p. 224, empowerment of team members to come to effective solutions is a way to improve care and engender a shared commitment to continuous improvement.

How does one use the theory to improve care?

As a quality improvement champion, you encourage your team members to embrace improvement and support your quality improvement journey:

- Look at the intrinsic and extrinsic motivations;
- Start small;
- Look for early adopters;
- Have a sponsor to link to the organization's mission;
- Develop a strategic imperative for change.

Communication by the board or senior leaders to champion improvement can enable clinical teams to feel supported in adopting a different approach.

John Kotter proposed that to develop a change process, one needs to go through eight steps, each of which aims to build the will for change (Figure 11.2):

1. The first step is to create a sense of urgency, so that team members can see why the change is required.
2. Then one needs to build the team for change—the guiding coalition.
3. Any change requires a vision—a direction to where the change is going, which will be better than the current state—this is the strategic vision.
4. Then to develop changes, one needs innovators and early followers.
5. Leaders must then enable staff to act to take down barriers to change by giving staff agency to make changes.

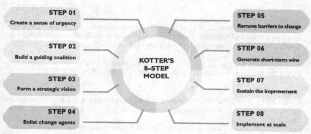

Figure 11.2 Kotter's change theory.
Adapted from Kotter, J. (2012).

6. To keep up morale and the will for change, the change process should generate short-term wins that give the team encouragement and demonstrate that change is worthwhile.
7. Maintaining quality improvement gains (also referred to as sustainability) must be built into the system, so that change will continue into the future.
8. Finally, when all is tested and seen to work, change must be implemented at scale.
   In Box 11.3 actions an application of Kotter's theory is demonstrated.

Box 11.3 Case study: Kotter's change theory during the COVID-19 pandemic

During the COVID-19 pandemic, a sense of urgency was created, coalitions were built across sectors, and solutions were tested and then implemented at scale.

We can use Kotter's 8-step process for leading change in order to help frame the change management processes during the COVID-19 pandemic:
1. *Create a sense of urgency*: the COVID-19 pandemic created a sense of urgency, given its largely unknown nature.
2. *Build a guiding coalition*: politicians, administrators, and frontline providers mobilized to guide efforts.
3. *Form a strategic vision and initiatives*: the guiding coalition envisioned prioritizing essential services, while being cognizant of not overwhelming the healthcare system.
4. *Enlist a volunteer army*: healthcare workers courageously volunteered to design, trial, and support new initiatives, treatments, and policies.
5. *Enable action by removing barriers*: healthcare workers empowered one another to critically reflect on their usual practices and to provide care that deviated from the norm to increase safety and decrease morbidity and mortality.
6. *Generate short-term wins*: daily successes were tracked, celebrated, and rewarded to boost morale.
7. *Sustain acceleration*: by consolidating changes through dynamic policies and protocols and consistently grounding daily work in the vision, momentum was sustained.
8. *Institute change*: institutionalizing change is ongoing, with its long-term effects unknown.

Further reading

Harrison, R., Fischer, S., Walpola, R.L., et al. (2021). Where do models for change management, improvement and implementation meet? A systematic review of the applications of change management models in healthcare. *Journal of Healthcare Leadership*, 13(13), pp. 85–108. doi: 10.2147/jhl.s289176.

Lukas, C.V., Holmes, S.K., Cohen, A.B., et al. (2007). Transformational change in health care systems. *Health Care Management Review*, 32(4), pp. 309–20. doi: 10.1097/01.hmr.0000296785.29718.5d.

References

Hall, J.N. (2021). The COVID-19 crisis: aligning Kotter's steps for leading change with health care quality improvement. *Canadian Medical Education Journal*, 12(1), pp. e109–10. doi: 10.36834/cmej.71165.

Kotter, J.P. (2012). *Leading Change*. Boston, MA: Harvard Business School Press.

How to build a quality team

What is the quality issue?

As is the theme of this chapter, the most important element in quality improvement is the people involved in undertaking, driving, and sustaining the change. When embarking on a project, engaging the right people is crucial to its success, and it is worth taking the time and trouble to build that team from the start.

What is the theory?

The Institute for Health Improvement recommends building a quality team, ensuring there is one member in each of the following roles shown in Table 11.1.

The optimal size of the quality team is between five and eight people, although diversity, fulfilling the above roles, and patient representation remain more important.

Table 11.1 Quality team members

Clinical leadership	A team needs someone with enough authority to be able to test and implement a change, and with the clinical experience and oversight to understand any consequences the change may have on other parts of the system
Technical expertise	A team member with in-depth knowledge of the processes or area involved. A further technical expert in the area of improvement methods is also valuable to ensure the right things are measured and interpreted effectively
Day-to-day leadership	The lead for the quality improvement team oversees the data collection and implementation of change on a daily basis. They must work closely with the other team members and understand the impact of the team's activities on the organization as a whole
Patient	Including a patient representative will ground the proposed change with the lived experience of the patients in the way care is delivered and received
Project sponsorship	This does not necessarily mean monetary sponsorship, but rather someone who can act as a link with senior management and, if needed, provide resources or overcome barriers to implementing improvements

Adapted from ℰ https://www.ihi.org.

How does one use the theory to improve care?

Take time to build your team carefully and deliberately with the right mix of people from the start. It can be tempting to get 'stuck in' to making changes that you are passionate about, but without the right team around you, the project is less likely to yield long-lasting results.

As a quality team leader, consider trying to 'work yourself out of a job', by making sure that it is the people who have the most to gain from the changes and are actively involved in the change who 'own' the change. This is particularly important if you are not a permanent member of the team such as a non-consultant hospital doctor. Frontline ownership also encourages staff to recognize their own capacity and potential to effect change.

Reference

Institute for Healthcare Improvement (2019). *How to improve. Science of improvement: forming the team.* Available at: ℅ https://www.ihi.org/resources/Pages/HowtoImprove/default.aspx (accessed 10 September 2023).

How to manage resistance to change

What is the quality issue?

Managing resistance to change is a challenge as resistance can impede the improvement process.

- Expect to have some resistance as, if there is no opposition, people may not be engaging.
- Resistance can be a response to prolonged exposure to occupational stressors, so try to understand why there is resistance.
- Resistance can be due to experience of improvement projects that did not work well.
- Initiatives to tackle resistance to change are focused on individuals rather than on taking a systems approach to the problem.

Why is this important for quality of health and healthcare?

- Resistance can cause workplace conflicts, which, in turn, cause demotivation, stress, health issues, absenteeism, and sick leave.
- Resistance can prevent good improvement work from being done if it cannot be managed effectively.
- If resistance is not embraced, insights and learning from people's reasons for resistance can be missed.

What is the theory?

There are several ways in which one can address the potential for resistance to change:

1. One can apply the hierarchy of needs discussed earlier to understand the reasons for resistance.
2. The use of de Bono's 'Six Thinking Hats' can ensure that the proposed change is viewed from different perspectives. As indicated in Figure 11.3, the process is thinking in parallel of all different aspects of the proposed project, so that resistance to change is channelled into a positive experience and is dealt with as part of the change planning process.

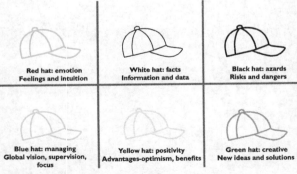

Red hat: emotion Feelings and intuition	**White hat: facts** Information and data	**Black hat: azards** Risks and dangers
Blue hat: managing Global vision, supervision, focus	**Yellow hat: positivity** Advantages-optimism, benefits	**Green hat: creative** New ideas and solutions

Figure 11.3 The 'Six Thinking Hats' of de Bono.
Adapted from de Bono, 2016.

The different members of the team take turn to examine the project from different perspectives, so that all views are accommodated and buy-in is facilitated.

How does one use the theory to improve care?

One can take the following preventive mechanisms to understand and manage resistance to change:

- Clarify roles, responsibilities, and authorities, so that everyone knows what is expected of them;
- Define the criteria for resource allocation for different processes, so that the results and resources allocated are adequately linked;
- Create mechanisms for proactively detecting potential knowledge gaps among staff and then provide the necessary training to enable the staff to perform the tasks assigned successfully;
- Ensure that there are clear communication channels for all, with a feedback loop to allow continual modifications of the process in response to the feedback.

In Box 11.4 the application of frontline ownership and 'liberating structures' is described.

> **Box 11.4 Case study: frontline ownership and 'liberating structures'**
>
> Engaging people in the improvement process is always the first step to success. The concept of frontline ownership was developed in Canada, with the view that if the frontline staff owned the improvement process and defined its outcomes and what has to be done to achieve the outcomes, then success is more likely. This builds on the theories of Deming, as well as on the microsystem theory.
>
> The approach involves providing frontline staff who are delivering the service with the agency to make changes and develop change. This is also similar to how Lean works.
>
> 'Liberating structures' is a series of techniques that can be used to engage with frontline team members to empower them to make change (available at: https://www.liberatingstructures.com, accessed 10 September 2023). The aim is to provide clinical teams with intuitive ways to disrupt the way in which they work and come up with new ideas. Like de Bono's thinking hats, the aim is to think laterally and come up with solutions that otherwise may not have been considered.

Further reading

Zimmerman, B., Reason, P., Rykert, L., Gitterman, L., Christian, J., and Gardam, M. (2013). Frontline ownership: generating a cure mindset for patient safety. *Healthcare Papers*, 13(1), pp. 6–22. Doi: 10.12927/hcpap.2013.23299.

Reference

De Bono, E. (2016). *Six Thinking Hats*. London: Penguin Life.

How to engage to maintain quality improvement gains

What is the quality issue?

A key challenge in all improvement projects is ensuring they are sustained after the end of the project. This requires buy-in from the people who have been part of the project and from others who may come after the project has ended. This requires the new process to be hardwired into the system. Creating supportive environments where there is shared decision-making and staff feel they can take responsibility for improvements in quality of care is key to successful and sustainable quality improvement.

Why is this important for quality of health and healthcare?

Quality improvement takes time, and its value is in the fact that it can make processes better and result in improved outcomes. However, it can also lead to increased work and improvement fatigue and burnout, unless it is well planned. One can pre-empt this by careful planning and stakeholder engagement from the start of the project.

What is the theory?

Two frameworks are offered to assist you in preventing project fatigue.

The Highly Adoptable Improvement Model (Hayes and Goldmann, 2018) proposes that there is an interplay of several factors which will determine whether or not an intervention will be successfully sustained.

- Does the *design* of the intervention make it easier to do one's work?
- How *complex* is the intervention? If it is simple and easy to do, it is likely to be accepted.
- Do the staff believe the intervention will make a difference (i.e. belief in the *efficacy* and potential benefit of the intervention)?
- Was there *co-design* at every stage of the process with the end user—the staff who are being asked to make the change?
- Does the intervention *align* with the culture, goals, and objectives of the clinical team, and not create competing priorities?
- Are there *resources*, both human and physical, to implement and will the intervention fit in with the current workflow?

This is represented in Figure 11.4, which indicates that if the above criteria are met, there will be success. If not, there will be a cycle of burnout and change fatigue.

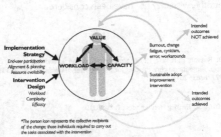

Figure 11.4 Highly Adoptable Improvement Model.
With permission from Chris Hayes.

The model is aligned with the sustainability (maintaining quality improvement gains) model that was developed by the NHS Institute for Innovation and Improvement. This has an interplay of 11 factors, as indicated in the Figure 11.5.

In this model, staff factors include leadership, behaviours, and culture, as well as the need for training. Process factors include measurement of the process, adaptability and credibility of the intervention, and then organizational factors such as having the resources and infrastructure and fitting with the goals of the organization.

Both models provide you with a framework against which to measure the progress of your project.

Creating supportive environments where there is shared decision-making and staff feel they can take responsibility for improvements in quality of care is key to successful and sustainable quality improvement.

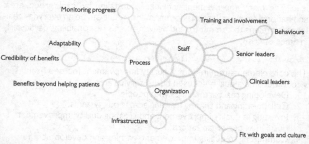

Figure 11.5 The NHS sustainability model.
🔗 https://www.england.nhs.uk/improvement-hub/wp-content/uploads/sites/44/2017/11/NHS-Sustainability-Model-2010.pdf.

Further reading

Doyle, C., Howe, C., Woodcock, T., *et al.* (2013). Making change last: applying the NHS Institute for Innovation and Improvement sustainability model to healthcare improvement. *Implementation Science*, 8, p. 127. Doi: 10.1186/1748-5908-8-127.

References

Hayes, C.W. and Goldmann, D. (2018). Highly Adoptable Improvement: a practical model and toolkit to address adoptability and sustainability of quality improvement initiatives. *The Joint Commission Journal on Quality and Patient Safety*, 44(3), pp. 155–63. Doi: 10.1016/j.jcjq.2017.09.005.

Maher, L., Gustafson, D., and Evans, A. (2010). *Sustainability model and guide*. Available at: 🔗 https://www.england.nhs.uk/improvement-hub/wp-content/uploads/sites/44/2017/11/NHS-Sustainability-Model-2010.pdf (accessed 10 September 2023).

Sharing learning

What is the quality issue?

A significant part of quality improvement is valuing our collective knowledge, wherever it comes from. Arming everyone with the proper knowledge and skills is at the centre of development, so that everyone can act on their design thinking ideas for improvement.

Why is this important for quality of health and healthcare?

By building your own quality improvement knowledge and skills, as well as increasing the quality improvement capacity and capability of local teams and organizations, this will give you the skills to respond readily to acute or emergency situations.

Improving the quality of healthcare we deliver is a valued responsibility of all staff within the health service. Everyone in our service is an expert in their area of work, and our managers and leaders must enable all staff to lead. The many improvement activities undertaken by local, group, area, and national teams reflect this commitment. Yet, it can be an everyday challenge for teams to commit to, and deliver on, this responsibility, particularly in times of crisis.

How does one use the theory to improve?

The core elements required for a quality improvement-focused health service to become a quality-focused health service are:

1. Developing real partnerships with people;
2. Collaborating and sharing learning across our systems;
3. Investing in quality improvement and creating quality improvement posts in all our organizations;
4. Committing to quality improvement learning and development for all staff;
5. Working on relationships and culture, so that staff feel valued and their input is encouraged;
6. Working with our leaders and managers to create a work environment where staff are enabled to work on improving care;
7. Using measurement for improvement approaches to better understand our data;
8. Ensuring we have quality at the centre of our management and governance of healthcare;
9. Working to integrate services;
10. Partnering with communities, so that we contribute to improving the social issues that profoundly affect health outcomes.

In Box 11.5 actions to support QI learning are provided.

1. Allocate protected time to meet with the person you are supporting.
2. Use appreciative inquiry to facilitate the development of agency.
3. Explore the identified areas for development, with the aim being that everyone reaches the level of 'confidence' which is appropriate for them.
4. Discuss the best development options available.
5. Contact your local quality and patient safety department to explore learning opportunities available in your area.
6. Agree a development plan with the person you are supporting.

Coaching for quality improvement

Quality improvement is a difficult task and often teams may not persevere as they proceed on the journey of improvement. A quality improvement coach is a person who provides both technical and psychological support to the quality improvement team. This may take the form of mentoring the team or coaching by providing technical advice to the team at regular project surgery. In Table 11.2, the steps needed in the quality improvement coaching process are provided.

Table 11.2 A coaching framework

Techniques to use	Use appreciative inquiry as your questioning technique to facilitate the team's thought processes to identify solutions and actions, rather than taking a directive approach
	Explain the purpose for your session and your role in supporting quality improvement activities
	Guide the direction of the work and future thinking
	Encourage ongoing work and future projects
	Recognize and praise what they are doing well
	Teach technical information and its use in this context
Introduction	Set the scene, present introductions, and explain the process. Ask a few direct questions; for example, 'Tell me about your quality improvement project'
	Focus on the basics of the project
Quality improvement basics Project prioritization	How was the project defined and chosen? What was the relevance of the problem? Are there baseline data? Are patients involved? Aim:
	• What is the aim of the project? Is it realistic? Is it SMART?
	Project charter and work plan:
	• How do you keep the project on track?
	Causal analysis:
	• How did you decide what the root causes to your problem were? Did you study the process with a process map? Did you analyse your findings with a fishbone diagram and Pareto?

(Continued)

Table 11.2   (Contd.)

	Theory of change: • Is there a hypothesis for change in a driver diagram? Measurement: • What measures do you have? • How do you display data? • How regularly do you review performance? • Does the project have the right information to make decisions? Teamwork: • Who are on the team? • Is it multidisciplinary? Is there a team leader? • How frequently does the team meet? • Is there patient representation? Is there a sponsor? • Have you assessed stakeholders?
Common challenges	The team has no time to meet: • Integrate quality improvement work into other meetings The team does not know the nature of the problem: • Map the current steps in the process flowchart to identify missed steps, waste, and rework; brainstorm all potential reasons for why something is or is not happening (cause and effect/fishbone); narrow the potential causes with actual causes The team has too many solutions: • Narrow down the reasons for the problem and identified gaps: 'Do you know what to do?'; 'Do you know how to do it?'; 'Do you have the necessary equipment and tools to do it?'. Match one solution to one identified reason, and test on a small scale
Use of data	Does the team show effective use of data to set priorities and drive improvement efforts? Do they use visual displays of data to review trends and determine whether improvements are successful? Are changes tested with PDSAs?
Documentation	Review data, work plans, flowcharts, etc.
Closure	Ask: 'Is there anything else I can help you with today?' Thank the team for sharing their learning Provide positive feedback, and identify the next steps and clarifications

Adapted with permission from Coaching for Quality Improvement (HealthQual 2021).

Reference

HealthQual (UCSF Institute for Global Health Sciences) (n.d.). *Coaching for quality improvement: a guide for implementing coaching strategies to spread QI knowledge and skills in low and middle income countries.* Available at: ℛ https://healthqual.ucsf.edu/sites/g/files/tkssra931/f/coachingtoolkit-complete_printable_updated%20%282%29.pdf (accessed 10 September 2023).

Top tips

In an improvement programme, remember to:
- Distribute leadership;
- Create a safe environment that invites change;
- Create a vision for the change process and a common purpose;
- Respect what works and make the future state attractive;
- Be creative and use the different tools available to obtain buy-in and active participation in the change process;
- Make the process attractive—people are often scared of change.

Summary

- If you invest time in developing the will for change, then the resistance to change will diminish.
- The improvement team must involve people who are part of the process and include patients or their representatives.
- Co-design and co-production are essential if you are to have success—people will often have the solutions to their problems and challenges if you empower them.
- The psychology of change is 90% of the work—if you have people's hearts, then it is likely the improvement will follow.
- Learning is an integral part of the process, and coaching for improvement will bring sustainable success.

Further reading

Maben, J., Ball, J., and Edmondson, A. (2023). *Workplace Conditions* (Elements of Improving Quality and Safety in Healthcare series). Cambridge: Cambridge University Press.

Mannion, R. (2022). *Making Culture Change Happen* (Elements of Improving Quality and Safety in Healthcare series). Cambridge: Cambridge University Press.

The Lens of Appreciation of Systems

Key points

- An understanding of how a system works is an essential component of quality improvement.
- There are different types of systems, varying in complexity, each composed of people and processes interacting to achieve a desired (or sometimes undesired) outcome.
- Healthcare is considered a complex adaptive system, defined by the relation of its component parts—dynamic, adaptive, and constantly changing—with the emergence of new behaviours and solutions.
- Clinical teams constitute a microsystem and most improvement takes place within the microsystem.
- Analysis of how a system is operating is the first step in quality improvement.

Introduction to systems

'A system is more than the sum of its parts; it is an indivisible whole.'
Russell L. Ackoff (1973) 'Science in the systems age: beyond IE, OR and MS' in: Operations
Research Vol 21, pp. 664

What are systems in healthcare?

In our working and personal lives, we encounter errors, lapses in quality, problems, barriers, and challenges. Have you ever considered how and why these occur? Is it by chance? Is it an isolated event? Has the error/problem you have encountered occurred as a consequence of another action or inaction?

The seventeenth-century poet John Donne stated, *'No man is an island.'* We wonder if he knew that he was acknowledging that we are all part of a system reliant on, and affected by, one another and our environment.

- The basis of quality improvement is understanding the system and its interacting parts as much as we can.
- In everyday life and in the way we work, understanding how the system works is the first step towards improving the system.
- In the case study shown in Box 12.1, we can ask whether the owners of the coffee shop plan their system to ensure that their customers get the correct order, or not.

Box 12.1 Example of a system in day-to-day life

You have just finished a busy shift at work and stop by your local coffee shop to pick up a takeaway coffee before your drive home. You place your order at the till—a medium Americano with no milk or sugar. You pay for your coffee and wait for it to be prepared. The coffee shop is crowded and noisy; it is rush hour, with many local workers having the same idea as you.

You think you hear your order being called, and pick up the cup at the end of the counter and exit the building. Once outside, you take a sip from your cup, and you realize the sweet milky contents of the cup is not what you ordered.

You return to the coffee shop and hear several people complaining to the barista that they have received the wrong order.

- This is comparable to medicine where we, as clinicians, study the human body and the different systems within the body and how they interact, as indicated in Box 12.2.

As discussed in ⊙ Chapter 3, the study of systems is the foundation of quality improvement and patient safety. Rather than focusing on individual performance, we now look at how the individual performs within and with the system.

In this chapter, we describe different types of systems and then provide you with a way to analyse the system in which you work. Only then will you be able to improve processes and then outcomes.

Box 12.2 Systems in clinical care

The concept of systems is not new in medicine. We can consider the body to be a complex adaptive system made up of many smaller systems that are interdependent on one another to deliver a healthy life, and one cannot easily function without each of them being in good working order and interacting to produce the desired outcome. For example, for an athlete this is essential and the respiratory, cardiovascular, neurological, and musculoskeletal systems must interact to produce peak performance.

An athlete is continually doing a quality improvement project on a specific system to improve performance.

And most of our patients present with clinical symptoms when one or more of their systems start to malfunction. For example, the neurological system is dependent on a well-functioning cardiovascular system, which is dependent on a well-functioning haematological system, etc. All our clinical interventions are focused on improving how the different systems in the body work and interact. The healthcare system is no different—complex and made up of many interacting microsystems.

Why is there a system quality problem?

'Every system is perfectly designed to get the results it gets.'

W. Edwards Deming. https://deming.org/

- Systems in healthcare have often developed organically, without thought as to how they will best work or fit.
- Originally, the healthcare system was simple, involving a doctor and a patient.
- The growth of the healthcare system responded to the increase in scientific knowledge and the ability to treat disease.
- While good clinical outcomes have always been the aim of clinicians, the evolving complexity of disease management has not always been matched with changes in healthcare organization so as to guarantee quality outcomes.
- Outcomes are dependent on how we work within systems.
  - Major patient safety failures have been attributed to how the systems operate.
  - Healthcare systems have been shown to be inefficient in many ways, including waiting and with lists, delays to access, and economic and carbon waste.
- Understanding the system in which you work is a prerequisite of any quality improvement endeavour.
- To understand your system, various tools and conceptual frameworks have been developed, which help to visualize and understand the system you are trying to improve.
- Differing conceptual frameworks may fit your system better than others, and this chapter will help you identify which tools and models might best fit your system, and aid in your quality improvement work.
- Often one does not know how complex a system is until one attempts to implement change. The diagnosis phase is key to understanding the extent of complexity.

Why is system theory important?

Understanding systems theory and recognizing the type of system you are trying to improve. or the type of system within which you exist, are important skills. This is because the approach to managing change in these different types of systems can differ greatly.

As noted above, clinicians are taught to be systems thinkers as we progress in through clinical training.

- The study of anatomy, physiology, pathology, and pathophysiology is in essence the study of a complex adaptive system—the human body.
- As we consider why one system of the body is not working, we also consider how this impacts other systems. For example, cardiac failure impacts other systems (e.g. respiratory, renal) and the functioning of the total system (body) as a whole.

This concept of system thinking transfers to how we organize ourselves in society and how we have organized healthcare.

- Traditionally, we have three or four major systems, from primary to secondary to tertiary and then to quaternary care. Each of these very large systems will be composed of component parts, organized in different ways.
- Each will have a different culture, which will impact the way they work and the outcomes achieved.

In the United Kingdom, the National Health Service (NHS) in each country is a complex system with many interacting parts.

- Improving clinical outcomes and the experience of people who access the system for care requires an understanding of how the system works.
- In quality improvement, we recognize the enormity of this challenge; we therefore break down the system into manageable parts.

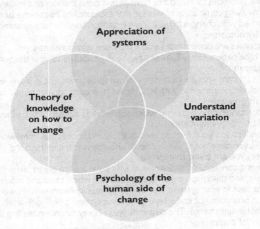

Figure 12.1 Lenses of Profound Knowledge.

What is the theory?

In quality improvement, the approach to systems is based mainly on the theories of Donabedian and Deming. Deming's theory of Profound Knowledge (⊙ Chapter 3) placed *appreciation for a system* as a core component which must be understood in order to improve (Figure 12.1).

The first step is to understand the types of system that exist and then to be able to analyse how your system is functioning to achieve desired outcomes.

Further reading

Best, A., Greenhalgh, T., Lewis, S., Saul, J.E., Carroll, S., and Bitz, J. (2012). Large-system transformation in health care: a realist review. *The Milbank Quarterly*, 90(3), pp. 421–56. doi: 10.1111/j.1468-0009.2012.00670.x.

Clarkson, J., Bogle, D., Dean, J., et al. (2017). *Engineering better care: a systems approach to health and care design and continuous improvement*. London: Royal College of Physicians. Available at: ⅊ https://raeng.org.uk/media/wwko2fs4/final-report-engineering-better-care-version-for-website.pdf (accessed 10 September 2023).

Kaplan, G., Bo-Linn, G., Carayon, P., et al. (2013). Bringing a systems approach to health. *NAM Perspectives*. Discussion paper. Washington, DC: National Academy of Medicine. Available at: ⅊ https://doi.org/10.31478/201307a (accessed 10 September 2023).

Martin, L.A. and Mate, K. (2018). *IHI innovation system*. IHI White Paper. Boston, MA: Institute for Healthcare Improvement. Available at: ⅊ https://www.ihi.org/resources/Pages/IHIWhitePapers/IHI-Innovation-System.aspx (accessed 10 September 2023).

Sampath, B., Rakover, J., Baldoza, K., Mate, K., Lenoci-Edwards, J., and Barker, P. (2021). *Whole system quality: a unified approach to building responsive, resilient health care systems*. IHI White Paper. Boston, MA: Institute for Healthcare Improvement. Available at: ⅊ https://www.ihi.org/resources/Pages/IHIWhitePapers/whole-system-quality.aspx (accessed 10 September 2023).

Types of systems

A system can be defined as an interdependent group of items, people, or processes with a common purpose. Systems range in complexity in a continuum from simple to chaotic. In Table 12.1, different types of systems we encounter in our daily activities are explained.

Table 12.1 Types of systems

System	Characteristic
Simple 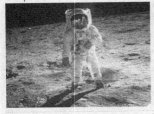	In a simple system, if you do X, the result will be Y. For example, if you place a slice of bread in a toaster and switch it on, it results in toasted bread
Complicated 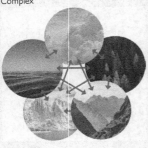	A complicated system has multiple structures and processes, operating in series or in parallel. These systems are linear and deterministic, making analysis and prediction possible. An example of a complicated system is putting a man on the moon. While this endeavour is daunting, it is made up of many simple systems working together
Complex 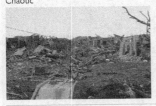	In a complex system, there are many more 'unknowns'. For example, our climate is a complex system consisting of several subsystems and components, the atmosphere, the ocean, and terrestrial ecosystems, etc. All of these systems/components interact to create our climate, but they are more than a sum of their parts. Complex systems are non-linear, which makes prediction difficult. Other examples include raising a child or the behaviour of economies
Chaotic	In a chaotic system, there is no immediately known relationship between cause and effect. An example would be a natural disaster or an emergency. The priority is to establish stability, and the aim is to bring the situation/system back from chaotic to complex

Types of systems

Healthcare is made up of all of these systems. Several theories have been developed to help understand systems in order to facilitate quality improvement. They range from very simple models and frameworks to complex theories. Here we will identify some of the most applicable theories in the healthcare context and provide examples of how they can be applied.

The Cynefin framework proposes sorting the types of systems with which we are confronted into five domains, each of which demands a different approach to leading quality improvement projects: simple, complicated, complex, chaotic, and disordered (Kurtz and Snowden, 2003).

Simple systems

Simple systems are stable and have clear relationships between cause and effect (Box 12.3).
- There are relatively few components and they are highly interrelated.
- In these systems, it is often easy to identify the correct thing to do in order to achieve a desired outcome.
- Consensus among stakeholders is also achieved more easily than in more complicated systems.

Box 12.3 Example of a simple system in healthcare

An example of a simple system in the healthcare context is the medical admission of a patient from the emergency department.
- The patient is seen by the emergency physician, who decides the patient needs to be reviewed by the medical admitting team, who then assess the patient and decide to admit to the hospital or not.
- If the patient is admitted, then the admissions office locates a bed for the patient in the hospital, and the patient is transferred to the ward.

This is a simple system. However, as anyone who works in healthcare will recognize, it is not without its inefficiencies or pitfalls. The end goal of identifying those who need inpatient medical treatment and providing that care is not in dispute from any of the participants in the system.

Complicated systems

In complicated systems, while there is a clear relationship between cause and effect, this may not be evident to all participants in the system, and there may be multiple 'right' ways to do things (Box 12.4).
- There can be many components to the system, but interrelatedness between components is low.
- In order to understand how the system works, analysis is required before improvement efforts can be made.
- This requires expertise at the service delivery level to help decide which of a number of options is the best one to take.
- This reliance on expertise makes stakeholders prone to entrained thinking, which can cause resistance to novel ideas.
- As a result, decision-making can be slow and recognizing that 'perfect is the enemy of good' can be the best way forward if paralysis by analysis develops.

Electronic health records (EHRs) are an example of a complicated system.
- Held up as a panacea in healthcare systems where work continues to be done on paper, the successful deployment of an EHR is, in practice, extremely challenging.
- EHRs are required to be used by all healthcare professionals in the hospital, from doctors to nurses to physiotherapists to dieticians and so on.
- Yet each job role has differing requirements from the EHR.
- The interface presented to the doctor who wants to have fast access to a patient's diagnostic imaging and laboratory results is different to the interface that the dietician needs to be presented with in order to do their job efficiently.

Complex adaptive systems

'A complex adaptive system is a dynamic network of agents acting in parallel, constantly reacting to what the other agents are doing, which in turn influences behaviour and the network as a whole.'

Holland, J.H., 1992

When we zoom out and begin to look at the macrosystem level, be it the hospital level or even the regional or national healthcare system, considerable complexity emerges that makes studying these systems challenging. One way of looking at these systems is to look at them as a complex adaptive system. In Box 12.5 the NHS is described as an example of such a system.

A practical set of statements that can be derived from complex adaptive system theory as it applies to healthcare systems are as follows:
- Accept the system as complex with many patterns and relationships between elements (departments, units, hospitals, services, etc.), in which cause and effect cannot always be ascribed.
- Deconstructing the system to understand it better is sometimes not possible.

The English National Health Service (NHS) is a complex adaptive system. It consists of a wide range of participants, including health and social care professionals, administrators, managers and policymakers, and patients and their families.

These individuals interact from within multiple organizations (such as trusts, hospitals, general practices, and community mental health teams) in an interrelated manner to deliver patient care. From the perspective of the patient, the boundaries between systems are indistinct, as they are referred from one service to another on their patient journey.

Each organization is capable of changing how it operates to best meet local challenges and how to deploy centrally allocated resources in order to meet the healthcare needs of the local population.

- Acknowledge that what has happened before is not necessarily predictive of future events.

When you reflect on these statements from the perspective of an improver, by using QI methods to try to understand, map, and analyse a system to undertake some improvement effort, these statements can, at first, seem quite demoralizing.

Having the ability to recognize that your system is a complex adaptive system is an important first step, as it helps to avoid some of the improvement pitfalls that can be encountered.

The characteristics of complex adaptive systems are listed in Table 12.2 (Health Foundation, 2010). As you analyse the system within which you work, ask whether your system is characterized by some or all of the following principles.

Table 12.2 Characteristics of complex adaptive systems

Characteristic	Definition	Healthcare example
Constituted relationally	This means that they are more defined by the relationships between elements rather than by the elements themselves Individual elements of the system respond only to contiguous elements of the system and have no impression or visibility of how the whole system is behaving	Much of how we work is about relationships that are not always defined by a process (e.g. referrals across systems from one specialty to another are not a simple linear), knowing the person can make it easier
Radically open	The boundaries between systems are indistinct, and many agents act across boundaries or within different systems concurrently	This is more evident with chronic care where a person may have many different specialties involved (e.g. for a person with diabetes)
Determined contextually	The identity and function of each element are defined by the context in which it exists Any element of the system is affected by, and can affect, multiple other elements or systems	In improvement, this is key—different solutions are dependent on context. A good example is the Matching Michigan initiative for central line infections (see ➲ Chapter 5)
Adaptive capabilities	Elements can react dynamically to prevailing local conditions	An example is how the system reacts to increased demand (e.g. in the emergency department) and the rest of the system has to adapt dynamically

Table 12.2 (Contd.)

Characteristic	Definition	Healthcare example
Dynamic processes	There is non-linearity where small changes can bring about large effects	Often if one improves a process in one area, there are unintended consequences in others; for example, improving assessment in the emergency department can lead to long waits for admissions, increased discharges, and then increased readmissions
Complex causality	Novel qualities can emerge unexpectedly	This is a feature of our health system where new solutions are constantly found for "wicked" problems, as demonstrated by the COVID-19 crisis

Chaotic systems

Chaotic systems are characterized by high turbulence where there are no clear cause-and-effect relationships (Box 12.6).

- Leaders in this environment do not have time to wait for evidence or data-based feedback on the correct course of action.
- There is an imperative to *act* to establish order, to *sense* where the stability lies, and to *respond* to turn the chaotic system into a complex system.
- When complex systems are operating at the edge of control and further complexity or pressure on the system is introduced, the system can break down into a chaotic state.
- Mitigation measures can be taken to prevent this degradation such as clearing the emergency department waiting room of non-urgent presentations in advance of an anticipated influx of patients from a major incident.

Box 12.6 Example of a chaotic system

Disaster response during a major incident, such as a commuter train derailment, can be thought of as a chaotic system.

- There is a requirement to make decisions quickly, under pressure, in order to mitigate the effects of the evolving situation.
- The first *act* decided upon by leaders at the scene is extrication of the injured from the train, followed by rapid triage of injuries using a traffic light system.
- This action converts the chaos of hundreds of injured people who require care into a hierarchy of needs, allowing prioritization of resource allocation to those who would benefit the most.

A potentially chaotic system has been termed by the United States military as living in a VUCA world—*Volatile, Uncertain, Complex*, and *Ambiguous*.

The coronavirus disease 2019 (COVID-19) pandemic has demonstrated this concept and often chaotic responses. In this situation, the steps to follow are:

- Pay attention to detail, which is the foundation of highly reliable systems, and even more so in a crisis.
- Consider the needs of the people involved (i.e. pay attention to the challenges facing the frontline staff and the public).
- Be transparent with a good communication programme, as informed people are less stressed.
- Think out of the box to create innovative solutions and link up with people in other sectors, as together solutions can be found (Nembhard *et al.*, 2020).

The challenge for us in healthcare and in quality improvement is how to take advantage of system models and use the knowledge to improve the system in which we work.

- Use linear models, design, and engineering rules for simple and complicated systems.
- Appreciate the limitations of these approaches, as the broader healthcare system is complex, adaptive, and at times chaotic.
- Apply the principles of working within complex adaptive and chaotic systems to guide decisions.

References

Health Foundation (2010). *Complex adaptive systems*. Available at: ℘ https://www.health.org.uk/publications/complex-adaptive-systems (accessed 10 September 2023).

Kurtz, C.F. and Snowden, D.J. (2003). The new dynamics of strategy: sense-making in a complex and complicated world. *IBM Systems Journal*, 42(3), pp. 462–83.

Nembhard, I.M., Burns, L.R., and Shortell, S.M. (2020). Responding to Covid-19: lessons from management research. *NEJM Catalyst*, 17 April 2020. doi: 10.1056/CAT.20.0111.

Further reading

Braithwaite, J. (2018). Changing how we think about healthcare improvement. *BMJ*, 361(361), p. k2014. doi: 10.1136/bmj.k2014.

Braithwaite, J., Churruca, K., Ellis, L.A., *et al.* (2017). *Complexity science in healthcare: aspirations, approaches, applications and accomplishments. A white paper*. Sydney: Australian Institute of Health Innovation, Macquarie University. Available at: ℘ https://www.mq.edu.au/__data/assets/pdf_file/0012/683895/Braithwaite-2017-Complexity-Science-in-Healthcare-A-White-Paper-1.pdf (accessed 10 September 2023).

Braithwaite, J., Churruca, K., Long, J.C., Ellis, L.A., and Herkes, J. (2018). When complexity science meets implementation science: a theoretical and empirical analysis of systems change. *BMC Medicine*, 16, p. 63. doi: 10.1186/s12916-018-1057-z.

Carroll, A. (2021). The Irish healthcare system as a complex adaptive system. *Irish Medical Journal*, 114(4), p. 332.

Fraser, S.W. and Greenhalgh, T. (2001). Coping with complexity: educating for capability. *BMJ*, 323(7316), pp. 799–803. doi: 10.1136/bmj.323.7316.799.

Holland, J.H. (2010). *Adaptation in Natural and Artificial Systems: An Introductory Analysis with Applications to Biology, Control, and Artificial Intelligence*. Cambridge, MA: MIT Press.

Lipsitz, L.A. (2012). Understanding health care as a complex system. *JAMA*, 308(3), p. 243. doi: 10.1001/jama.2012.7551.

Plsek, P.E. and Greenhalgh, T. (2001). Complexity science: the challenge of complexity in health care. *BMJ*, 323(7313), pp. 625–8. doi: 10.1136/bmj.323.7313.625.

Plsek, P.E. and Wilson, T. (2001). Complexity science: complexity, leadership, and management in healthcare organisations. *BMJ*, 323(7315), pp. 746–9. doi: 10.1136/bmj.323.7315.746.

Wilson, T., Holt, T., and Greenhalgh, T. (2001). Complexity science: complexity and clinical care. *BMJ*, 323(7314), pp. 685–8. doi: 10.1136/bmj.323.7314.685.

Application of theory to practice

Structure–process–outcome (SPO) model

As noted in → Chapter 3, Donabedian's SPO model aimed to link the structure and processes of a system to outcomes. The model suggests that the quality of a system can be determined by examination of its structure, processes, and outcomes (Figure 12.2; Box 12.7).

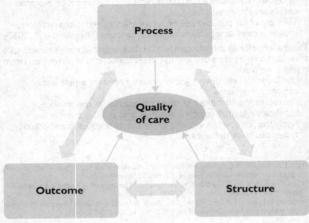

Figure 12.2 The Donabedian system.

Box 12.7 Application of Donabedian theory

You are a general practitioner working in a small practice in a rural community. You have made several referrals to the dermatology service in the local tertiary referral centre for patients. The majority of these referrals have been for expert opinion and investigation of suspected malignant melanoma and occasionally other skin carcinomas.

- You have noticed that some patients are receiving appointments whereas others are not, and this does not seem to depend on the underlying suspected diagnosis.
- This has resulted in delays to accessing expert care for a number of patients, leading to poorer outcomes.
- You decide to review your process in making the referrals.
- When you believe a referral is necessary, you send a letter to the dermatology department and await a response.
- You realize that you have no way of tracking if the referrals have been received and processed by the dermatology department.

- When you contact the dermatology clinic, they advise you that there is an electronic referral system that facilitates all referrals and that the fields requested on the online booking form are designed to capture all the appropriate information to allow for stratification of patients in terms of acuity.
- Currently, your practice does not have access to an electronic referral system. However, by a simple change to your structure (registering as a clinician on the online referral system) and process (submitting all referrals electronically), your patients will be triaged and reviewed in a timely manner.

Microsystem theory

We need to remind ourselves: 'Who does this system serve?' Often in healthcare, systems and processes develop and evolve to serve the needs of healthcare providers, be they frontline or in administrative functions. This can occur at the expense of the service user, through unintended consequence or failure to see the service from the perspective of the patient.

In clinical microsystem theory (Figure 12.3), understanding the service user's perspective, expectations, and desired health outcome must come first, as this is the jumping-off point from which all other activity must occur. This approach holds true for any improvement effort, regardless of the framework being used.

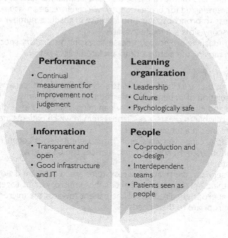

Figure 12.3 Microsystem theory.
Adapted with permission from Nelson et al. 2008.

- A clinical microsystem is formed whenever a patient interacts with a healthcare provider and information about the patient and their health needs is exchanged with the provider.
- It is the smallest replicable unit of healthcare delivery. For example, a patient attends an outpatient department for a consultation with a respiratory specialist, has some tests ordered, and attends a follow-up visit to plan ongoing treatment.
- This interaction can be broken down into inputs, outputs, feedback loops, and processes, allowing us to draw a schematic of the microsystem.
- This interaction does not happen in isolation, and the patient will have initially been referred following an interaction with their own general practitioner, which, in itself, is its own microsystem.
- If the patient requires an intervention as a result of the consultation in outpatients, say a bronchoscopy, they will then enter another microsystem in the bronchoscopy suite of the hospital. The results of the bronchoscopy will be communicated to collections of related microsystems that interact to wrap around the patient to meet their healthcare needs.
- The patient perceives the pathway on which they have been as a continuum of care; yet they have been passed from one microsystem to another in a manner appropriate to their needs.

When we work to improve the performance of one microsystem, heed must be paid to the other microsystems that interact with it.

- For example, if quality improvement work is undertaken to increase the number of patients seen in a session in the respiratory outpatient department, and metrics indicate that 20% of patients seen in this service are referred for bronchoscopy, we can foresee an issue with access to bronchoscopy if no increase in absolute number of bronchoscopy slots are made available.
- This well-meaning project to increase access to respiratory specialists results in moving the bottleneck to a related microsystem.

Mesosystems

Microsystems that are closely related to serve defined healthcare needs of a shared population of patients are referred to as mesosystems.

- Effective and efficient dialogue between microsystems is essential and must be reliable to create a resilient system in which patients' healthcare needs are met in a timely manner.
- For example, cancer services, emergency percutaneous coronary intervention systems, and obstetric services can be seen as mesosystems.
- In these services, the related microsystems are in constant dialogue with one another, and the mesosystem ties these microsystems together and ensures appropriate direction of the patient towards the microsystem most appropriate to their needs.

How can the microsystem theory be put to use?

(See ➔ Chapter 17.)

- At its core the clinical microsystem theory approach involves giving those at the interface with service users (patients and their families) the autonomy to problem-solve and improve services (Box 12.8).
- As such, clinicians are best positioned to redesign and implement healthcare delivery systems, as they are most likely to understand the needs and expectations of patients.

The approach is summarized as follows.

Box 12.8 The microsystem approach

The approach is similar to how we approach and treat patients:
1. Organize a team
2. Assess your microsystem;
3. Make a diagnosis;
4. Treat your microsystem.

Adapted from Assessing and diagnosing your microsystem. https://clinicalmicrosystem.org/knowledge-center/workbooks

Organize an improvement team

(See ➔ Chapter 10.)

- A team should be assembled with representatives from all disciplines that are active within the microsystem, including patients and their families, as well as medical, nursing, administrative, managerial, and other supporting roles.
- The team should meet weekly, and communicate and engage with staff to help drive projects.
- Active engagement with service users (patients and their families) must be a core consideration of the leadership team.

Assess how your microsystem works

(See ➔ Chapter 17.)

To assess the 'as is' state of your microsystem, a tool called 'The 5Ps' can be used to assess it. The 5Ps are explained in Table 12.3, and implementation is demonstrated in ➔ Chapter 17.

Table 12.3 The 5Ps assessment tool

Purpose (see ➔ Chapter 1)	Ask every person in your microsystem the question: 'Why does this microsystem exist?'. Use this exercise to define a statement of common purpose in which everyone believes.

Table 12.3 (*Contd.*)

Patients (see ⊃ Chapter 8)	Gather relevant knowledge about your patients. • What is their lived experience of the service they receive (e.g. waiting times, satisfaction, complaints, compliments)? • What resources are used (e.g. tests, procedures)?
Professionals (see ⊃ Chapter 10)	Create a comprehensive picture of your microsystem. • Who does the work? • What is their lived experience of doing the work to achieve the common purpose of the microsystem? • What they think of the microsystem? • What works well? (e.g. Learning from Excellence). • Do they feel psychologically safe? Do they have the tools and technology to do their job?
Processes (see ⊃ Chapter 13)	Processes are how work is undertaken to achieve outcomes. You should try to identify which processes work well and which work less well. To know your processes, you need to be able to map them, so process flow diagrams should be developed to help visualize processes.
Patterns (see ⊃ Chapter 13)	Patterns are present in work, although we may not always be aware of them. These need to be measured and displayed, so all can see how they are performing on their processes. Is there variation in the following agreed processes and in the desired outcomes represented in run charts and/or safety crosses?

Make a diagnosis

Once the assessment of the microsystem is complete, the team should review the analysis and agree on a theme for improvement. Based on this assessment, an aim statement should be agreed upon, which defines what is to be improved, in what timescale, and how making changes is expected to benefit the microsystem.

Treat your microsystem
(See ⊃ Chapter 17.)

Use the model for improvement (Plan–Do–Study–Act (PDSA) cycles) to test theories of change.

Follow-up and sustain improvements
(See ⊃ Chapters 15 and 18.)

Develop metrics to monitor key indicators of microsystem performance based on the thematic area of improvement. Quality improvement dashboards can be used in staff common areas to keep all staff informed of unit performance on an ongoing basis.

Systems theory and human factors

Integration of the systems theory and human factors is a powerful way to address safety and quality of healthcare. Healthcare systems are created for humans and delivered by humans. Therefore, it is logical that the system is designed around the needs and characteristics (factors) of humans.

- Focus on the people receiving and delivering care is essential to a person-centred care model for healthcare systems.
- Human factors and ergonomics (HFE) have their origins in industrial manufacturing and complex activities such as aviation.
- HFE examines and designs work systems to improve efficiency and safety by combining biological sciences (anatomy, physiology, psychology) with design, engineering, and organizational knowledge.
- It focuses on assessing how the system can be adapted and optimized to make the most of human traits, skills, and capabilities to improve quality, efficiency, and safety.
- HFE considers the role of human cognition and behaviour in complex systems, with the aim of creating adaptive capacity or resilience.

In the field of patient safety, the combination of the Donabedian's approach and the microsystem is represented in the Systems Engineering Initiative for Patient Safety (SEIPS) model (Figure 12.4) that is discussed in ⊃ Chapter 14.

- The SEIPS model builds on Reason's 'Swiss cheese model' and Donabedian's SPO framework.
- The model was created by using research on industrial engineering human factor principles and focuses on the three environments which contribute to patient safety: physical, social, and biological.
- Most importantly, it emphasizes how human interactions within the system contribute to the functioning and safety of the system.
- The most recent iteration SEIPS 3.0 adds a new focus on the journey taken by both the patient and the caregiver(s) as being key to patient safety.
- The assessment of the work system is very similar to the 5Ps assessment of the microsystem analysis, with the HFE perspective added on how the individuals in the system interact with one another, their environment, and the tools and technology needed to complete their work.
- The assessment of processes and feedback loops is an essential component of all improvement safety analysis of variation in the system.
- Examples of the application of SEIPS are given in ⊃ Chapter 14.

Signposting

Institute for Excellence in Health and Social Systems. Available at: ℵ https://clinicalmicrosystem. org/ (accessed 10 September 2023).Sheffield Microsystem Coaching Academy. Available at: ℵ https://www.sheffieldmca.org.uk (accessed 10 September 2023).

Further reading

Ayanian, J.Z. and Markel, H. (2016). Donabedian's lasting framework for health care quality. *New England Journal of Medicine*, 375(3), pp. 205–7. doi: 10.1056/nejmp1605101.

Carayon, P. and Perry, S. (2020). Human factors and ergonomics systems approach to the COVID-19 healthcare crisis. *International Journal for Quality in Health Care*, 33(Supplement_1), 1–3. doi: 10.1093/intqhc/mzaa109.

Carayon, P., Schoofs Hundt, A., Karsh, B.-T., et al. (2006). Work system design for patient safety: the SEIPS model. *Quality and Safety in Health Care*, 15(suppl 1), pp. i50–8. doi: 10.1136/qshc.2005.015842.

Carayon, P., Wooldridge, A., Hoonakker, P., Hundt, A.S., and Kelly, M.M. (2020). SEIPS 3.0: human-centered design of the patient journey for patient safety. *Applied Ergonomics*, 84, p. 103033. doi: 10.1016/j.apergo.2019.103033.

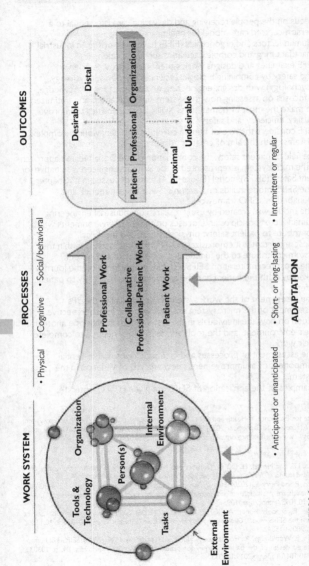

Figure 12.4 SEIPS 2.0.

WORK SYSTEM

- Organization
- Internal Environment
- Person(s)
- Tools & Technology
- Tasks
- External Environment

PROCESSES

- Physical
- Cognitive
- Social/behavioral

Professional Work

Collaborative Professional-Patient Work

Patient Work

OUTCOMES

Distal

Desirable

Organizational

Professional

Undesirable

Patient

Proximal

ADAPTATION

- Anticipated or unanticipated
- Short- or long-lasting
- Intermittent or regular

Donabedian, A. (1988). The quality of care. *JAMA*, 260(12), p. 1743. doi: 10.1001/jama.1988.03410120089033.

Godfrey, M.M., Nelson, E.C., Wasson, J.H., Mohr, J.J., and Batalden, P.B. (2003). Microsystems in health care: part 3. Planning patient-centered services. *The Joint Commission Journal on Quality and Safety*, 29(4), pp. 159–70. doi: 10.1016/s1549-3741(03)29020-1.

Holden, R.J. and Carayon, P. (2021). SEIPS 101 and seven simple SEIPS tools. *BMJ Quality and Safety*, 30(11), p. 901–10. doi: 10.1136/bmjqs-2020-012538.

Mohr, J. (2004). Integrating patient safety into the clinical microsystem. *Quality and Safety in Health Care*, 13(suppl 2), pp. ii34–8. doi: 10.1136/qshc.2003.009571.

Wasson, J.H., Anders, S.G., Moore, L.G., *et al.* (2008). Clinical microsystems, part 2. Learning from micro practices about providing patients the care they want and need. *The Joint Commission Journal on Quality and Patient Safety*, 34(8), pp. 445–52. doi: 10.1016/s1553-7250(08)34055-0.

References

Holden, R.J., Carayon, P., Gurses, A.P., *et al.* (2013). SEIPS 2.0: a human factors framework for studying and improving the work of healthcare professionals and patients. *Ergonomics*, 56(11), pp. 1669–86. doi: 10.1080/00140139.2013.838643.

Nelson, E.C., Godfrey, M.M., Batalden, P.B., *et al.* (2008). Clinical microsystems, part 1. The building blocks of health systems. *The Joint Commission Journal on Quality and Patient Safety*, 34(7), pp. 367–78. doi: 10.1016/s1553-7250(08)34047-1.

Learning healthcare systems

The financial cost of healthcare delivery is constantly increasing due to the complexity of clinical work, drug and equipment development, cost recoupment, and further subspecialization of clinicians.

- Many healthcare systems are approaching zero-sum scenarios with respect to funding, due to resource constraints, where the cost of new innovative treatments must be found from within current budgetary limits.
- Furthermore, what is known as the 60-30-10 challenge has persisted for decades, despite the quality revolution (Braithwaite et al., 2020). This observed ratio states that 60% of care is evidence- or consensus-based, 30% is waste or work of low value, and 10% is harmful to patients.
- Value-based healthcare seeks to deliver the best possible care for the lowest cost.
- In order to evolve our healthcare systems towards this goal, implementation of what are known as learning healthcare systems (LHS) may help to provide the solution.
- LHS are defined as systems where 'Science, informatics, incentives, and culture are aligned for continuous improvement and innovation, with best practices seamlessly embedded in the delivery process and new knowledge captured as an integral by-product of the delivery experience' (Institute of Medicine, 2011).
- Strategy for the use of an LHS framework has three core components which must be present, as indicated in Table 12.4.
- These core components are then utilized in a learning cycle that is at the heart of LHS and, in many ways, are analogous to PDSA cycles. The learning cycle consists of three core processes (Figure 12.5):
  - Gathering data on how practice has performed—the 'P2D' phase;
  - Converting data to knowledge—the 'D2K' phase;
  - Applying knowledge to influence practice—the 'K2P' phase.
- These cycles can occur as fast or as slowly as is required, and at any scale—be it at the microsystem, mesosystem, or macrosystem level.
- Fundamentally though, LHS goals cannot be achieved or sustained without adequate governance, financing, and accountability mechanisms.
- Healthcare generates huge amounts of data continuously. However, these data are simply noise if they are not interrogated in a considered manner.

Table 12.4 Key elements of learning health systems

Foundational elements	Clinical data Information technology, including artificial intelligence and machine learning Evidence standards and practice guidelines Patient engagement
Characteristics	Care-driven learning Person-centredness Networked leadership
Collaborative actions	Clinical effectiveness research Best practices Value incentives

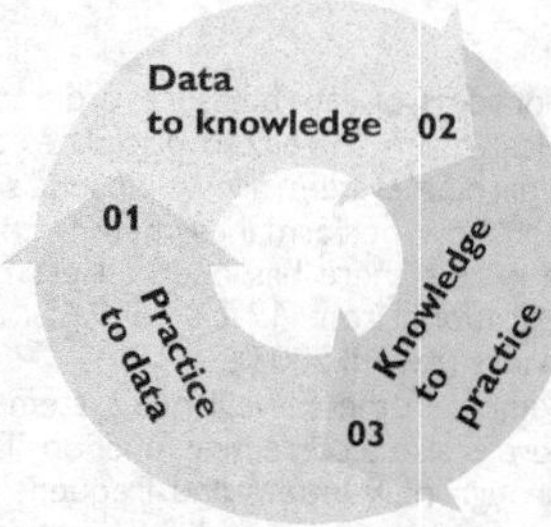

Figure 12.5 Learning cycles in learning healthcare systems.

- In the P2D phase, practice-based data are collected, often requiring the help of IT experts and data scientists. Ensuring the right data can be collected requires design of data collection systems that are user-friendly and intuitive and that integrate into normal workflows. This ensures that sustainability of data collection is possible.
- In the D2K phase, the data gathered in the conduct of patient care, from research projects or quality improvement, are converted into knowledge that can inform and drive improvement projects. Not only is knowledge garnered from 'hard' data important, but attention should also be paid to knowledge gathered from service users and providers, based on their shared experience of the system.
- The K2P phase is where skills in quality improvement can be leveraged to make changes and assess their impact on the system. As change is at the heart of this phase, organizational-level removal of barriers to change, creating a corporate culture of urgency for change, and engaging key stakeholders are of utmost importance. Changes may be piloted to assess their impact before scale-up is considered.

In Box 12.9 an example of how a learning health system can work is provided.

Box 12.9 Case study: LHS implementation

Learning healthcare systems in action

An example of a learning healthcare system is Washington State's Surgical Care and Outcomes Assessment Program (SCOAP). It is a grassroots, voluntary quality improvement collaborative, initially set up in 10 hospitals undertaking appendicectomies, bariatric surgery, and colorectal operations.

It now has 60 hospitals participating that undertake vascular, Interventional Radiology (IR), spinal, high-risk cancer, and gynaecology surgeries. It is a peer-to-peer collaborative among surgeons who use a combination of evidence base, experience, and common sense to develop a set of quality metrics with direct links to optimal surgical care—for example, improving glycaemic control perioperatively or improved diagnostic imaging use in patients with suspected appendicitis.

(Continued)

Box 12.9 (Cont'd.)

A panel of over 50 process-of-care measures are tracked and extended out beyond the surgical realm to related disciplines such as pathology and radiology. This learning system allows hospitals to drive process improvement based on how performance metrics compare with other hospitals. Within the group, there has been an estimated reduction in post-operative complications from 17.7% to 9.6%, and an estimated US$67.3 million in savings (Kwon, 2003).

Interestingly, in addition, in the surveillance system gathering data on patient outcomes, there is also a correcting function. This uses education and peer support through newsletters and frequent peer-led meetings where the focus is on sharing of clinical best practice, change management, and improvement projects that have yielded results.

The validity of the tracked process-of-care measures is also kept under constant review, allowing the system to adapt dynamically to innovations in healthcare technology and changes in best practice, guided by the evidence base.

Kwon, S., Florence, M., Grigas, P., Horton, M., Horvath, K., Johnson, M., Jurkovich, G., Klamp, W., Peterson, K., Quigley, T., Raum, W., Rogers, T., Thirlby, R., Farrokhi, E.T. and Flum, D.R. (2012). Creating a learning healthcare system in surgery: Washington State's Surgical Care and Outcomes Assessment Program (SCOAP) at 5 years. *Surgery*, 151(2), pp. 146–152. doi: 10.1016/j.surg.2011.08.015.

Signposting

The Learning Healthcare Project. *Learning healthcare system*. Available at: ✍ https://learninghealth careproject.org/background/learning-healthcare-system/ (accessed 10 September 2023).

Further reading

Budrionis, A. and Bellika, J.G. (2016). The learning healthcare system: where are we now? A systematic review. *Journal of Biomedical Informatics*, 64, pp. 87–92. doi: 10.1016/j.jbi.2016.09.018.

Menear, M., Blanchette, M.-A., Demers-Payette, O., and Roy, D. (2019). A framework for value-creating learning health systems. *Health Research Policy and Systems*, 17(1), p. 79. doi: 10.1186/s12961-019-0477-3.

Platt, J.E., Raj, M., and Wienroth, M. (2020). An analysis of the learning health system in its first decade in practice: scoping review. *Journal of Medical Internet Research*, 22(3), p. e17026. doi: 10.2196/17026.

Pomare, C., Mahmoud, Z., Vedovi, A., et al. (2021). Learning health systems: a review of key topic areas and bibliometric trends. *Learning Health Systems*, 6(1), p. e10265. doi: 10.1002/lrh2.10265.

References

Braithwaite, J., Glasziou, P., and Westbrook, J. (2020). The three numbers you need to know about healthcare: the 60-30-10 Challenge. *BMC Medicine*, 18(1), p. 102. doi: 10.1186/s12916-020-01563-4.

Foley, T., Horwitz, L., and Zahran, R. (2021). *Realising the potential of learning health systems*. London: Health Foundation.

Institute of Medicine (2011). *Roundtable on value and science-driven health care: the learning health system and its innovation collaboratives: update report*. Washington, DC: Institute of Medicine.

Top tips

When starting your improvement project, ask:
- Which microsystem will be affected by the project?
- Which other systems affect the processes I want to improve?
- Who are the people in the system—patients and people providing care?
- Do I know how work is done to achieve outcomes?
- How do we measure performance of the system?
- What changes are needed to improve the performance and then the outcomes of the system?

Summary

- Systems thinking is central to quality improvement.
- Deming places the understanding of how systems work at the core of improvement and change.
- Systems are made up of people who determine how that system will operate.
- Systems vary in complexity—from simple to complicated, complex, and chaotic.
- Healthcare systems are now regarded to be complex adaptive, characterized by ever-changing relationships and interactions to achieve outcomes.
- In healthcare, systems are composed of many interacting clinical microsystems which deliver care.
- If a person has a chronic condition with different needs, then they will require several microsystems to interact to deliver the outcomes required.
- Quality improvement requires the study of the components of a clinical microsystem—that is, the people, environment, organization, and tasks to be undertaken, the tools and technology needed to complete the task, as well as the processes followed to achieve outcomes.

The Lens of Understanding Variation

Key points

- The understanding of variation is the foundation of quality improvement.
- Failure to differentiate between common cause variation and special cause variation can have unintended consequences and may create a barrier to effective improvement.
- Variation in a process can be identified by a process map and by analysing the process with an Ishikawa diagram and a Pareto chart.
- Measurement of variation is illustrated on a statistical process control (SPC) chart or a run chart.

Introduction

Variation is one of the Lenses of Profound Knowledge (see ➔ Chapter 3). The understanding of variation and how it impacts clinical outcomes is the focus of this chapter. Variation is part of daily life and part of the fabric of healthcare. If we want to improve the quality of care and the outcomes achieved, it is essential that we understand variation and know how to manage it in a way that can lead to improvement. As discussed in ➔ Chapter 12, healthcare delivery consists of a large number of interacting systems, processes, and people. Variation exists within each of these components:

- *Systems*: the way in which we design and deliver services varies;
- *Processes*: we have many different processes to achieve outcomes;
- *People*: clinicians have different skills;
- Patients present with different clinical conditions at different stages of disease, at different times of the day;
- The beliefs and attitudes of healthcare workers and patients differ.

All of these types of variation come into play when we consider how to ensure that variation does not have an impact on the quality of care delivered and received, both of which may have an impact on clinical outcomes and the experience of healthcare workers and patients.

How do different people see variation?

Different people in a system may have alternative ways of seeing variation (Neuhauser et al., 2011).

- Healthcare managers generally are concerned with performance over time. They want a stable process to produce outcomes and this can be demonstrated on a statistical process control (SPC) chart.
- Clinical researchers are interested in the impact of an intervention on different populations. They want to control the variation, so that the impact of the intervention can be measured, and they use a randomized controlled trial.
- Patients are interested in their individual needs and how they differ from the generalizable inference of longitudinal studies and standardized treatments.
- Although healthcare can be viewed as a 'mass production' system, in which one has to decrease variation, this overlooks the fact that individual patient needs may also vary. With increasing patient complexity, healthcare might be better viewed as a 'mass bespoke' system, in which the majority of planning is performed prior to offering choices and options that comply with the agreed standards of care and are person-centred.

An appreciation of these different views is important when one is undertaking an improvement project.

Reference

Neuhauser, D., Provost, L., and Bergman, B. (2011). The meaning of variation to healthcare managers, clinical and health-services researchers, and individual patients. *BMJ Quality and Safety*, 20(Suppl 1), pp. i36–40. doi: 10.1136/bmjqs.2010.046334.

Why is the study of variation important?

Why is the study of variation important?

The presence of variation is not, in itself, good or bad, as it will always be present. Inspection is often based on this interpretation of variation.

If one observes a process or outcomes, one can plot these on a Gaussian or bell curve. This will provide an understanding of the variation. As indicated in Figure 13.1, there is a normal distribution and often quality assurance will concentrate on decreasing the 'bad' performance, rather than focusing on how to have all care delivered within a range that is above the desired standard.

In quality improvement, the focus is on shifting the bell curve and narrowing the distribution between 'bad' and 'good', so that all of the distribution falls within the defined measure of good.

To achieve this shift in distribution requires a deep understanding of the variation in performance and outcomes, and what changes need to be made to shift the distribution (Gawande, 1996).

Whenever we receive a service or buy a product, we want it to be of the same quality every time, and not dependent on either the person delivering the service or the system that has been designed to deliver the service. For example, if one goes to a restaurant, one expects the quality of the food to be consistently reliable. The quality should not depend on the person making the food.

Likewise, in healthcare, patients expect the quality of care to be the same, and not person-dependent. Variation is a problem when it has a negative impact on clinical outcomes. Experiences may differ; however, it would be expected that there is no variation in what is delivered as per the prevailing evidence.

Deming (1986) proposed that it is the identification of variation that provides the opportunities for improvement. A vital purpose of quality

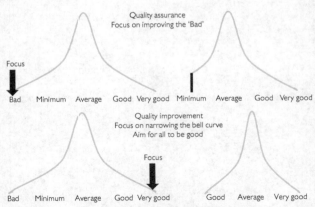

Figure 13.1 Bell curve quality assurance and quality improvement.
Adapted from Balestracci and Medical Group Management Association, 2015.

improvement is to identify the variation that is present within processes, as this may impact the clinical outcomes that are achieved. In this chapter, we discuss variation and how management of variation is the focus of most improvement programmes.

Further reading

Gawande, A. (2004). The bell curve. *The New Yorker*. Available at: ஃ https://www.newyorker.com/magazine/2004/12/06/the-bell-curve (accessed 10 September 2023).

Nolan, T.W., Perla, R.J., and Provost, L.P. (2016). Understanding variation 26 years later. *Quality Progress; Milwaukee*, 49(11), pp. 28–37. Available at: ஃ https://www.apiweb.org/images/PDFs/understanding-variation26-years-later.pdf (accessed 10 September 2023).

Nolan, T.W. and Provost, L.P. (1990). Understanding variation. *Quality Progress*, pp. 70–8. Available at: ஃ https://www.apiweb.org/UnderstandingVariation.pdf (accessed 10 September 2023).

References

Balestracci, D.; Medical Group Management Association (2015). *Data Sanity: A Quantum Leap to Unprecedented Results*. Englewood, CO: Medical Group Management Association.

Deming, W.E. (1986). *Out of the Crisis*. Cambridge, MA: MIT Press.

Types of variation

> 'Decisions made without knowledge of common and special causes often lead to increased variation, poor performance and mis-attributed credit or blame.'
>
> (Nolan, Perla, Provost, 2016)

Shewhart defined two types of variation, both of which occur in healthcare systems (Nolan et al., 2016).

- *Common cause variation* arises due to inherent variation within a system. This variation is caused by unknown factors and/or factors intrinsic to a system that result in a predictable, but random, variation over time. It is neither 'good nor bad', but rather an indication of a stable system, for example:
  - Arrival times of people to the emergency department;
  - Seasonal presentations of infectious diseases;
  - Turnaround times for laboratory tests.
- *Special cause variation* occurs due to variation outside a system. This variation is not predictable and is non-random. The variation can be explained and is due to changes in external or environmental factors, for example:
  - A bus accident leading to increased presentations to an emergency department;
  - Increase in staffing absences in March 2020 due to the onset of coronavirus disease 2019 (COVID-19);
  - The impact of the COVID-19 pandemic on waiting times for elective surgery.
- Common cause variation can be differentiated from special cause variation using an SPC. Common cause variation will lie within the expected standard deviation for that factor within a system, whereas special cause variation will lie outside of this limit.

(See ⊃ Chapter 2.)

- Variations in patient care are not necessarily wrong and can be 'warranted'. Indeed, given the unique differences between individual patients, a degree of variation is to be expected and can be an important component of patient-centred care.
- Natural variation, such as the prevalence of some infections or characteristics of individuals or populations, is a normal phenomenon.
- However, if a variation in care cannot be explained by differing patient characteristics or circumstances, then it is deemed unwarranted. This type of variation may lead to harm. Identifying and understanding drivers of unwarranted variation within a system can reveal opportunities for improvement.
- Much of the inequity in outcomes, as discussed in ⊃ Chapter 5, can be due to unwarranted variation in the provision of care to people with disadvantaged backgrounds.
- The drivers underlying unwarranted variation are often complex and multifactorial. Potential factors contributing to unwarranted variation

include differing professional behaviours, professional uncertainty, environmental circumstances, and patient preferences.

• Potential strategies to address unwarranted variation include developing objective clinical guidelines and protocols, sharing best practice principles among healthcare professionals, and using big data to gain insight into health systems.

• For example, the NHS RightCare programme (available at: ℘ https://www.england.nhs.uk/rightcare/, accessed 10 September 2023) aims to tackle unwarranted healthcare variation in England by developing a wide range of resources that are freely available to everyone, with the goal of optimizing value of care at both individual and population levels.

• Management of unwarranted variation requires an understanding of the complexity of decision-making, beliefs, and attitudes of patients and clinicians, and requires reflection and shared decision-making. (Atsma et al., 2020).

Signposting

There are several atlases of variation that demonstrate variation in clinical outcomes across regions and countries:

Atlas of Variation (Office for Health Improvement and Disparities). Available at: ℘ https://fingert ips.phe.org.uk/profile/atlas-of-variation (accessed 10 September 2023).

Atlases (NHS RightCare). Available at: ℘ https://www.england.nhs.uk/rightcare/rightcare-resour ces/atlas/ (accessed 10 September 2023).

Scottish Atlas of Healthcare Variation (Public Health Scotland). Available at: ℘ https://www. isdscotland.org/products-and-services/scottish-atlas-of-variation/introduction/ (accessed 10 September 2023).

Dartmouth Atlas of Health Care (Dartmouth Atlas Project). Available at: ℘ https://www.dartmou thatlas.org (accessed 10 September 2023).

Further reading

Berwick, D.M. (1991). Controlling variation in health care. *Medical Care*, 29(12), pp. 1212–25. doi: 10.1097/00005650-199112000-00004.

Stoecklein, M. (2015). *Understanding and misunderstanding variation in healthcare: case study*. Available at: ℘ https://createvalue.org/wp-content/uploads/Understanding-and-Misunderstanding-Variation-in-Healthcare.pdf (accessed 10 September 2023).

Wennberg, J.E. (2002). Unwarranted variations in healthcare delivery: implications for academic medical centres. *BMJ*, 325(7370), pp. 961–4. doi: 10.1136/bmj.325.7370.961.

References

Atsma, F., Elwyn, G., and Westert, G. (2020). Understanding unwarranted variation in clinical practice: a focus on network effects, reflective medicine and learning health systems. *International Journal for Quality in Health Care*, 32(4), pp. 271–4. doi: 10.1093/intqhc/mzaa023.

Nolan, T.W., Perla, R.J., and Provost, L.P. (2016). Understanding variation 26 years later. *Quality Progress; Milwaukee*, 49(11), pp. 28–37. Available at: ℘ https://www.apiweb.org/images/PDFs/understanding-variation26-years-later.pdf (accessed 10 September 2023).

How is variation illustrated?

Variation within clinical systems is context-dependent.

- If one wants to improve outcomes for patients, one needs to identify the type of variation that exists and apply the right intervention to manage it.
- Understanding variation within a system is achieved by observing a process and measuring the variation within it over time.
- Analysis of the causes of variation provides opportunities for improvement.
- Variation is illustrated on a run chart or an SPC chart.

Run charts

- Run charts are a useful tool for graphically representing data in a simple way to assess trends over time. They are easy to construct and interpret (Figure 13.2), and do not require any detailed knowledge of statistics. They are very helpful for detecting improvement signals early, even with limited amounts of data.
- Data can be *continuous* and take on changing values on a continuous scale, such as length of stay and attendances in clinic, or in units of time.
- Data can be absolute or *discrete* (e.g. pressure ulcer or not, arrived on time or arrived late, attended clinic or did not attend, alive or dead, etc.).
- Time is plotted on the x-axis, and data measurements in which we are interested are plotted on the y-axis.
- The median is the middle number of the data points.
- A number of simple rules can be used to interpret run charts, which help to detect non-random patterns emerging in the data as set out in Table 13.1 and Figure 13.3.

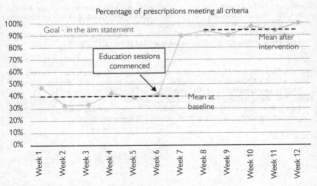

Figure 13.2 Construction of a run chart.

Table 13.1 Rules for run charts

Shift	Six or more consecutive data points either all above or all below the median line. This suggests a non-random pattern
Trend	Five or more consecutive data points either going up or going down
Astronomical point	Suggests that there is a special cause that needs to be investigated
Run	A series of data points that fall either above or below the median. One counts the number of times the data points line connecting the data points cross the median and add 1
	Reference tables can be used to determine the expected number of runs for a given data set. Too many or too few runs may indicate a non-random pattern which warrants further investigation

Interpretation of a Run Chart: Shift, Trend & Astronomical Data

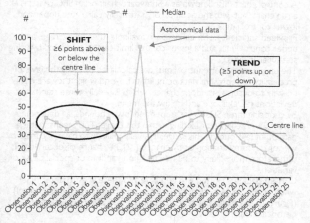

Figure 13.3 Run chart rules.

© Clinical Excellence Commission 2023.

In Box 13.1 the application of a run chart to the documentation of vital signs is illustrated.

An everyday clinical example of run charts can be seen when observing patients' vital sign charts. We are very familiar with reviewing patients' vital signs, which are plotted multiple times a day on a visual chart. By connecting the dots for each of the measurements, we have actually created a run chart.

As expected, there is a degree of random variation within the normal range for each vital sign (e.g. fluctuation between 60 and 100 for the heart rate of a typical adult, for which 80 beats per minute is the median). Each of the run chart rules can then be applied when analysing these charts. This will provide an early indication of a patient potentially becoming unwell if multiple readings are trending in the wrong direction (e.g. the heart rate and respiratory rate trending upwards as an early sign of evolving sepsis).

Statistical process control charts

- A control chart (also known as a Shewhart chart or an SPC chart) is like a run chart, but with the addition of statistically calculated upper and lower control limits.
- Provided sufficient historical data are available, then an average, an upper control limit, and a lower control limit can be calculated by using statistical analysis.
- The upper and lower control limits are calculated by using the laws of probability to represent data point limits beyond which they are highly unlikely to occur by random chance, which is usually three standard deviations (SDs) above and below the mean.
- By choosing three SDs as the upper and lower bounds, all data points have a 99.7% chance of landing within this range. This means that if a data point falls outside this range, it is very unlikely to have occurred by way of random variation or by chance (<0.3% chance of occurring). It is therefore more likely to be due to a non-random or special cause of variation.
- Current data are plotted and compared to these lines to determine whether the process variation is either consistent with (i.e. in control) (Figure 13.4) or unpredictable (out of control) relative to these historical data.

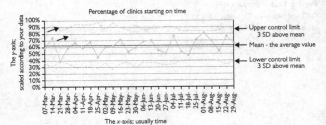

Figure 13.4 Statistical process control: normal variation.

- Unpredictable process variation therefore suggests that the process may be affected by special causes of variation. Having identified an 'out-of-control' signal on the chart, it should be marked and the underlying cause of this variation should be investigated, so that any necessary adjustments can be made (Figure 13.5).

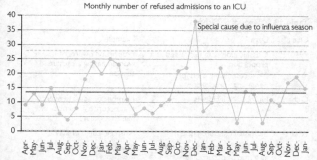

Figure 13.5 Statistical process control: special cause outlier.

- The SPC chart can be used in a variety of different sectors to good effect, including industrial processing and healthcare. Its emphasis on early detection and prevention of problems offers a distinct advantage over other quality tools.
- This early identification allows for a shift from detection to prevention of defects. They can be used to help reduce costs, to identify sources of delay within a process, and to improve customer satisfaction.
- Common cause variation is indicated if the data points are within the control limits.
- As with run charts, there are rules to follow that indicate when there is statistically significant improvement, and the mean and control limits can then be recalculated.
- Special cause variation is present if one of the rules in Table 13.2 applies.

Table 13.2 Rules for SPC charts

Rule 1	1 point outside the ± 3 sigma control limits
Rule 2	6 or more consecutive points steadily increasing or decreasing
Rule 3	8 successive consecutive points above or below the central line
Rule 4	2 out of 3 successive points beyond the ± 2 sigma limits
Rule 5	15 consecutive points within ± 1 sigma on either side of the central line

- Each SD above or below the mean is referred to as a sigma, and there are three sigmas (SD) below and above the mean when we choose three SDs as the upper and lower bounds.
- There are different types of SPC charts (Table 13.3), depending on the data, and more can be obtained from the specialized signposted links. In most cases, you will use a run chart in your project or a P SPC chart.

Table 13.3 Types of SPC charts

Chart	Data	Example
P chart	Classification data expressed as a proportion Most commonly used for percentage proportions	Proportion of pregnant women having a caesarean section
C chart	Number of incidents	Number of adverse events that occur (e.g. number of falls that occur)
I chart	Individual measurements	Average length of stay
U chart	Number of incidents expressed as a rate of occurrence	Number of falls per 1000 inpatients

In Figure 13.6 a trend and in Figure 13.7 a run on a statistical process control chart are illustrated.

It is important to:
- Establish a stable baseline before the intervention;
- Have a defined outcome measure;
- Describe the quality improvement design clearly, so it is understood;
- Use the correct SPC chart to be able to infer an effect of the intervention on the outcome (Marang-van de Mheen and Woodcock, 2022).

Using an SPC chart can be challenging for the novice. However, the references below and the signposted links can support you in using the P chart. If

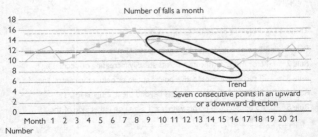

Figure 13.6 Statistical process control trend.

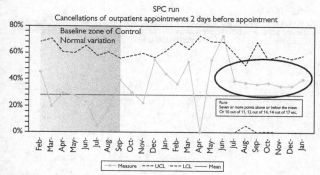

Figure 13.7 Statistical process control run.

other charts are required, consult with the data expert in your organization. Examples will be provided in ⏵ Chapter 17.

Signposting

Run charts and SPC charts

Healthcare Improvement Partnership (HQIP): Run Chart Rules and Table Instructions – HQIP https://www.hqip.org.uk/wp-content/uploads/2016/03/Template-8-Run-chart-rules-and-table.pdf (accessed 10 September 2023).

Clinical Excellence Commission New South Wales (2023) Run chart reference https://www.cec.health.nsw.gov.au/CEC-Academy/quality-improvement-tools/run-charts (accessed 10 September 2023).

NHS Institute for Innovation and Improvement (2009): A guide to creating and interpreting run and control charts. https://www.england.nhs.uk/improvement-hub/wp-content/uploads/sites/44/2017/11/A-guide-to-creating-and-interpreting-run-and-control-charts.pdf (accessed 10 September 2023).

Institute for Healthcare Improvement(IHI) (2023): Run chart tool. https://www.ihi.org/resources/Pages/Tools/RunChart.aspx (accessed 10 September 2023).

NHS England Improvement (2023): Statistical process control tool. https://www.england.nhs.uk/statistical-process-control-tool/ (accessed 10 September 2023)

American Society for Quality (ASQ) Control chart tool (2023). https://asq.org/quality-resources/control-chart (accessed 10 September 2023).

Clinical Excellence Commission New South Wales (2023): Control charts. https://www.cec.health.nsw.gov.au/CEC-Academy/quality-improvement-tools/control-charts (accessed 10 September 2023).

NHS Scotland (2017): Statistical Process Control - https://www.isdscotland.org/health-topics/quality-indicators/statistical-process-control/_docs/Statistical-Process-Control-Tutorial-Guide-180713.pdf (accessed 10 September 2023

Further reading

Benneyan, J.C., Lloyd, R.C., and Plsek, P.E. (2003). Statistical process control as a tool for research and healthcare improvement. *Quality and Safety in Health Care*, 12(6), pp. 458–64. doi: 10.1136/qhc.12.6.458.

Ogrinc. G. (2021). Measuring and publishing quality improvement. *Regional Anesthesia and Pain Medicine*, 46(8), pp. 643–9. doi: 10.1136/rapm-2020-102201.

Perla, R.J., Provost, L.P., and Murray, S.K. (2011). The run chart: a simple analytical tool for learning from variation in healthcare processes. *BMJ Quality and Safety*, 20(1), pp. 46–51. doi: 10.1136/bmjqs.2009.037895.

Provost, L.P. and Murray, S.K. (2022). *The Health Care Data Guide: Learning from Data for Improvement*. Hoboken, NJ: John Wiley & Sons.

Reference

Marang-van de Mheen, P.J. and Woodcock, T. (2022). Grand rounds in methodology: four critical decision points in statistical process control evaluations of quality improvement initiatives. *BMJ Quality and Safety*, 32(1), pp. 47–54. doi: 10.1136/bmjqs-2022-014870.

studying variation by understanding the process

Studying variation by understanding the process

- Process mapping helps to elucidate the 'real-life' processes, systems, and contexts within which improvement interventions are implemented (Antonacci et al., 2018).
- Process mapping aims to gain a holistic understanding of the process being studied. It allows individual steps in a system to be considered, which may have been overlooked previously. It can also help to identify weak points within a system.
- Where unwarranted variation has been identified in a process, process maps can be used to better understand the causes of this variation and allow changes to be made to improve the consistency of the process.
- Process mapping can assist in understanding work as done, rather than work as imagined.
- Process mapping involves several steps:
  - Identifying the scope of the process (e.g. how an outpatient clinic operates, how a patient with stroke is managed in the emergency department);
  - Identifying the people involved in the process;
  - Involving the people in the process in studying how the process works;
  - Gathering information on the process by observing how it works;
  - Identifying and ordering each step in the process;
  - Generating a process map to illustrate each step;
  - Measuring each step where appropriate;
  - Analysing the process map to look for variation, steps that are duplicated or not needed as they do not add value, and who has responsibility for each step of the process.
- Process mapping can be a team-building exercise to assess how work is done rather than as imagined.
- The first step may be using Post-it notes to illustrate each step of the process and then transfer to a formal process map.
- Standard nomenclature is used when constructing a process map (Figure 13.8). The most common ones used are:

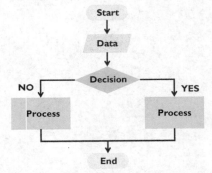

Figure 13.8 Nomenclature for process maps.

- Start and end points;
- Action points;
- Decision points;
- Direction arrows.

A process map with swim lanes can define how a process has hand-offs and different people or systems in the process have their own responsibilities (Figure 13.9).

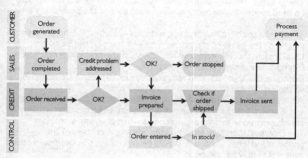

Figure 13.9 Swim lane process map.

Signposting

NHS Institute for Innovation and Improvement (2005) Process mapping, analysis and redesign. https://www.england.nhs.uk/improvement-hub/wp-content/uploads/sites/44/2017/11/ILG-1.2-Process-Mapping-Analysis-and-Redesign.pdf (accessed 10 September 2023).
NHS England (2023) Conventional process mapping. https://www.england.nhs.uk/wp-content/uploads/2021/12/qsir-conventional-process-mapping.pdf (accessed 10 September 2023).

Reference

Antonacci, G., Reed, J.E., Lennox, L., and Barlow, J. (2018). The use of process mapping in healthcare quality improvement projects. *Health Services Management Research*, 31(2), pp. 74–84. doi: 10.1177/0951484818770411.

Analysing processes

Analysis of the causes of variation in a process can be undertaken by using the Ishikawa diagram and/or careful use of the '5 Whys' to understand the root causes of the problem, and then by using the Pareto chart to demonstrate the important factors that need to be addressed.

The 5 Whys

- The '5 Whys' is a tool adopted from the Lean methodology, which can be used to identify the root causes of each part of the problem in a process.
- Identify the problem in a process, and then ask why it is a problem until you reach the cause of the problem on which action can be taken.
- Usually after the fifth Why, the root cause of the problem is reached. Examples are provided in ➲ Chapter 17.
- Combine this approach with appreciative inquiry (see ➲ Chapter 10), so the experience for the team is a positive one.
- Although this tool is used widely, it has the potential to be too simplistic in the analysis of the root cause of a problem. Different clinical teams could come up with different outcomes when analysing a problem.
- The '5 Whys' therefore must be used within the context of the problem and when used, one should be careful not to close down other causes that may be present.

Ishikawa diagrams

- An Ishikawa diagram, also known as fishbone or cause-and-effect diagram, is constructed after a problem and the contexts and processes relating to it have been identified.
- These diagrams are essentially visual illustrations of possible explanations or hypotheses that could explain, or contribute to, the problem under review. This is a form of root cause analysis (Murtagh Kurowski et al., 2015).
- Ishikawa diagrams, like process mapping, are best constructed as part of a team-brainstorming exercise.
- Improvement teams can then investigate whether the most convincing explanations do indeed contribute to the problem.
- These problems can then be addressed as part of improvement initiatives.
- Each part of the fishbone represents the different elements of the work system or microsystem, as indicated in ➲ Chapter 12. For example, one can use the Systems Engineering Initiative for Patient Safety (SEIPS) work system model's categories of people, environment, organization or management, tasks, technology, and processes to be the six bones of the diagram. Each of these will have associated factors that influence the outcome.
- In Figure 13.10, an example of a fishbone for medication errors shows the different factors that are involved, each of which can be an opportunity for improvement.

Prescribing errors

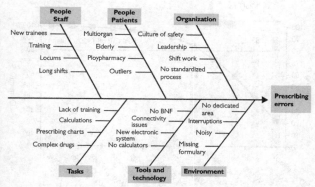

Figure 13.10 Ishikawa diagram for prescribing errors. BNF, British National Formulary.

Pareto analysis

- Once one has analysed the causes of a problem by using the Ishikawa diagram, one then uses the Pareto chart to decide where to concentrate one's improvement activities.
- The Pareto principle dictates that 80% of effects come from 20% of causes. Its origins are rooted in economics, but it can also be applied to improvement.
- Pareto analysis is a ranked comparison of weighted factors relating to a problem that an improvement intervention aims to address. It aims to identify those factors that contribute most to the problem.
- In essence, Pareto analysis involves three elements:
  - All factors contributing to a problem (e.g. blood samples lost, blood samples taken incorrectly) ordered by the magnitude of their contribution (e.g. number of times these errors occurred over a time period);
  - Contributions of individual factors expressed numerically (e.g. as a percentage of the total);
  - A calculation of the contribution of each contributor as a cumulative percentage.
- These elements can be easily entered in software, such as Excel, to yield a Pareto diagram.
- A Pareto diagram helps to identify the top factors relating to a problem that, if addressed, have the highest likelihood of resulting in an improvement, as shown in Figure 13.11.

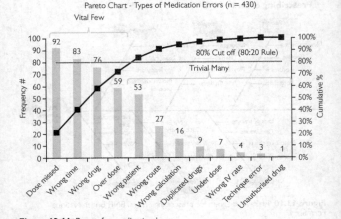

Figure 13.11 Pareto for medication harm.
© Clinical Excellence Commission 2023.

Signosting

NHS England (2023): (accessed 10 September 2023)
Cause and Effect (Fishbone). https://www.england.nhs.uk/wp-content/uploads/2021/12/qsir-cause-and-effect-fishbone.pdf
Pareto https://www.england.nhs.uk/wp-content/uploads/2022/01/qsir-pareto.pdf
Pareto Chart tool. https://www.england.nhs.uk/pareto-chart-tool/
Using five whys to review a simple problem. https://www.england.nhs.uk/wp-content/uploads/2022/02/qsir-using-five-whys-to-review-a-simple-problem.pdf
Card, A.J. (2017). The problem with '5 whys'. *BMJ Quality and Safety*, 26(8), pp. 671–7. doi: 10.1136/bmjqs-2016-005849.

Further reading

Antonacci, G., Reed, J.E., Lennox, L., and Barlow, J. (2018). The use of process mapping in healthcare quality improvement projects. *Health Services Management Research*, 31(2), pp. 74–84. doi: 10.1177/0951484818770411.
NHS Institute for Innovation and Improvement (2005). *Improvement leaders' guide. Process mapping, analysis and redesign.* https://www.england.nhs.uk/improvement-hub/wp-content/uploads/sites/44/2017/11/ILG-1.2-Process-Mapping-Analysis-and-Redesign.pdf (accessed 10 September 2023)
NHS Institute for Innovation and Improvement (2005). *Improvement leaders' guide. General improvement skills.* https://www.england.nhs.uk/improvement-hub/wp-content/uploads/sites/44/2017/11/ILG-1.1-Improvement-Knowledge-and-Skills.pdf (accessed 10 September 2023)

Reference

Murtagh Kurowski, E., Schondelmeyer, A.C., Brown, C., Dandoy, C.E., Hanke, S.J., and Tubbs Cooley, H.L. (2015). A practical guide to conducting quality improvement in the health care setting. *Current Treatment Options in Pediatrics*, 1(4), pp. 380–92. doi: 10.1007/s40746-015-0027-3.

Top tips

Summary

Top tips

- Once a problem has been identified, study the variation in the process that leads to the outcome by observing it directly.
- Ask the people who work in the process to assist in defining each step of the process, so that you identify work as done rather than work as imagined.
- Analyse the process with a root cause analysis, and illustrate it on a fishbone diagram.
- Organize the causes on a Pareto chart to identify which ones will be the focus of your project.

Summary

Variation is one of the Lenses of Profound Knowledge. Common cause variation occurs as a natural part of a system and is what the system has been designed to deliver. Special cause variation is an event that occurs due to factors outside the natural running of the processes in a system.

Warranted variation in healthcare is provided to meet the individual characteristics of the patient. Unwarranted variation is variation that does not benefit the clinical outcome or experience of the patient.

Run charts and SPC charts are used to illustrate variation, and the study of processes allows us to identify and analyse variation.

The Lens of Knowledge

Methods used in quality improvement

Key points

- The methods for improvement are all derived from the different Lenses of Profound Knowledge
- The theory of knowledge includes ways to test ideas, predict what may or may not happen, test the prediction against what happened, and to learn
- The Model for Improvement asks three questions on aim, measurement of the impact of the intervention and what changes will be tested using a Plan-Do-Study-Act cycle
- Lean and Six Sigma focus on decreasing waste and variation in process.
- Theory of constraints allows analysis of bottlenecks in the system that impede the process.
- Experience-based co-design is a method to include providers and receivers of care in the design of the process.
- Improvement collaboratives are structured learning systems to accelerate learning between improvement teams.
- Human factors can provide a framework to analyse systems and processes

Introduction

In ⊃ Chapter 3, the theories underlying the Science of Improvement were discussed. Three Lenses of Profound Knowledge have been discussed:

- ⊃ Chapter 10 discussed the *Lens of Psychology* and the ways in which you can build will for change;
- ⊃ Chapter 12 discussed the *Lens of Systems* and the need to understand systems and how they operate to ensure change can take place;
- ⊃ Chapter 13 discussed the *Lens of Variation* and how understanding processes provides the opportunity for improvement.

In this chapter, we explore the *Lens of Knowledge*, that is, understanding how change takes place.

The Science of Improvement has resulted in different change methodologies being developed, all of which base their change process on the four lenses of improvement.

- They are all appropriate in different contexts. Some organizations may choose one over another.
- The key is to have a method that one uses consistently.
- All are based on having a reliable measurement system, which will be discussed in ⊃ Chapter 15.

The methods are based on the concepts of testing ideas and predicting what will happen, as shown in Figure 14.1. Application of the theory and method will be discussed in ⊃ Chapters 17 and 18.

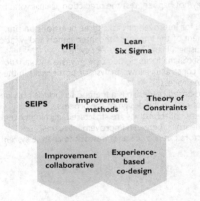

Figure 14.1 Methods used in quality improvement.

Model for Improvement

Model for Improvement

What is the theory?

The Model for Improvement (MFI), developed by Associates in Process Improvement, is probably the most widespread of the methods used in healthcare. The MFI is designed to combine quality improvement (QI) thinking and QI doing. It consists of three questions and a cycle (Figure 14.2). It has been designed as a practical way to apply Deming's System of Profound Knowledge (SOPK) to improve quality (see ➔ Chapter 3; Table 14.1).

The MFI is advantageous because:

- It condenses a complex and comprehensive theory into an accessible practical model;
- It facilitates an iterative and adaptive approach to change;
- It promotes stepwise progress through the breakdown of large and complex quality problems into smaller, more manageable building blocks of change.
- Prior to applying the MFI, the first steps in the improvement process are to identify a problem and study the system producing the problem— usually with a process map, and then by Ishikawa analysis and with a Pareto chart, as discussed in ➔ Chapter 13.
- Once the problem is identified, a SMART aim statement is developed (see ➔ Chapter 17).
- The next step is to choose a set of measures that will be used in the project (see ➔ Chapter 15).
- Finally, a change programme is undertaken, incorporating tests of changes using the Plan–Do–Study–Act (PDSA) cycle (see ➔ Chapters 3 and 18).

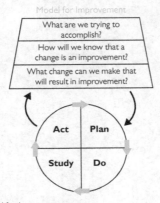

Figure 14.2 Model for Improvement.
Reproduced with permission from Associates in Process Improvement; http://www.apiweb.org/

Table 14.1 Aligning the Model for Improvement with the System of Profound Knowledge

Model for Improvement	System of Profound Knowledge
What are we trying to achieve?	Psychology: a shared aim is a powerful tool for aligning goals and behaviours for change
How will we know that a change is an improvement?	Variation: measurement is an objective statistical way for evaluating the effectiveness of any change effort
What change can we make that will result in an improvement?	Systems: change ideas emerge from a deep and broad understanding of the care system producing the quality problem
PDSA cycle	Theory of knowledge: the PDSA cycle facilitates a learning approach through testing change as its epistemological basis

PDSA, Plan–Do–Study–Act.

Limitations of the Model for Improvement

- Application of the MFI can be variable, with low scientific evidence of its improvement impact.
- Improvers sometimes struggle to scale their change ideas appropriately for a test of change. A simple rule of thumb is that the test of change can never be too small, but it can be too big. Useful learning from larger complex changes can be harder to harvest, with goodwill easier to lose when efforts do not meet the desired outcome.

See ⊃ Chapters 17 and 18 for practical examples on use of the MFI.

Signposting

NHS Improving Quality (2014). *First steps towards quality improvement.* Available at: ⊗ https://www.england.nhs.uk/improvement-hub/wp-content/uploads/sites/44/2011/06/service_improvement_guide_2014.pdf (accessed 10 September 2023).

Further reading

Crowl, A., Sharma, A., Sorge, L., and Sorensen, T. (2015). Accelerating quality improvement within your organization: applying the Model for Improvement. *Pharmacy Today*, 21(7), pp. 79–89. doi: 10.1016/s1042-0991(15)30278-4.
Langley, G.J., Moen, R.D., Nolan, K.M., Nolan, T.W., Norman, C.L., and Provost, L.P. (2009). *The Improvement Guide*, 2nd edition. San Francisco, CA: Jossey-Bass.
Reed, J.E. and Card, A.J. (2016). The problem with Plan–Do–Study–Act cycles. *BMJ Quality and Safety*, 25(3), pp. 147–52. doi: 10.1136/bmjqs-2015-005076.

Lean and Six Sigma

What is the theory?

Lean and Six Sigma are distinct, but related, approaches to improving quality. These approaches, also derived from the work of Deming, were originally developed to guide improvement of quality in manufacturing. In practice, Lean and Six Sigma are often applied together to improve overall quality in different ways.

Lean

Lean, which emerged from the Toyota Production System, employs standardized methodologies and tools to continuously improve quality through elimination of waste. Its focus is on removing non-value-added elements or processes.

The core principles of Lean are about value creation for the customer or receiver of the service, who may change at different points in the process (Box 14.1).

Box 14.1 Lean principles

Value is defined by the needs of the patient.

Value stream is identifying and mapping all of the steps and processes necessary to create what the patient needs.

Flow is ensuring that all necessary steps and processes run smoothly and without waste.

Pull is the system realizing value, with patient demand driving further service (i.e. the person is not pushed through the process).

Perfection is continuously seeking improvement and spread of efficiency. Perfection in Lean identifies eight types of waste (Table 14.2).

Lean healthcare focuses on creating value in every step of the process, and value can be for the patient or members of the clinical team. Table 14.2 gives the different types of wastes. This will resonate with clinicians in training, as many of their activities do not add value to their learning, the patient, or the clinical process.

The Lean theory is particularly useful for process-driven QI projects in healthcare, with the aim of improving efficiency as these methodologies support the identification, measurement, and removal of waste.

Several Lean methods are shown in Table 14.3.

The 5S Model (Figure 14.3; Box 14.2) applies Lean principles to optimize workspaces for maximum efficiency, effectiveness, and safety.

Table 14.2 Categorizing waste in healthcare

Waste type	Healthcare example
Waiting	A surgical team waiting for a patient to arrive at the operating theatre to begin surgery
Inventory	Excess vaccine is ordered and expires before it can be administered
Transportation	A patient must be transported from one hospital to another for coronary angiography
Unused talent	A doctor spending significant amounts of time looking for test results
Motion	A long walk from the consultation room to the waiting room to get the next patient
Defects	Surgical gloves that rip easily when putting them on
Overproduction	Emergency departments treating minor illnesses
Processing	Ordering additional unnecessary tests on a blood sample

Table 14.3 Selected Lean methods

Method	Description
Gemba walk	Gemba refers to the place *where work is actually being done or where value is being created*. One goes to see how work is done rather than work as imagined
Kaizen	Making continual improvements using the PDSA cycles
Kaizen event	A workshop over a few days to identify and resolve problems
Andon	Fixing a problem in real time when identified
5 Whys	To identify the root cause of a problem
Value stream mapping	Assessing the value added by each step in a process. This requires analysis of the process and noting the value for the different parts of the process
Waste reduction	Removing steps that do not add value
Zero defect	Eliminating defects moving to Six Sigma

PDSA, Plan–Do–Study–Act.

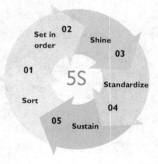

Figure 14.3 Lean 5S.

- *The Problem*: in a hospital, there is a resuscitation trolley on each ward. Each trolley has a different design, with different drawers and equipment. As emergencies are rare on some wards, the trolley is also used to store other items. When an emergency arises, the medical team responding often loses valuable time in assessing and treating the patient as they search for essential equipment.
- *Sort*: remove non-essential equipment from the resuscitation trolley.
- *Set in order*: order the equipment as it will be required, based on frequency of use (e.g. a designated drawer for airway, breathing, circulation, etc.), with items arranged according to size, from left to right and clustered as required (e.g. a pack for intravenous cannulation).
- *Shine*: ensure the resuscitation trolley is reordered as required after use, and checked regularly so that all items are ready for use.
- *Standardize*: make this approach routine, and ensure that all resuscitation trolleys in the hospital are arranged and maintained in this way.
- *Sustain*: continue to maintain resuscitation trolleys in this way into the future through training and adoption of a standard operating procedure.

Six Sigma

Six Sigma, which originated from Motorola, uses a more data-driven approach to improving quality. It refers to a statistical concept and aims to reduce the number of defects and amount of variation within a system to negligible levels. DMAIC (Figure 14.4) is a key project methodology. DMAIC stands for:

- *Define* the system, the problem, and the goals;
- *Measure* key processes and outcomes;
- *Analyse* the data to build an understanding of the problem to inform optimal improvement;
- *Improve* processes by making data-informed changes;

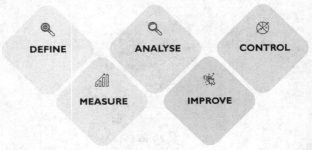

Figure 14.4 DMAIC Six Sigma.

- Control the changed processes through monitoring (using statistical process control charts (cross-reference to chapter 13 currently page 290)) and acting before control limits are breached.

Six Sigma emphasizes the importance of sustained effort, committed leadership, and measurement with a strong statistical underpinning.

Limitations of Lean and Six Sigma

- Originally developed within the manufacturing industry, Lean and Six Sigma assume a product-dominant logic where the contribution of patients to co-creating the service of healthcare is not explicitly recognized.
- Six Sigma requires a relatively high level of statistical literacy that may require specialist support.

Signposting

Virginia Mason Institute. *What is Lean healthcare?* Available at: ℘ https://www.virginiamasoninstitute.org/what-is-lean-health-care/# (accessed 10 September 2023).

Further reading

Ahmed, S. (2019). Integrating DMAIC approach of Lean Six Sigma and theory of constraints toward quality improvement in healthcare. *Reviews on Environmental Health*, 34(4), pp. 427–34. doi: 10.1515/reveh-2019-0003.

Mahmoud, Z., Angelé-Halgand, N., Churruca, K., Ellis, L.A., and Braithwaite, J. (2021). The impact of lean management on frontline healthcare professionals: a scoping review of the literature. *BMC Health Services Research*, 21(1), p. 383. doi: 10.1186/s12913-021-06344-0.

NEJM Catalyst (2018). *What is Lean healthcare?* Available at: ℘ https://catalyst.nejm.org/doi/full/10.1056/CAT.18.0193 (accessed 10 September 2023).

Scoville, R. and Little, K. (2014). *Comparing Lean and quality improvement*. IHI White Paper. Cambridge, MA: Institute for Healthcare Improvement. Available at: ℘ https://www.ihi.org/resources/Pages/IHIWhitePapers/ComparingLeanandQualityImprovement.aspx (accessed 10 September 2023).

Theory of Constraints

What is the theory?

The Theory of Constraints (TOC) is a production optimization approach, based on the premise that all production systems are limited by their greatest constraint (Goldratt and Cox, 2016).

The theory can be applied in healthcare where the optimal use of resources is constantly under pressure.

- A constraint is a production 'bottleneck' of any sort.
- By addressing the most significant constraint, production or activity throughput can be increased and will be limited only by the next most significant constraint.
- The theory proposes that this focus on constraints alone (as opposed to whole system change) offers a relatively efficient path towards improvement.
- Key measures when applying the TOC include:
  - Throughput (the rate of production or processing);
  - Inventory (facilities, equipment, work in progress);
  - Operating expense (cost of production, including labour, utilities, etc.).

There are five steps in the TOC, as shown in Figure 14.5 and Table 14.4.

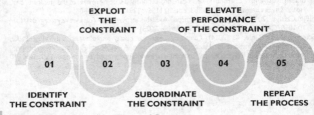

Figure 14.5 Process of the Theory of Constraints.

Table 14.4 The five steps of the Theory of Constraints applied to healthcare

Step	Healthcare example
1. Identify the system constraint The physical, process, or policy element limiting production	Production is assessing patients in an emergency department. The constraint may be the availability of clinical staff to assess arriving patients
2. Decide how to exploit the constraint Maximize production through the constraining element without large-scale or expensive change	Rearrange the way in which the staff work by giving a new role to nurses in assessing minor illnesses, so that doctors can concentrate on sicker patients

Table 14.4 (*Contd.*)

Step	Healthcare example
3. Subordinate everything else Adjust other elements of the system to match and support the maximum output of the constraint	Rearrange the rota to match the demand with supply of available clinical staff
4. Elevate the constraint If steps 2 and 3 have not been successful in 'breaking' the constraint, consider major system change or investment	Employ new staff or redeploy staff from other wards to ensure sufficient staff are available to meet the demand
5. Return to step 1 Repeat the process with the next most significant constraint to achieve continuous improvement	Having eased the constraint of demand and supply for assessment, begin the process again to address the constraint of waiting for clinical investigations

Limitations of the Theory of Constraints

* There is a paucity of scientific evidence on its magnitude of effect and failure to recognize possible roles of frontline workers in finding solutions.
* The TOC orientates around a linear process mindset, as opposed to complex adaptive systems.

Signposting

Theory of Constraints Institute. Available at: ℅ https://www.tocinstitute.org/what-is-the-goal.html (accessed 10 September 2023).

NHS England (2023) Theory of constraints. Available at: https://www.england.nhs.uk/wp-content/uploads/2021/12/qsir-theory-of-constraints.pdf (accessed 10 September 2023).

Reference

Goldratt, E.M. and Cox, J. (2016). *The Goal: A Process of Ongoing Improvement.* Abingdon: Routledge Taylor And Francis Group. Copyright.

Further reading

Bacelar-Silva, G.M., Cox, J.F. and Rodrigues, P.P. (2020). Outcomes of managing healthcare services using the Theory of Constraints: A systematic review. *Health Systems*, pp. 1–16. doi.org/10.1080/20476965.2020.1813056.

Experience-based co-design

What is the theory?

Experience-based co-design (EBCD) is a design-driven improvement methodology.

- EBCD encompasses a structured approach to the establishment of a partnership for improvement between those receiving and those providing care.
- This partnership is generated through shared understanding, ideation, and creative vision for improvement.
- The established structure underpinning the process creates a psychologically safe environment for this partnership to flourish (Table 14.5).
- EBCD builds design for improvement from a foundation of shared care experience and perspectives.
- This is achieved by gathering, sharing, and learning from the care experiences of others.
- A structured approach is used to record perspectives offered independently by both clinicians and patients.
- Recordings are collated before being shown to the wider improvement stakeholder group. Through watching and learning from the perspectives of others, a shared picture of a quality problem is created.
- From this base, design thinking approaches are then applied to unlock ideas from all stakeholders within the group to inform improvement. The group then shares how ideas for improvement are prioritized.
- Improvements in quality are owned and celebrated together.

Table 14.5 Experience-based co-design

Why	1. Design principles and techniques are used to improve experience from the perspective of the service user
	2. Through partnership, patients and clinicians are empowered to make changes
	3. The approach provides rich qualitative insights and can be tailored to a variety of care settings
How	1. Use observation to appreciate how care happens daily
	2. Interview and record the experiences of patients, carers, families, and clinicians
	3. Edit the interviews to create a film
	4. Meet with clinicians and agree on the elements that they are happy with to share with patients
	5. Show the film to patients
	6. Identify improvement areas with patients
	7. Hold a joint meeting of patients and clinicians to share experiences and agree on improvement priorities
	8. Organize structured design groups composed of patients and clinicians to drive improvement
	9. Celebrate improvements in safety together

Why is experience-based co-design important for quality improvement?

QI needs to take into account the lived experience of the people who work in the service and those who receive the care.

Strengths of EBCD include:

- The ethos of partnership building between clinicians and patients;
- The ability to draw perspectives from a wide array of viewpoints;
- The focus on using this shared picture of a quality problem as a basis for a future design that will work better for all.
- In Box 14.3 an application of experience-based co-design is described.

Box 14.3 Case study of application of experience-based co-design

Following feedback from a number of patients, a psychiatry department decided to embark on a quality improvement project in the outpatient clinic using experience-based co-design. They formed a quality improvement team composed of a consultant, a registrar, a clinical nurse specialist, and an administrative manager. They also recruited the quality lead from the local hospital for support, as she had prior experience in using this approach.

To begin, the quality improvement team went to the outpatient clinic to observe how care was usually being provided. They adopted an ethnographic approach, standing back to look at the work 'as is' done. They took time to elicit perspectives and discuss experiences with patients and clinicians alike. They were surprised to notice many things that had not occurred to them before such as where delays seemed to occur and how patients interacted with staff.

Staff members from across the department were then recruited to record interviews, in which they shared their views on how the clinic functioned. Patients with a variety of backgrounds, conditions, and experiences were also invited to record interviews. These interviews were edited into two short films: one of patient perspectives and one of staff views. The quality improvement team then arranged a departmental meeting to view the staff film. Issues raised were discussed and narrowed down to three areas for improvement: to improve clinic timeliness; to reduce non-attendance rates; and to increase shared decision-making in care planning. The quality improvement team also arranged a meeting of the patient contributors and showed them the patient film.

After watching the film, a structured discussion highlighted three priority areas for improvement: more listening by clinicians; focus on what matters to the patient when planning treatment; and greater comfort while waiting to be seen (e.g. softer chairs and/or fewer windows open in winter).

Following these individual group meetings, a meeting of staff and patients was then arranged. At this meeting, both groups watched the patient video. Clinicians were struck by the candour, honesty, and keen observations of the patients. Some of the feedback was hard to hear, but all seemed very fair. Patients and staff were then split into smaller groups of eight, and had the opportunity to discuss the film, its themes, and areas that had been identified as priorities for improvement during previous meetings.

(Continued)

Box 14.13 (Contd.)

All outcomes of these smaller group discussions were then brought back to the wider group, with three priority areas for co-design chosen: clinic flow; clinic comfort; and shared decision-making, with a focus on what matters to the patient. Patients and staff were then invited to join the group, aiming to tackle the issue that interested them the most. Subsequent co-design workshops revealed novel solutions to long-standing issues, with change and improvement in these areas driven by all stakeholders.

Limitations of experience-based co-design

- As a particularly structured approach, EBCD can be relatively resource- and time-intensive, with less adaptability to evolving quality problems, compared to less linear improvement approaches. Briefer approaches incorporating fewer steps have been proposed.
- While comprehensive, the method is complex and requires strong facilitation skills. This may require recruitment of external expertise.

Signposting

The Point of Care Foundation (n.d.). *EBCD: Experience-based co-design toolkit*. Available at: ⌖ https://www.pointofcarefoundation.org.uk/resource/experience-based-co-design-ebcd-tool kit/ (accessed 10 September 2023).

Improvement collaboratives

What is the theory?

A 'collaborative' is a structured programme in which individuals or multidisciplinary teams from different settings come together to work on improving a specific quality problem.

- There is a shared interest over a defined period (e.g. nursing teams from acute and long-stay residential care settings working to prevent pressure ulcers over a 12-month period).
- Collaboratives can follow an established structure (e.g. Institute for Healthcare Improvement, 2003, Fig. 2) or a more emergent improvement approach (e.g. community of practice).
- Improvement collaboratives usually focus on learning and applying a formal QI method (e.g. the MFI to achieve improvement).

Why are collaboratives important for quality improvement?

- The spread of improvement ideas is often difficult, so the improvement collaborative can act as a vehicle to spread improvement ideas and solutions at scale.
- Collaboratives can be:
  - Designed with the aim to achieve higher reliability in the implementation of a known best evidence-informed practice (e.g. care bundle to prevent ventilator-associated pneumonia); or
  - Used to iteratively test, learn, and share improvements in care situations where less robust evidence exists (e.g. respiratory teams working to improve acute care for patients with chronic obstructive pulmonary disease across different settings; Box 14.4).

In the case study below an example of how a collaborative can be operationalized is demonstrated (Box 14.4).

> ### Box 14.4 Case study: the Irish National COPD Improvement Collaborative
>
> #### The problem
> Chronic obstructive pulmonary disease (COPD) is characterized by chronic, slowly progressive decline in lung function, with only partially reversible airflow obstruction, systemic manifestations, and increasing frequency and severity of exacerbations. COPD can result in frequent hospital admissions and premature death. COPD is the fourth leading cause of death in Ireland, with marked variation in hospital performance.
>
> #### The collaborative: setup
> - A scoping literature review and consultation process involving a wide range of stakeholders on acute care COPD change interventions.
> - A successful pilot in two hospital sites.
> - Spread with 18 consultant-led, multidisciplinary respiratory teams from 19 hospitals across Ireland participated in a 15-month Royal College of Physicians of Ireland (RCPI)- and Health Service Executive (HSE)-led National COPD Collaborative learning programme.

Box 14.4 (Contd.)

- The programme followed an adapted version of the Institute for Healthcare Improvement (IHI) Breakthrough Series Collaborative Model, with the aim of improving care during an acute exacerbation of COPD (AECOPD) in the following areas.

The objective: to improve
1. Access to respiratory specialist review.
2. Compliance with admission clinical bundle.
3. Use of standardized, evidence-based assessment e.g. Dyspnoea, Eosinopenia, Consolidation, Acidaemia and atrial Fibrillation (DECAF) Score.
4. Adherence to best practice at hospital discharge.

The collaborative: process
- COPD collaborative teams attended five mandatory full-day face-to-face learning sessions with quality improvement faculty support.
- 'Action periods' aimed to develop and implement locally appropriate tests of change towards a global goal of improved care for acute COPD presentations.
- Teams submitted a monthly data set (anonymous patient data relating to measures within the COPD care pathway).
- Learning sessions included team- and network-building opportunities, COPD best practice expert talks, and patient and carer narratives.
- Teams learnt quality improvement methodology, with practical exercises, data review and analysis, opportunities to share site-specific learning, and an element of fun.
- All teams tested COPD pathway improvements for patients at admission, assessment, and discharge through redesign of current pathways or implementation of new processes.

The collaborative: outcomes
Improvements were site- and context-specific for each site, based on the problems that they had identified as needing improvement most urgently. Overarching these site-specific initiatives, based on tracking almost 2000 patient episodes, during the National COPD Improvement Collaborative:
- Overall length of stay (median) reduced from 6.75 days to 5 days (a 1.75-day reduction);
- Patient prescription review prior to discharge increased by 200% (from 25% to 75%);
- Inhaler technique training prior to discharge increased by 63% (from 55% to 89%);
- Time to respiratory specialist review reduced from a median of 25 hours to 13 hours;
- Standardized assessment using the DECAF score and documented spirometry diagnosis increased significantly.

What are the key elements of a collaborative?

Improvement collaboratives can vary in different contexts. However, there are fundamental components, as indicated in Table 14.6.

Table 14.6 The anatomy of a collaborative

Components	Processes	Involvement
Expert planning (panel, committee, or steering group)	Collection of new data for QI	Leadership involvement/outreach
Demonstrable organizational commitment	Review of data and feedback	Training by subject matter experts
Learning sessions (in-person or online)	Expert support with data analysis and feedback	Training by QI experts
Action periods (e.g. PDSA cycles between learning sessions)	Teams implement and test	Training for non-QI team members (i.e. for those not directly part of the collaborative, but affected by its remit)
Coordinating/teaching faculty	Ensure the faculty can provide the required improvement and subject matter information	Patients, families, and carers (individually or support groups)
Multidisciplinary QI teams	Active involvement at all levels of the collaborative	Teams should include all members to ensure engagement and ownership
QI team calls (between and among teams)	Use an effective communication plan to spread learning	Include all forms of contact—SMS
Asynchronous support (email and other learning resources)	Provide real-time responses to queries	Aimed at all members and across teams

PDSA, Plan–Do–Study–Act; QI, quality improvement.
Data from Nadeem et al., 2013.

Benefits of the improvement collaborative methodology

- Fostering connections and network building (across sites, professions, and disciplines).
- Rapidly sharing lessons from different approaches and contexts.
- Sharing leadership for improvement.
- Enhancing motivation and commitment to an aim.
- Generating friendly competition between teams.
- Improving performance accountability and transparency.
- Greater acceptance and use of objective data for improvement.
- New team-based norms in recognizing and approaching quality problems.

Mixed evidence exists on the overall effectiveness of improvement collaboratives, drivers of success and failure, and what the most effective collaborative approach entails.

Limitations of the collaborative methodology

- Collaboratives designed only to focus on technical fixes are less likely to succeed than those that work simultaneously to build strong social ties.
- Collaboratives should be designed to take the local context into account (see the case study of Matching Michigan, Box 4.3 in ⟳ Chapter 4, p. 82).
- In Box 14.5 tips on how to have a successful collaborative are listed.

Box 14.5 Collaborative top tips

1. Align with system priorities: successful recruitment, lasting commitment, and achieving the aim often depend on how the purpose of the collaborative matches to professional and organizational goals.
2. Flatten the healthcare hierarchy: create a space and an environment that is safe for interprofessional interaction and input from all (consider using liberating structures – Chapter 11, p. 15).
3. Embrace a culture of learning: harvest and share learning that arises from all sites on an ongoing basis in as many ways as possible (e.g. posters, presentations, social media, etc.).
4. Let data drive improvement: find ways to share data between sites, provide regular feedback, and allow safe comparisons to drive performance; for example, consider semi-anonymized and collaborative aggregate data sets).
5. Patient perspectives: involve patients, family members, and carers in all aspects of design, delivery, and evaluation.
6. Robust evaluation: include rigorous evaluation at all stages, from design through delivery to outcome.
7. Improve the improvement: use improvement methodology to continuously improve how the collaborative runs and delivers improvement.
8. Celebrate: learning, celebrate collaboration, and celebrate success. This is a key tool for lasting culture change and sustainability.

Signposting

Institute for Healthcare Improvement (2003). *The Breakthrough Series: IHI's collaborative model for achieving breakthrough improvement.* IHI Innovation Series white paper. Boston, MA: Institute for Healthcare Improvement. Available at: ℘ https://www.ihi.org/resources/Pages/IHIWhitePapers/TheBreakthroughSeriesIHIsCollaborativeModelforAchievingBreakthroughImprovement.aspx (accessed 10 September 2023).

Health Foundation (2014). *Improvement collaboratives in health care.* Evidence scan. Available at: ℘ https://www.health.org.uk/sites/default/files/ImprovementCollaborativesInHealthcare.pdf (accessed 10 September 2023).

Further reading

Martin, G. and Dixon-Woods, M. (2022). *Collaboration-Based Approaches* (Elements of Improving Quality and Safety in Healthcare series). Cambridge: Cambridge University Press. doi: 10.1017/9781009236867.

Rohweder, C., Wangen, M., Black, M., et al. (2019). Understanding quality improvement collaboratives through an implementation science lens. *Preventive Medicine*, 129, p. 105859. doi: 10.1016/j.ypmed.2019.105859.

Wells, S., Tamir, O., Gray, J., Naidoo, D., Bekhit, M., and Goldmann, D. (2017). Are quality improvement collaboratives effective? A systematic review. *BMJ Quality and Safety*, 27(3), pp. 226–40. doi: 10.1136/bmjqs-2017-006926.

Zamboni, K., Baker, U., Tyagi, M., Schellenberg, J., Hill, Z., and Hanson, C. (2020). How and under what circumstances do quality improvement collaboratives lead to better outcomes? A systematic review. *Implementation Science*, 15(1), p. 27. doi: 10.1186/s13012-020-0978-z.

References

Institute for Healthcare Improvement (2003). *The Breakthrough Series: IHI's collaborative model for achieving breakthrough improvement*. IHI Innovation Series white paper. Boston, MA: Institute for Healthcare Improvement. Available at: ⚲ https://www.ihi.org/resources/Pages/IHIWhitePapers/TheBreakthroughSeriesIHIsCollaborativeModelforAchievingBreakthroughImprovement.aspx (accessed 10 September 2023).

Nadeem, E., Olin, S.S., Hill, L.C., Hoagwood, K.E., and Horwitz, S.M. (2013). Understanding the components of quality improvement collaboratives: a systematic literature review. *The Milbank Quarterly*, 91(2), pp. 354–94. doi: 10.1111/milq.12016.

Improvement through human factors

What is the theory?

- 'Human factors and ergonomics is an evidence-based scientific discipline and profession that uses a design-driven systems approach to achieve two closely related outcomes of performance and wellbeing' (Chartered Institute of Ergonomics and Human Factors, 2018).
- Human factors focus on the interface and interactions between humans, work systems, and technology. It draws on many disciplines, including psychology, physiology, social sciences, engineering, design, and behavioural economics.
- As a discipline, it is applied in many industries and can be particularly effective in healthcare.
- To achieve improvement, a human factors approach can leverage a systems mindset to understand how care is provided through observation, measurement, and discussion.
- This allows effective and practical redesign of the system, with the needs, abilities, and natural limitations of human beings in mind.
- This can be achieved through the redesign of:
  - Work settings (e.g. environment, layout, furniture, etc.);
  - Work processes (e.g. tools, software, etc.);
  - Work interactions (e.g. huddles, checklists, etc.).

How can human factors be incorporated in quality improvement?

- As discussed in ⊙ Chapter 12, The Systems Engineering Initiative for Patient Safety (SEIPS) model is an example of human factors designed specifically for healthcare, namely the improvement of patient safety.
- It uses the Donabedian construct and proposes a socio-technical approach to improving care that involves a complex work system.
- The work system includes patients, a care team, care tasks, tools and technologies, organizational culture, and a physical environment, operating within an external social environment.
- The work system performs processes that result in outcomes for patients, caregivers, clinicians, and the wider healthcare organization.
- Evolution and adaptation within the work system are informed by feedback for learning and continuous improvement.
- SEIPS can be applied and used practically to understand, design, and implement system changes for improvement through the application of tools (Table 14.7).

Table 14.7 SEIPS 101 tools

Tool	Use
PETT scan	To identify the people, environments, tools, and tasks within a system. Can be further applied to examine barriers and facilitators
People map	To identify the people involved in the system and how they interact. Can be further applied to develop 'personas'

Table 14.7 (*Contd.*)

Tool	Use
Tasks and tools matrices	To identify and describe the work tasks and associated tools within a system. Can be further applied to examine mismatches between tasks to be completed and available tools
Outcomes matrix	To identify relevant outcomes and their measures. Can be further applied to assist in balancing outcomes for different stakeholders
Journey map	To illustrate a process over time, including dynamic interactions with other people, tasks, tools, and environments. This is a type of process map (Chapter 17)
Interactions diagram	To depict relevant and important interactions between work system components. Can be further applied to compare sets of interactions (e.g. between settings, teams, or approaches)
Systems story	To share a narrative highlighting how work systems, processes, and outcomes are related. Can be further applied by using powerful storytelling techniques

PETT, people, environment, tools, and tasks.
Holden and Carayon, 2021.

Limitations of human factors

- The SEIPS model requires an understanding of human factors theories.
- In healthcare, to date, human factors have been applied mainly to improvement of patient safety and has been slow to penetrate other areas for QI.
- In Box 14.6 the SEIPS model is applied to a clincal situation.

Box 14.6 SEIPS in action

In the emergency department (ED), a senior house officer (SHO) administers a dose of penicillin to a patient known to have a penicillin allergy. The patient suffers an anaphylactic reaction requiring emergency care and admission to the intensive care unit. Fortunately, the patient survives. The doctor in question blames themselves for causing this harm but is encouraged by their supervising consultant to review factors contributing to this incident using the SEIPS model. Here is what they discovered.

Tools and technology
- Patient not wearing allergy alert bracelet—had fallen off and was not replaced.
- Inconspicuous placement of allergy status on paper-based drug chart.

Task
- Prescription was instructed by a different senior doctor without prior knowledge of patient allergies.

(Continued)

Box 14.6 (Contd.)

- Lack of a standardized approach for administration of intravenous medication by doctors.
- Relatively infrequent execution of task (usually done by nurses).
- Administration occurred in corridor due to lack of protected space.
- Allergy status check not performed prior to administration.
- Medication checks not completed with another member of staff—nobody immediately available.

Environment

- Night-time—lights were turned down in the department.
- High volume of patients, with trolleys lining the corridor—wards at full capacity.
- High noise levels (beeping monitors, large numbers of staff and patients).

Organizational

- Understaffed department and high workload.
- Long shift patterns.
- Suboptimal ratios of doctors to nurses, with changing roles and responsibilities depending on staff availability.
- Varying practice in administration of intravenous medication.
- Variable senior supervision and access to advice.
- Patient not known to doctor.

Individual

- Twelfth hour of shift.
- Fifth consecutive night shift.
- No opportunity for a break in preceding 5 hours.
- Case immediately preceding this incident had involved an emotionally charged interaction with a patient family following a tragic death.

Assessment

In addition to this review, the SHO worked with colleagues to create a people map illustrating the different personas involved in the administration of medication in the ED. The process was mapped, and an interactions diagram created. The SHO also used their experience from this incident to tell a systems story that further highlighted the complexity of this system. This tool also assisted in securing senior departmental support and buy-in for improvement.

Following the review and application of the SEIPS tools, rather than blaming the SHO who administered the drug, the department used the SEIPS model to redesign the work system, so that prescribing and administration of medications could be safer.

Further reading

Carayon, P. and Perry, S. (2021). Human factors and ergonomics systems approach to the COVID-19 healthcare crisis. *International Journal for Quality in Health Care*, 33(Suppl 1), pp. 1–3. doi: 10.1093/intqhc/mzaa109.

Carayon, P., Schoofs Hundt, A., Karsh, B.-T., et al. (2006). Work system design for patient safety: the SEIPS model. *Quality and Safety in Health Care*, 15(suppl 1), pp. i50–8. doi: 10.1136/qshc.2005.015842.

Carayon, P., Wooldridge, A., Hoonakker, P., Hundt, A.S., and Kelly, M.M. (2020). SEIPS 3.0: human-centered design of the patient journey for patient safety. *Applied Ergonomics*, 84, p. 103033. doi: 10.1016/j.apergo.2019.103033.

Holden, R.J., Carayon, P., Gurses, A.P., *et al.* (2013). SEIPS 2.0: a human factors framework for studying and improving the work of healthcare professionals and patients. *Ergonomics*, 56(11), pp. 1669–86. doi: 10.1080/00140139.2013.838643.

O'Connor, P. and O'Dea, A. (2021). *An introduction to human factors for healthcare workers*. Dublin: Health Services Executive. Available at: https://www.hse.ie/eng/about/who/nqpsd/qps-incident-management/incident-management/a-guide-to-human-factors-in-healthcare-2021.pdf (accessed 10 September 2023).

References

Chartered Institute of Ergonomics and Human Factors (2018). *Human factors in health and social care*. Available at: https://ergonomics.org.uk/resource/human-factors-in-health-and-social-care.html (accessed 10 September 2023).

Holden, R.J. and Carayon, P. (2021). SEIPS 101 and seven simple SEIPS tools. *BMJ Quality and Safety*, 30(11), pp. 901–10. doi: 10.1136/bmjqs-2020-012538.

Top tips

- Choose an appropriate improvement methodology for the quality problem, rather than making the problem fit a particular method.
- Improvement methods can be combined to tackle different types of quality problems; for example, process improvement can be achieved using the Lean methodology through co-design of changes tested by using PDSA cycles.
- Be aware of, and acknowledge, the limitations of different improvement approaches to maintain objectivity and scientific support for QI as an endeavour.

Summary

- Improvement methods seek to practicalize and operationalize the improvement theory. Many of these theories have been adapted from other industries and disciplines.
- Organizations may choose one improvement method over another, but usually they are all derived from the theories of Donabedian, Shewhart, Juran, and Deming.
- Improvement methods can be applied individually or in combination to different types of quality problems, so as to achieve improvement.

Chapter 15

Strategies for measurement

Key points

- Measurement is the foundation of quality improvement.
- It is important to develop a robust measurement plan, so that the impact of the intervention can be proved.
- Measures in quality improvement differ from those for judgement in audit and those for new knowledge in research.
- Time series analysis using either run charts or statistical process control charts are the best way to demonstrate improvement over time.
- Measurement results should be illustrated by using a range of methods, so that a wider audience is reached.

Measurement for improvement

'Without data, you're just another person with an opinion.'

W. Edwards Deming, Out of a Crisis

Why is measurement important in healthcare?

In healthcare, we measure constantly so that we can make a diagnosis and then monitor a response to an intervention. Measuring data is essential for us to know if an intervention makes a difference. For example, if a person presents with symptoms of diabetes, we take baseline blood tests, which we will then monitor over time when we commence therapy. We will not know if there is improvement over time without comparing data to the baseline measurement.

Measurement in quality improvement (QI) is no different to measurement in clinical practice. In this chapter, we will consider how to develop a measurement plan that includes baseline measurements and measurement over time in a time series analysis. We will build on the study of variation, as discussed in ⮕ Chapter 13, where you were shown how to look for variation within the processes of the system in which you work, and will show how to illustrate this variation on a run chart or a statistical process control (SPC) chart.

In all improvement methods discussed in ⮕ Chapter 14 (Model for Improvement, Six Sigma, DMAIC, and Lean 5S), measurement is an essential component. Failure to develop a measurement strategy and a plan is often the reason why QI fails to be sustainable or to spread to new contexts.

In addition, deficiencies in measurement undermine the evidence base for QI interventions. It is important that the process of measurement is designed to provide reliable evidence of the fidelity of the intervention (Box 15.1).

Box 15.1 Key actions for fidelity of measurement

- Develop a measurement plan.
- Define the operational definition of the measures and their purpose—that is, what is it aiming to measure, and will it demonstrate that the outcome is the result of the intervention?
- Use standardized measures, where possible.
- Ensure reliable collection, analysis, and interpretation of data.
- Develop capacity and capability for measurement.
- Include patient stories as part of the data.
- Data should tell a story.

How do we use measurement in quality improvement?

The purpose of measurement in QI is to understand how a system is working and then to be able to monitor improvement over time. Measurement for improvement differs from measurement for judgement (audit) and measurement for new knowledge (research), as shown in Table 15.1.

Table 15.1 Different types of measurement

	Audit	Research	Improvement
Aim of measurement	To assess how a system is performing over a defined period	To determine new knowledge	To demonstrate improvement over time
Hypothesis	None	Fixed	Changes with new knowledge
How one measures	All data	Sufficient data to power the study	Data as required for the project
Type of data	Counts all data over a period	One large test and before and after data	Sequential tests over time
Bias	No action	Control/eliminate	Manage bias
Duration of data collection	Over a defined period	Determined by the research question	Short interval PDSA cycles with prediction of what will happen
Statistics	None	p-value t-test Confidence intervals	SPC
Display	Bar charts, pie charts, tables	Tables	Run charts, SPC charts, safety cross

PDSA, Plan–Do–Study–Act; SPC, statistical process chart.
From Solberg et al., 1997

Often a mixed measurement approach is taken by combining qualitative and quantitative measures (e.g. measures of activity with measures of patient experience).

Sources of data in the healthcare setting

Several sources of data exist within contemporary healthcare settings. Deciding on which data to measure depends on the nature of the improvement project, the ease with which data can be measured, and the validity and reliability of available data.

- *Administrative data* often relate to coding systems in healthcare jurisdictions and can be readily available. These figures tend to have limited clinical data.
- *Healthcare records* provide detailed data about a patient's journey through healthcare service interaction(s). These data are usually entered by healthcare professionals and can be paper-based or

electronic. Institutional review board approval and/or patient consent is usually needed to draw on clinical data from healthcare records.

- *Patient-generated data* include formal surveys of patient experience (quantitative or qualitative) of a healthcare service and informal data gathered during day-to-day interactions.
- *Improvement data* are data collected for an improvement project. These should be granular, including data on tests of change.

Further reading

Mendlowitz, A., Croxford, R., MacLagan, L., Ritcey, G., and Isaranuwatchai, W. (2020). Usage of primary and administrative data to measure the economic impact of quality improvement projects. *BMJ Open Quality*, 9(2), p. e000712. doi: 10.1136/bmjoq-2019-000712.

Reference

Solberg, L.I., Mosser, G., and McDonald, S. (1997). The three faces of performance measurement: improvement, accountability, and research. *The Joint Commission Journal on Quality Improvement*, 23(3), pp. 135–47. doi: 10.1016/s1070-3241(16)30305-4.

Challenges in measurement for improvement

Challenges in measurement for improvement

As discussed in ⊕ Chapter 12, healthcare is made up of many different systems that interact in a complex manner. Therefore, as one implements changes, it is difficult to attribute the cause and effect or fidelity of the intervention in a linear manner—unlike a randomized controlled trial.

The challenges facing clinical teams undertaking QI initiatives and the need to collect reliable data are immense (Woodcock et al., 2021).

- Good data collection takes time and this is not always available.
- Those involved in a QI project may not be trained in data collection.
- Understanding of the methods to analyse the data may not be commonplace.
- Healthcare is a complex adaptive system, and linear inferences are difficult to make in QI.
- In clinical research, data collection is within a controlled environment (i.e. enumerative research where random samples are taken to make an inference); in QI, the focus of data collection is analytical within a constantly changing environment and prediction of future performance is important (Provost, 2011).
- This makes inferences more difficult to make and there may be different initiatives at the same time, and proving which one had an impact can be complex.
- Sampling for data collection may not be well defined.
- Context plays an important part in QI and is often not taken into account; for example, what an intervention is and how it works are not easy to explain (Dixon-Woods, 2014).
- Detailed measurement plans may not be routine, and not adhered to if they are. They may not be aimed at the medium to longer term.
- Selected measures may not be sensitive to the needs of the outcomes and may not measure what was intended. For example, the desired outcome may be to improve the patient experience by improving efficiency of the service (e.g. decreasing waiting times). However, the experience may be worse if the throughput is too fast.
- Operational definitions are often difficult to define.
- If Plan–Do–Study–Act (PDSA) cycles are undertaken, reliability of the methodology is not guaranteed as the methodology may not be followed as required (Reed and Card, 2016).
- Relevance of the measures to patients and clinicians may not always be ensured. Frontline ownership of measures is important (Mountford and Shojiana, 2012).
- Etchells and Trbovich (2023) highlight five issues to be addressed: knowing why the innovation may work; understanding how to measure change; the complexity of assigning fidelity; recognizing the lag time for the impact of an intervention to have an effect; and accounting for possible unintended consequences. In Box 15.2 the challenges of measurement in a quality improvement project are discussed.

These challenges can be addressed with a detailed and focused measurement plan that is developed with clinicians and patients. The plan should mitigate each of the challenges listed above.

John is the new registrar on the care for the elderly ward. He notices that there is variation in the length of stay of the patients and wonders whether or not he could improve this. Before he starts the improvement project, he realizes that there are some issues to be addressed.

- *People*: there are several teams and each has different priorities.
- *Patients*: they differ in diagnoses and social issues, and the processes do not seem to be uniform in treating their conditions.
- *Context*: although he tackled a similar project in his last post, he is not sure whether the same interventions would work here.
- *Operational definitions*: defining the length of stay and of the different factors that may affect this has not been undertaken in this department before.
- *Time*: he does not have the capacity to do the project by himself as he works shifts. He knows about data collection, but no one else in the team does.

John realizes that by listing these issues, he can work to address them before starting on the project.

Further reading

Dixon-Woods, M. and Martin, G.P. (2016). Does quality improvement improve quality? *Future Hospital Journal*, 3(3), pp. 191–4. doi: 10.7861/futurehosp.3-3-191.

Shah, A. (2019). Using data for improvement. *BMJ*, 364, p. l189. doi: 10.1136/bmj.l189.

References

Dixon-Woods, M. (2014). *The problem of context in quality improvement*. London: Health Foundation. Available at: https://www.health.org.uk/sites/default/files/PerspectivesOnContextDixonWoodsTheProblemOfContextInQualityImprovement.pdf (accessed 10 September 2023).

Etchells, E. and Trbovich, P. (2023). Five golden rules for successful measurement of improvement. *BMJ Quality and Safety*, bmjqs-2023-016129. Advance online publication. Available at: https://doi.org/10.1136/bmjqs-2023-016129 (accessed 10 September 2023).

Mountford, J. and Shojania, K.G. (2012). Refocusing quality measurement to best support quality improvement: local ownership of quality measurement by clinicians: Table 1. *BMJ Quality and Safety*, 21(6), pp. 519–23. doi: 10.1136/bmjqs-2012-000859.

Provost, L.P. (2011). Analytical studies: a framework for quality improvement design and analysis. *BMJ Quality and Safety*, 20(Suppl 1), pp. i92–6. doi: 10.1136/bmjqs.2011.051557.

Reed, J.E. and Card, A.J. (2016). The problem with Plan–Do–Study–Act cycles. *BMJ Quality and Safety*, 25(3), pp. 147–52. doi: 10.1136/bmjqs-2015-005076.

Woodcock, T., Liberati, E.G., and Dixon-Woods, M. (2021). A mixed-methods study of challenges experienced by clinical teams in measuring improvement. *BMJ Quality and Safety*, 30(2), pp. 106–15. doi: 10.1136/bmjqs-2018-009048.

Measurements used in improvement

- As discussed in ⊃ Chapter 14, the most commonly used framework for guiding improvement work is the Model for Improvement, in which measurement is a key step once the aim of the project has been determined.
- As changes do not always result in an improvement, measurement is essential to demonstrate that an improvement has been achieved.
- Choosing what to measure is a very important step. You need to consider whether the measures you have selected are correctly measuring what you intended them to measure, and that they can be used to answer your desired question through analysing the data.
- Always consider the population and whether or not you should segment the data to account for differential impact on different population groups (Hirschhorn et al., 2021).
- Once you have decided what to measure, it is important to also consider how you are going to measure it and who will do the measurement.
- Measurement can be in the form of both quantitative and qualitative measures, depending on the circumstance. A combination of these is often useful.
- Collecting baseline data is an important step, which is sometimes overlooked. This helps us to better understand our current system performance and allows us to evaluate whether the changes have led to an improvement.
- Unlike audits, the process of measurement should not be overly onerous or time-consuming.
- Small tests of change ideas, PDSA cycles, allow you to analyse emerging data quickly, which can then be fed back to adapt the interventions accordingly.
- It is important that the chosen measures cover the aim of the project and the domain of quality.
- If key endpoints are recorded and reviewed as part of business as usual, change can become inevitable. Planning for automated data to be readily available is essential in future planning.

Six types of measures that are essential in improvement are shown in Table 15.2.

In Box 15.3 the application of different types of QI measures are considered.

Table 15.2 Types of measures in improvement

Type	Characteristic	Example
Outcome	What happens to the person or system	Decreasing central line infections
Process	How the system and the processes in the system are working to achieve the outcome	Adherence to the components of a care bundle for line infections
Balancing	Unintended consequence of the intervention	Increased readmission rate in a project aimed at decreasing the length of stay Improved patient satisfaction
Economic cost (see ➲ Chapter 7)	Determines the cost-effectiveness of the improvement	Increased or decreased cost
Climate change (see ➲ Chapter 6)	The impact the project intervention has on the environment	Decreased or increased use of carbon
Equity (see ➲ Chapter 6)	Has every person or patient in the project had equitable benefit?	Segment the data as per population
Patient-reported measures (see ➲ Chapter 8 and 16)	What is the quality of outcomes or experience from the perspective of the person receiving care?	Measure patient-reported outcome measures (PROM) and patient-reported experience measures (PREM)

Box 15.3 Example of types of measures used in improvement

Consider an improvement intervention on a busy paediatric ward where it has been noted that a number of avoidable medication errors have been taking place each week, a common occurrence in any healthcare setting.

An improvement project was developed, with the global aim of reducing the rate of medication errors occurring on the ward. We have seen that the first step is to develop this into a SMART aim statement. As a first phase of the project and to make it achievable, the team decided to focus on reducing prescribing errors first, a key component of medication errors which can be easily measured, given the clear prescribing guidelines available. The aim statement was to increase compliance with medication prescribing guidelines from a baseline of 39% to over 90% for patients on the paediatric ward within a 3-month period.

Let us consider a number of different measures that could be used for this project by using some of the headings above:
- Outcome measures: days between medication adverse events;
- Process measures: percentage of prescriptions that fully complied with the prescribing guidelines (i.e. dose, frequency, etc.);
- Balancing measures: time in minutes saved by pharmacist and by doctors—financial saving due to time saved.

Further reading

Clarke, J., Davidge, M., and James, L. (2017). *The how-to guide for measurement for improvement* 2. Available at: ✒ https://www.england.nhs.uk/improvement-hub/wp-content/uploads/sites/44/2017/11/How-to-Guide-for-Measurement-for-Improvement.pdf (accessed 10 September 2023).

Martin, L.A., Nelson E.C., Lloyd R.C., and Nolan, T.W. (2007). Whole system measures. IHI Innovation Series white paper. Cambridge, MA: Institute for Healthcare Improvement. Available at: ✒ https://www.ihi.org/resources/Pages/IHIWhitePapers/WholeSystemMeasuresWhitePaper.aspx (accessed 10 September 2023).

Shah, A. (2019). Using data for improvement. *BMJ*, 364(189), p. l189. doi: https://doi.org/10.1136/bmj.l189.

Reference

Hirschhorn, L.R., Magge, H., and Kiflie, A. (2021). Aiming beyond equality to reach equity: the promise and challenge of quality improvement. *BMJ*, p. n939. doi: 10.1136/bmj.n939.

Qualitative measurement

Although less easily measurable and tracked prospectively over time, qualitative data are as important as quantitative data when guiding improvement interventions.

- Qualitative data are useful to obtain a deeper understanding of a multilayered clinical problem and to gain insight into subjective phenomena that are difficult to measure quantitatively.
- Qualitative data include peoples' opinions and feelings on a particular healthcare subject. This can be of staff or of patients and their families.
- Qualitative data can indicate '*what matters most*' to those affected by the problem being addressed.
- Qualitative data can range from simple surveys allowing free text responses to formal interviews and focus groups.
- PDSA cycles also make use of qualitative data, particularly in the 'Study' phase.

When considering using qualitative data, consider the following:
- How will the data be collected?
- Who will collect the data?
- Are the data collection methods and tools validated?
- When will the data be collected? For example, for patient satisfaction or experience, the response may change over time.
- How will the data be analysed?
- How will the respondents be given the results?

Qualitative data add to the tapestry of information needed to understand what really matters to people receiving or providing care (Box 15.4).

Box 15.4 Case study: measuring what really matters

When you consider the concept of what really matters, one needs to assess the measures through the lived experience of the people receiving care.

In a monograph from the Health Foundation, it has been proposed that we need to look at quality by using qualitative and quantitative data to measure four key issues that really matter to patients and their families:

- *Coordination of care*: is care arranged around the patient or the service?
- *Personalization of care*: as we standardize processes, ask whether we are personalizing care so it has meaning for the person who receives it.
- *Enabling people*: is the care we provide empowering people to manage their condition?
- *Dignity and respect*: are people treated with dignity and respect? What do they think of the care provided?

Measures such as patient-reported experience measures (PREM) and patient-reported outcomes measures (PROM) and qualitative patient data can assist in determining the person-centredness of your intervention.

CCollins, 2014.

Further reading

Dixon-Woods, M., Agarwal, S., Jones, D., Young, B., and Sutton, A. (2005). Synthesising qualitative and quantitative evidence: a review of possible methods. *Journal of Health Services Research and Policy*, 10(1), pp. 45–53. doi: 10.1258/1355819052801804.

Duddy, C. and Wong, G. (2023). Grand rounds in methodology: when are realist reviews useful, and what does a 'good' realist review look like? *BMJ Quality and Safety*, 32(3), pp. 173–80. doi: https://doi.org/10.1136/bmjqs-2022-015236.

Martin, G.P., Aveling, E.-L., Campbell, A., et al. (2018). Making soft intelligence hard: a multi-site qualitative study of challenges relating to voice about safety concerns. *BMJ Quality and Safety*, 27(9), pp. 710–17. doi: 10.1136/bmjqs-2017-007579.

References

Collins, A. (2014). *Measuring what really matters*. London: Health Foundation. Available at: https://www.health.org.uk/sites/default/files/MeasuringWhatReallyMatters.pdf (accessed 10 September 2023).

Developing your measurement plan

The decision on which measures to use will depend on the problem that has been identified and the process that has created that problem. The more time you spend on defining the measures for the project, the more likely you will be able to have reliable measures that demonstrate whether your improvement project has been successful or not.

The following steps can be used to assist in the development of a measurement plan (see Chapters 17 and 18):

- Identify a problem to be improved (i.e. an outcome that needs to be improved).
- Study the process that causes the current outcome.
- Collect baseline data on the processes and outcome.
- From the analysis of the process, identify the key process measures that need to be measured.
- Consider unintended consequences that may occur and whether they can be measured.
- Add measures for finance and climate change where possible.
- Segment the data to ensure the improvement is equitable.
- If personal experience is to be measured, consider qualitative measurement, in addition to quantitative measurement.

Important features of a measurement plan are:

- Making measurement easy to do;
- Deciding who is responsible for measurement;
- Choosing as few measures as is feasible, so that measurement is not a burden;
- Ensuring the measurement plan is robust and using a template as shown in Table 15.3;
- For each measure, giving a rationale as to why the measure is required for the project—and remembering that we do not collect 'just in case' data but must be sure we have sufficient data for the project;

Table 15.3 Example of a measurement plan for stroke service

Name and type of measure:	Type of measure:	Operational definition:	Collection:	Display:
Outcome	Quantitative	Precise definition	Who will collect data?	How will data be displayed?
process	(%, count, rate, etc.)	Include numerator and denominator	When will data be collected?	How will data be communicated?
Balancing	Qualitative	if a rate	Where will data be collected?	
Financial			How will data be recorded— manual or IT?	
Sustainable				
Equity				
Person-centred			Sampling method	

Table 15.3 *(Contd.)*

Outcome	Percentage	Percentage of people who had door-to-decision time to be under 30 minutes	Stroke nurse to collect (Emergency Department) ED data weekly on a manual form to be entered into the database Every patient with a stroke is included	Run chart displayed in the ED
Process measures	Time for each step of the process	Examples: • Time from arrival to triage • Time from triage to CT scan • Time from CT scan to decision	Sheet to be filled in at each stage of the process by the clinician in charge of that step in the process	Run charts displayed in ED
Balancing measures	Number	Increase or decrease in wait times for non-stroke patients	Measure by ED-led nurse on a weekly basis	Run charts displayed in ED
Financial	Euros	Cost-effectiveness assessment of impact of early diagnosis and treatment of stroke	Assessment by team on a monthly basis	Run charts of savings made

CT, computed tomography; ED, emergency department.

- Assessing whether statistical or methodology advice is needed to ensure the measurement plan is robust;
- Collecting baseline data and ensuring they have the same operational definition that will be used in the improvement project.

Further reading

Woodcock, T., Adeleke, Y., Goeschel, C., Pronovost, P., and Dixon-Woods, M. (2020). A modified Delphi study to identify the features of high quality measurement plans for healthcare improvement projects. *BMC Medical Research Methodology*, 20(1), p. 8. doi: 10.1186/s12874-019-0886-6.

How do we display measurement?

As the main purpose of data for improvement is to learn, we need to demonstrate the data in a way that facilitates learning.

- Visual displays of data over time can be particularly powerful at demonstrating the effects of our interventions, to determine whether interventions have led to an improvement, much more so than summary statistics.
- Data need to tell a story and therefore must have a versatile approach to display.
- The way data are displayed depends on the audience for whom they are intended.
- You may wish to display the same data in different ways, so that the impact is maximized.
- Always annotate the data, so that the audience for whom they are intended can see where there have been improvements.
- These visual displays are a very effective means of communication within and between teams, and can provide clear validation of the achievements made to date, which further motivates teams and conversely can act as a reality check where results have not met our expectations, offering us an opportunity to tailor our approach as needed.

Box plot

A box plot provides a way to illustrate the distribution of data to see whether there are outliers or whether data are symmetrical, tightly grouped, or skewed. It is a way to demonstrate variation among clinicians or services, and provides similar information to a bell curve. Fifty per cent of the data are in the box (Figure 15.1).

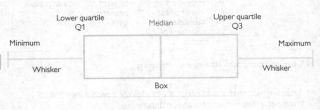

Figure 15.1 Box plot.

Scatter plot

A scatter plot is a graph used to look for relationships between two variables and is used when you have paired data (Figure 15.2).

- The variable to be controlled is on the horizontal axis, and the one that is expected to respond to the control is on the vertical axis.

The scatter plot helps you assess the strength of the relationship between two variables and whether the intervention is worthwhile or not.

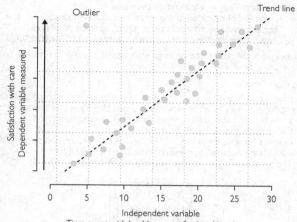

Figure 15.2 Example of a scatter plot.

Funnel plot

A funnel plot is a graphical method to evaluate healthcare quality by comparing hospital performances on certain outcomes (Figure 15.3).

- Funnel plots are often used in research to demonstrate differences between individuals, teams, or organizations and to see if there are outliers demonstrating special cause variation.
- A funnel plot is a form of scatter plot with control limits to assess the outliers. It takes the sample size into account (e.g. size of hospital or clinical ward).
- A funnel plot has four components:
  - The standard indicator, which indicates the performance on an outcome (e.g. the rate of falls on the y-axis);

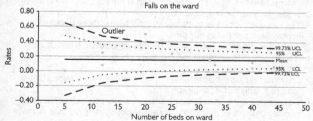

Figure 15.3 Example of a funnel plot.

- The sample size of each unit on the x-axis;
- A measure of precision of the certainty of the comparison;
- The upper and lower control limits to identify statistical differences. Outliers exceeding the control limits are special causes (Willik et al., 2020).

Funnel plots are often used on large-scale projects and is akin to the bell curve being on its side.

Safety cross

A safety cross is a visual demonstration of the presence or absence of an event (Figure 15.4). It can be motivating as one eliminates an adverse event (e.g. medication harm, deterioration, falls, pressure ulcers, etc.).

- Each square is for a day of the month.
- Green is for absence of the incident, and red for occurrence; amber is if the incident occurred but was not caused in the clinical area.
- The number of days between events is also recorded.

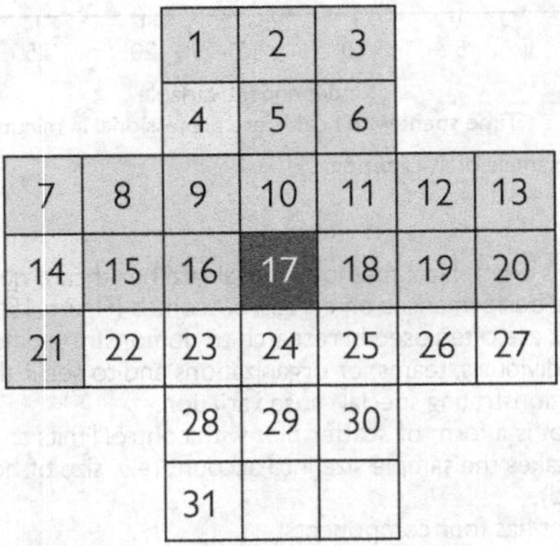

Figure 15.4 Safety cross.

Run chart

As discussed in Chapter 12, the run chart is the standard way in which we demonstrate improvement over time (Figure 15.5).

- The run chart allows us to demonstrate whether there has been an improvement or not in real time.
- A pen and paper, or Excel can be used to construct the run chart.
- It is important to annotate the run chart, so that it relays the story of the changes made.
- Data can take on different values on a continuous scale over a unit of time (e.g. length of hospital stay).
- Data can be aggregated into percentages of discrete categories (e.g. infected patients vs those not infected, clinics starting on time vs those not starting on time).

In Box 15.5 application of a run chart in a clinical improvement project is discussed.

Interpretation of a Run Chart: Shift, Trend & Astronomical Data

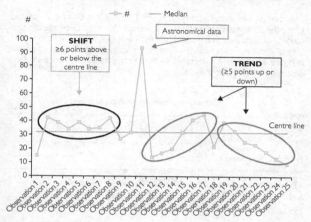

Figure 15.5 Run chart rules.
With permission of the CEC, New South Wales.
© Clinical Excellence Commission 2023.

Box 15.5 Run chart used in a quality improvement project in a clinical context

John is a house officer on a busy paediatric ward. The pharmacist Sean, who attends the ward rounds, complains that he must correct over 60% of the scripts (baseline data taken in weeks 1 and 2 prior to commencing the improvement initiative found that only 39% of prescriptions were fully compliant with guidelines at baseline, as shown in Figure 15.6). He says this is time-consuming and a danger to the patients.

John agrees to start an improvement project with Sean. They introduced a weekly huddle focusing on reducing medication errors (a 'druggle') to discuss all the prescribing errors. They set what they believe to be an achievable target of aiming to have at least 90% of scripts being fully compliant with prescribing guidelines.

Sean reviewed a sample of scripts on a weekly basis and documented the errors, arranged them into categories, and developed a Pareto chart, so he could explain which were the most important. John was responsible for engaging with the other doctors on the ward to ensure they would attend a weekly huddle, at which time the findings would be discussed. In order to engage the team further and to introduce an element of fun, a small prize-giving was held at week 4 of the project to help further motivate members and to celebrate success, recognizing that human factors are an important component of any successful improvement initiative.

(Continued)

Box 15.5 (Contd.)

A run chart must tell a story. In Figure 15.7, the run chart is annotated, giving the different interventions in a project aiming to decrease the prescribing of sedatives in a general practitioner's practice.

Finally, the run chart can demonstrate statistical significance, as shown in Figure 15.8, where a decrease in the caesarean section rate also demonstrated a significant p-value.

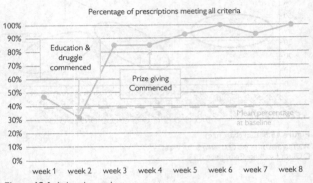

Figure 15.6 A druggle run chart.
Reproduced with from permission of Eoin Fitzgerald.

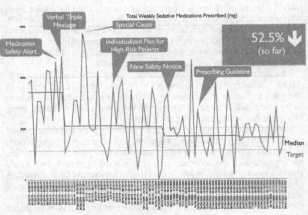

Figure 15.7 Run chart in a sedative reduction project.
© Clinical excellence Commission 2023.

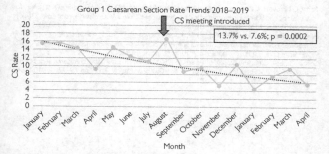

Figure 15.8 Run chart with *p*-value.

Reproduced with permission from David Crosby.

Statistical process control chart

Finally, SPC charts are used when you want to demonstrate statistical significance of your improvement. Details of how to use an SPC chart are provided in ⊃ Chapter 13.

Further reading

General

Gupta, M. and Kaplan, H.C. (2020). Measurement for quality improvement: using data to drive change. *Journal of Perinatology*, 40(6), pp. 962–71. doi: 10.1038/s41372-019-0572-x.

Ogrinc, G. (2021). Measuring and publishing quality improvement. *Regional Anesthesia and Pain Medicine*, 46(8), pp. 643–9. doi: 10.1136/rapm-2020-102201.

Scatter diagram

NHS England (2023) Scatter diagram (correlation) Available at https://www.england.nhs.uk/wp-content/uploads/2021/03/qsir-scatter-diagram.pdf **(accessed 10 September 2023)**

Funnel plots

Ilona, Holman, R., Peek, N., Ameen Abu-Hanna and Nicolette (2017). Guidelines on constructing funnel plots for quality indicators: A case study on mortality in intensive care unit patients. *Statistical Methods in Medical Research*, 27(11), pp.3350–3366. doi:https://doi.org/10.1177/0962280217700169.

Willik, E.M., Zwet, E.W., Hoekstra, T., *et al.* (2020). Funnel plots of patient-reported outcomes to evaluate health-care quality: basic principles, pitfalls and considerations. *Nephrology*, 26(2), pp. 95–104. doi: 10.1111/nep.13761.

Safety cross

Flynn, M. *Quality and safety—the safety cross system: simple and effective.* Available at: ℘ https://www.inmo.ie/MagazineArticle/PrintArticle/11155 (accessed 10 September 2023).

Run chart

Perla, R.J., Provost, L.P., and Murray, S.K. (2011). The run chart: a simple analytical tool for learning from variation in healthcare processes. *BMJ Quality and Safety*, 20(1), pp. 46–51. doi: 10.1136/bmjqs.2009.037895.

Shewhart Statistical Control Chart (SPC) chart

Marang-van de Mheen, P.J. and Woodcock, T. (2023). Grand rounds in methodology: four critical decision points in statistical process control evaluations of quality improvement initiatives. *BMJ Quality and Safety*, 32(1), pp. 47–54. doi: https://doi.org/10.1136/bmjqs-2022-014870.

Parry, G., Provost, L.P., Provost, S.M., Little, K., and Perla, R.J. (2021). A hybrid Shewhart chart for visualizing and learning from epidemic data. *International Journal for Quality in Health Care*, 33(4), p. mzab151. doi: 10.1093/intqhc/mzab151.

Perla, R.J., Provost, S.M., Parry, G.J., Little, K., and Provost, L.P. (2021). Understanding variation in reported covid-19 deaths with a novel Shewhart chart application. *International Journal for Quality in Health Care*, 33(1), p. mzaa069. doi: 10.1093/intqhc/mzaa069.

Soong, C., Bell, C.M., and Blackstien-Hirsch, P. (2023). 'Show me the data!' Using time series to display performance data for hospital boards. *BMJ Quality and Safety*, 32(2), pp. 69–72. doi: 10.1136/bmjqs-2022-014999.

Quality of measurement

Quality of measurement

The validity of the measures is dependent on ensuring each step of the measurement plan is implemented reliably. The spread and scale-up of any positive outcomes depend on good data quality. When conducting a quality analysis of your measurement plan, ask the following questions (based on Needham et al., 2009) (Box 15.6).

Constant attention to measurement quality will improve the outcome of the project.

Box 15.6 Data quality checklist

Planning
1. Are the aims of the project clearly stated?
2. Are there clear operational definitions of each measure?
3. Are the family of measures appropriate for the project?
4. Is data quality the main focus, rather than too much data?
5. Are data collected in a standardized way (e.g. with a data form or directly into the IT system), with clear procedures for collection?
6. Are staff trained to collect data?
7. Are there any ethical considerations for the use of data?
8. Will data be segmented to account for equity?
9. Are there measures for person-centred care and for sustainable quality improvement?

Collection
10. Is there accountability for data collection?
11. Are there quality assessments of data collection?
12. Is there a standardized data entry system with regular backup?
13. Is there a process for missing data both in measurement and in analysis?

Analysis
14. Is data analysis standardized with relevant expertise?
15. Is there a good reporting system for the data?
16. Have confounding factors been addressed?
17. Are the statistics reliable?

Reporting
18. Have the data illustration and reporting been decided?
19. How will the data be summarized?
20. How will data be reported to patients?

References

Needham, D.M., Sinopoli, D.J., Dinglas, V.D., et al. (2009). Improving data quality control in quality improvement projects. *International Journal for Quality in Health Care*, 21(2), pp. 145–50. doi: 10.1093/intqhc/mzp005.

Top tips

- Plan your measurement carefully before you start a project.
- Define each measure precisely—the 'operational definition'.
- Develop a comprehensive measurement plan, and do not make it too difficult to implement.
- Include a family of measures that reflect the different aspects of the project.
- Constantly assess the quality of data collection to ensure the final results are reliable.

Summary

Measurement is the foundation of clinical medicine and of QI. In QI, the focus is on prediction and learning. Data are collected in real time, so changes can be made as you implement the intervention.

In the past, the quality of data was variable, and results not easily transferable, as the context was not taken into account. A measurement plan and clear lines of responsibility for data collection, analysis, and quality control are required. Run charts and SPC charts are the preferred way to illustrate data.

Signposting

NHS Institute for Innovation and Improvement.(2008) The How-to guide for measurement for improvement. Available at: https://www.england.nhs.uk/improvement-hub/wp-content/uploads/sites/44/2017/11/How-to-Guide-for-Measurement-for-Improvement.pdf (accessed 10 September 2023)

NHS Scotland (2017) Handy guide to Measurement for Improvement. Available at: https://ihub.scot/media/5339/a46967-20171123-handy-guide-to-measurement-for-improvement-v1-0-3.pdf (accessed 10 September 2023)

NHS England (2019). Makin g Data Count. Available at https://www.england.nhs.uk/wp-content/uploads/2019/12/making-data-count-getting-started-2019.pdf (accessed 10 September 2023)

Further reading

Provost, L.P. and Murray, S.K. (2011). The Health Care Data Guide: Learning from Data for Improvement. San Francisco, CA: Jossey-Bass.

Measurement of person-centred care

Key points

- The views of patients are an essential component of the measurement strategy in either clinical work or improvement projects.
- There are many different ways to gather information from patients, including surveys, interviews, and focus groups.
- Patient satisfaction measures are subjective in that they reflect whether or not the expectation of the patient has been reached.
- Patient-reported measures are standardized measures to provide objective evidence of the patient's outcome or experiences.
- There are many challenges to introducing patient-reported experience or outcome measures and if these are addressed, then there can be benefits for patients as well as for clinical services.
- Clinician engagement is essential, as well as ensuring that collection of data and feedback is not burdensome on either the clinical staff or the patient.
- Reporting of data must be an integrated part of the process.
- Equity of access to the measurement system is essential.

Introduction

The rationale behind quality improvement is to improve outcomes for people receiving care (patients and their families) and to enable providers of care to deliver high-quality care in all its dimensions. The measurement of person-centred care (PCC) is an important part of the improvement process, as the person receiving care knows whether the experience and outcome of a healthcare intervention align with his or her values, preferences, and needs.

In Chapter 13, the study of variation in processes is discussed with methods to study the process and measure over time, reporting in a statistical process control (SPC) chart or a run chart. In Chapter 15, the development of a measurement strategy and plan is discussed, and in this chapter, the focus will be on the measurement of what matters to patients.

- High-quality healthcare requires people to provide information about how they feel, their symptoms, and the effects of their treatment outcomes, as well as their experience of care.
- Patient experience has been expanded to person, and now to human, experience and is defined by Wolf et al. (2021) as 'the experience of all interactions across the total continuum of care, without boundaries on the person's journey'.
- Introduction of the views of the patient as a person into routine clinical practice is a vital aspect of understanding and improving the quality of care.
- There can be a mismatch between the understanding of healthcare professionals and that of the patient as a person in preference for treatment and decision-making, and of the quality of care received.
- To ensure PCC and delivery of high-quality healthcare, it is important that services have a strategy to implement and measure PCC, so that an assessment can be made as to whether they are succeeding or not.
- Black and Jenkinson (2009) stated that 'patients offer a complementary perspective to that of clinicians, providing unique information and insights into both the humanity of care (such as dignity and respect, privacy, meeting information needs, waiting and delays, and cleanliness of facilities) and the effectiveness of health care'. The concept of humanity of care can be forgotten in the highly technical model of care that has been developed.

In Chapter 8, the concepts of PCC focused on the importance of understanding what really matters to people and comprehending their lived experience of the care processes, as well as their clinical condition, and co-producing solutions to improve care.

In this chapter, we will explore ways to measure patient-reported outcomes (PROs) in terms of their condition and patient-reported experience of the care received, so that a true reflection of the quality of care can be obtained. In all improvement projects, this dimension is required to ensure that the project has relevance to the people affected.

References

Black, N. and Jenkinson, C. (2009). Measuring patients' experiences and outcomes. BMJ, 339, p. b2495. doi: 10.1136/bmj.b2495.

Wolf, J.A., Niederhauser, V., Marshburn, D., and LaVela, S.L. (2021). Reexamining 'defining patient experience': the human experience in healthcare. Patient Experience Journal, 8(1), pp. 16–29. doi: 10.35680/2372-0247.1594.

Measuring patient experience and satisfaction

Different methods have been developed to assess the experience of patients. In Figure 16.1, the use of these methods is demonstrated.

- Each of these methods can be used to develop a comprehensive picture of patient experience and satisfaction.
- On reading the literature, it is clear that there has been interchangeable use of the terms of patient satisfaction and patient experience. This has led to confusion and a lack of validity of the reported measures.
- *Patient experience* can be considered to be a process measure which reflects the interpersonal aspects of quality of care received, with three main domains of: effective communication; respect and dignity; and emotional support. These domains are moderated by items such as facility environment, staffing wait times, and patient demographics (Larson et al., 2019).
- *Patient satisfaction* is an outcome measure of the patient's experience of care. Expectations are dynamic and can change and may be contextual (Larson et al., 2019).
- There has been a move away from satisfaction measures as expectations can be low, so meeting or exceeding the expectation may not be a good indicator of quality (Black and Jenkinson, 2009).
- The differences between experience and satisfaction are summarized in Box 16.1.

Reviews of the validity and reliability of patient satisfaction measures have shown that both are variable and that there is a need for standardization of measures. Therefore, it is recommended that patient experience measures, which have a stronger evidence base than patient satisfaction, are used (Anufriyeva, et al., 2020; Gill and White, 2009).

In Box 16.2 different methods of collecting data from patients is considered.

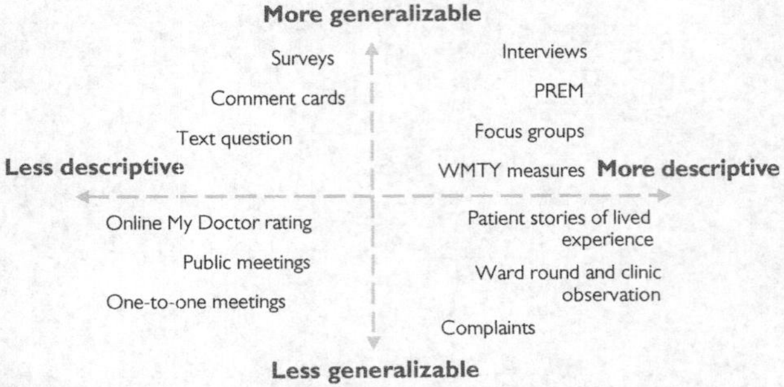

Figure 16.1 Measuring patient experience.

Based on DaSilva, D. (2013) Evidence Scan 18: Measuring patient experience. Available at: https://www.health.org.uk/publications/measuring-patient-experience (accessed 10 September 2023).

Box 16.1 Difference between experience and satisfaction

Patient satisfaction is focused on whether the expectations of the person receiving care for the service have been met. It is therefore more subjective and there is the potential for bias. It may use a rating scale, such as the Likert scale, to rate the satisfaction. Patient satisfaction surveys try to translate these subjective opinions into quantifiable data, which can lead to interventions if required.

Patient experience is focused on what happened in the episode of care and how the care was delivered and measured with validated and reliable objective measures.

For example, an *experience measure* may include a question asking a patient whether or not they were given discharge information from an admission, whereas a *satisfaction measure* would ask them how satisfied they were with the information they received.

Reference: Bull, C. (2021).

Box 16.2 Ways to collect data other than using questionnaires

So that the authentic lived experience of people is captured, a multifaceted approach needs to be undertaken. Each of the methods can be part of a quality improvement project.

- Novel *interviews* in different formats—face-to-face, via email, or web-based.
- *Focus groups* that come together to discuss a particular issue. This requires a clear purpose and careful moderation. Can be in person or virtual.
- *Citizen juries* where evidence is presented to the citizens who then decide on its value.
- *Photo elicitation interviews* to simulate a dialogue, usually in a research setting.
- *Video-reflexive ethnography* (*VRE*) recording healthcare encounters and then reviewing them to discover potential changes needed. Often used as part of experience-based co-design.

Prior *et al.*, 2020.

Challenges to address in measuring experience

The measurement of patient experience is complex, and several challenges should be addressed if you are to include them either in clinical practice or improvement projects (Table 16.1).

Table 16.1 Challenges in measuring patient experience

Challenge	Comment
When to administer the survey	This is often an issue—that is, whether it should be during, immediately after, or later—as different biases may be present. This is more of a problem with satisfaction scores and is dependent on the clinical condition being measured
Ranking of results	There is the temptation to rank and compare in a way that has no real meaning. Individual units or clinicians can measure scores over time, but for comparison purposes, the use of a funnel plot will allow outliers, both good and in need of improvement, in a non-judgemental way
The relationship between patient experience measures and clinical outcome	The correlation between experience ranking and outcome needs to be defined, as well as clinical outcomes that the clinicians identify.
Matching clinicians' perception of experience and outcome with that of the patient	The clinical assessment may differ as different perspectives are considered; for example, a hip replacement may be technically successful, but from the viewpoint of the patient, it may have added other challenges

Black and Jenkinson, 2009.

Patient-reported outcome and experience

The solution to the problem of bias is to use standardized, validated tools designed to provide a reliable result. Measurement tools have been developed to capture *patient-reported (health) outcomes* (PROs) and experience which are important to patients, which are known as *patient-reported outcome measures* (PROMs) and *patient-reported experience measures* (PREMs), respectively (Box 16.3).

Box 16.3 Definition of PROMs and PREMs

PROMs provide insight into the impact of an intervention or therapy on the patient, whilst PREMs provide insight into the quality of care during the intervention.

Patient-reported outcome measures (PROMs) are standardized, validated questionnaires measuring the patients' views of their health status.

Patient-reported experience measures (PREMs) are standardized, validated questionnaires measuring the patients' perceptions of their experience while receiving care.

PREMs can identify:
- The *relationship* aspects of experience—was what matters to them addressed? Did they receive emotional support, good communication, etc.?
- The *functional* aspects relating to timely, effective, and safe care, the environment, and facilities.

Box 16.3 *(Contd.)*

These two measurement domains tend to be associated with clinical care and experience. PREMs are therefore intended to be less prone to the influence of patient expectation.

Kingsley and Patel, 2017.

A patient-reported measure of safety (PMOS) has been developed and may perform a similar role as PREMs and PROMS in the future (Taylor et al., 2019).

One should also remember that there may be a subset of people who are not able to derive even average results from existing systems and we need to explore ways to determine their experience and outcomes.

Further reading

Beattie, M., Murphy, D.J., Atherton, I., and Lauder, W. (2015). Instruments to measure patient experience of healthcare quality in hospitals: a systematic review. *Systematic Reviews*, 4(1), pp.97–117. doi: 10.1186/s13643-015-0089-0.

Black, N., Varaganum, M., and Hutchings, A. (2014). Relationship between patient reported experience (PREMs) and patient reported outcomes (PROMs) in elective surgery. *BMJ Quality and Safety*, 23(7), pp. 534–42. doi: 10.1136/bmjqs-2013-002707.

Bull, C., Teede, H., Watson, D., and Callander, E.J. (2022). Selecting and implementing patient-reported outcome and experience measures to assess health system performance. *JAMA Health Forum*, 3(4), p. e220326. doi: 10.1001/jamahealthforum.2022.0326.

De Bienassis, K., Kristensen, S., Hewlett, E., Roe, D., Mainz, J., and Klazinga, N. (2021). Measuring patient voice matters: setting the scene for patient-reported indicators. *International Journal for Quality in Health Care*, 34(Suppl 1), ii3–ii6. doi: 10.1093/intqhc/mzab002.

References

Anufriyeva, V., Pavlova, M., Stepurko, T., and Groot, W. (2021). The validity and reliability of self-reported satisfaction with healthcare as a measure of quality: a systematic literature review. *International Journal for Quality in Health Care*. 33(1) doi: 10.1093/intqhc/mzaa152.

Black, N. and Jenkinson, C. (2009). Measuring patients' experiences and outcomes. *BMJ*, 339, p. b2495. doi: 10.1136/bmj.b2495.

Bull, C. (2021). Patient satisfaction and patient experience are not interchangeable concepts. *International Journal for Quality in Health Care*. 33(1). doi: 10.1093/intqhc/mzab023.

Gill, L. and White, L. (2009). A critical review of patient satisfaction. *Leadership in Health Services*, 22(1), pp. 8–19. doi: 10.1108/17511870910927994.

Kingsley, C. and Patel, S. (2017). Patient-reported outcome measures and patient-reported experience measures. *BJA Education*, 17(4), pp. 137–44. doi: 10.1093/bjaed/mkw060.

Larson, E., Sharma, J., Bohren, M.A., and Tunçalp, Ö. (2019). When the patient is the expert: measuring patient experience and satisfaction with care. *Bulletin of the World Health Organisation*, 97(8), pp. 563–9. doi: 10.2471/blt.18.225201.

Prior, S.J., Mather, C., Ford, K., Bywaters, D., and Campbell, S. (2020). Person-centred data collection methods to embed the authentic voice of people who experience health challenges. *BMJ Open Quality*, 9(3), p. e000912. doi: 10.1136/bmjoq-2020-000912.

Taylor, N., Clay-Williams, R., Ting, H.P., et al. (2019). Validation of the patient measure of safety (PMOS) questionnaire in Australian public hospitals. *International Journal for Quality in Health Care*, 32(Supplement 1), pp. 67–74. doi: 10.1093/intqhc/mzz097.

Developing a strategy for patient-reported measures

Challenges to be addressed in implementation

Although patient-reported measures have been available for many years, their use has been inconsistent and variable. To have a successful uptake and use of the measures either in clinical or improvement work, we need to address:

- A macrosystem organizational culture that places PCC as a priority and facilitates the use of patient-reported measures as part of the routine measures of the organization.
- At the mesosystem level of service, the domains of measuring performance need to include patient-reported measures, so that the implementation is not a burden.
- At the microsystem level, the frontline clinical teams need to be made aware of the use of patient-reported measures and supported, so that it is possible to implement.
- At the individual clinician level, where there is a lack of knowledge or understanding and, at times, scepticism on the value, education and support are required.

In addition, when planning the use of patient-reported measures, we need to ensure that the strategy addresses the challenge of equity, so that disadvantaged communities are not excluded:

- Language challenges are addressed;
- All challenged communities are included;
- The impact of demographics and patient characteristics is proactively managed.

Co-producing the introduction of the programme will help make PROMS and PREMS a desired introduction.

Implementation process

The implementation process has three steps, as delineated by Bull et al. (2022) (Table 16.2).

Table 16.2 Steps in the implementation of patient-reported experience measures

Steps	Action
Decide	Decide what you want to measure and why
	What is the purpose of the measurement?
	How will the information be used?
	Which measure is needed—a PREM or a PROM?
	How will patients be involved in measurement choice?
Choose the measure	Choose the measurement tool that will answer the question you are asking. This can be a generic or disease-specific measure. When choosing the measure, consider its validity, reliability, and responsiveness to change, as well as the context in which it is going to be measured. There are measurement repositories which can provide the information

Table 16.2 (Contd.)

Steps	Action
Implement	Develop an implementation plan that will address any barriers at each level
	Consider how the measurement links into an improvement programme
	How will patients be informed of the quality of care?
	How will you manage outliers?

In your improvement project, the use of PREMs and PROMs will be part of the measurement planning, as discussed in ➲ Chapter 15. Co-produce the plan with the patients and staff to ensure good uptake.

Signposting

Journal of Patient-Reported Outcomes Available at https://jpro.springeropen.com/ (accessed 10 September 2023).

Journal of Patient Experience. Available at https://journals.sagepub.com/home/jpx (accessed 10 September 2023).

COSMIN, COnsensus-based Standards for the selection of health Measurement INstruments. Available at: https://www.cosmin.nl/ (accessed 10 September 2023).

HCAHPS, Hospital Consumer Assessment of Healthcare Providers and Systems. Available at: https://hcahpsonline.org/en/ (accessed 10 September 2023).

ISOQOL, International Society for Quality of Life Research Available at: https://www.isoqol.org/ (accessed 10 September 2023).

ICHOM, International Consortium for Health Outcomes Management. Available at: https://www.ichom.org/ (accessed 10 September 2023).

PROQOLID, the Patient-Reported Outcome and Quality of Life Instruments Database Available at: https://www.qolid.org/ (accessed 10 September).

WHOQOL, Measuring Quality of Life Available at: https://www.who.int/tools/whoqol/whoqol-100 (accessed 10 September 2023).

EuroQol instruments, EQ-5D. Available at: https://euroqol.org/eq-5d-instruments/ (accessed 10 September).

OECD Patient-Reported Indicators Surveys (PaRIS). Available at: https://www.oecd.org/els/health-systems/paris.htm (accessed 10 September 2023).

Further reading

Kingsley, C. and Patel, S. (2017). Patient-reported outcome measures and patient-reported experience measures. *BJA Education*, 17(4), pp. 137–44. doi: 10.1093/bjaed/mkw060.

Reference

Bull, C., Teede, H., Watson, D., and Callander, E.J. (2022). Selecting and implementing patient-reported outcome and experience measures to assess health system performance. *JAMA Health Forum*, 3(4), p. e220326. doi: 10.1001/jamahealthforum.2022.0326.

Patient-reported outcome measures

PROs are focused on obtaining the outcomes from the viewpoint of the patient in an unbiased way. Key definitions are provided in Table 16.3.

Table 16.3 Definitions

Term	Description
Patient-reported outcome (PRO)	Any report of the status of a patient's health condition that comes directly from the patient without interpretation of the patient's response by a clinician or anyone else
Patient-reported outcome measures (PROMs)	PROMs measure the PROs, usually through self-report questionnaires to provide the patient's perspective on the outcome
Health status/health-related quality of life (HRQL)	The HRQL is determined by an individual's ability to perform the usual activities for age and social role. This goes beyond the illness, and deviation from normality represents a reduction in HRQL arising from a combination of measures, including symptoms and functioning, both objective and subjective. This yields a variety of scores in different domains of measurement
Overall quality of life (QoL)	'QoL is an individual's perception of their position in life in the context of the culture and value systems in which they live and in relation to their goals, expectations, standards and concerns' (World Health Organization, 2013) QoL is therefore driven by the individual's own identified human needs and the ability to satisfy these for fulfilment and satisfaction. For example, being able to walk may fulfil multiple functional needs such as independence, communication, and socialization ability. QoL measures are unidimensional and yield a single score

- PROs are used in conjunction with other clinical outcome assessment methods that complement biomarkers, measures of morbidity (e.g. disease status), burden of disease (e.g. hospitalization rates), and survival used in clinical studies to contribute to a full understanding of the quality of a healthcare intervention or management of a condition.
- PROs can be understood to contextualize the objective clinical assessment and signs, which often correlate poorly and are a reminder that biomarkers are often limited.
- PROMs are particularly important in conditions where there may be no clinical or biological markers to guide treatment (e.g. in irritable bowel syndrome (IBS) or depression).
- PROMs are the outcomes that often have the most importance to patients and their families, as they characterize the quality of life and function through the lens of the person receiving care, not through that of clinicians.

- With the move to integrated care models in which health and social care will be part of one continuum of care for the individual, especially those with long-term conditions, an integrated approach to reported outcomes can be developed. This will require considerable culture change, as well as an integrated data management system. Examples in the coronavirus disease 2019 (COVID-19) pandemic were use of PROs on unmet needs across health and social care in the United Kingdom, as well as symptom monitoring and tracking (Hughes et al., 2021).
- PROMs can be used as part of big data sets to develop health policy in the future (Calvert et al., 2015).

What does a 'good' PROM look like?

The PROM should inform an explicit PRO concept or construct, which should be clearly stated (Box 16.4). The commonly used domains include:
- Symptom measures that impact on the person;
- Function/activity limitations as a result of the condition or treatment.

Box 16.4 Characteristics of good PROM instruments

- Based on a sound theoretical model of what they measure with construct validity.
- Measures derived from direct patient input to ensure their relevance to the population.
- Possess adequate psychometric and scaling properties.
- Adequately sample or cover contents relevant to the construct assessed (content validity).
- Can assess patients across a broad spectrum of disease severity.
- Can demonstrate change.

Challenges specific to patient-reported outcome measures

When you select a PROM, Calvert et al. (2019) recommend an integrated approach, and attention given to the challenge of equity (Calvert et al., 2022). The identified challenges that need to be addressed are summarized in Table 16.4.

Table 16.4 Challenges specific to patient-reported outcome measures

Challenge	Description	Possible solution
Selection of the PROM	May not measure what really matters to patients and may not have cultural validity May not work across disease types	Need to have validity and acceptability to stakeholders, so that the PROM measures *what really matters*; best if the selection is co-produced with patients and other stakeholders. Use of data sets, such as the Patient-Reported Outcomes Measurement Information System (PROMIS) may help. https://www.promishealth.org/57461-2/

(Continued)

Table 16.4   (Contd.)

Challenge	Description	Possible solution
Ethical	Patients may not be informed about the purpose; feedback of data may not be reliable; inadequate response to concerns found in data	In setting up the programme, there must be a clear purpose on why the data are being collected, how they will be managed and fed back, and how patients will be supported
Data	How data are collected and integrated; whether all stakeholders accept them; how they will be used; data quality	Training and support and an integrated infrastructure are required
Logistics	IT systems may be incompatible, and data not integrated	An aspiration is for IT systems to be designed in an integrated way, so that the PROM is part of the electronic health record
Lack of coordination	Lack of coordination across subsets of data to make meaningful conclusions	On a national level, this is important for system-wide change as it is on an organizational level
Equity	Social determinants of health have a major impact on clinical outcomes. In setting up a PROM programme, the different groups may be disadvantaged (e.g. through poverty; lack of access to IT, IT literacy, and language; lack of representation in design, etc.)	In ⊙ Chapter 5, the challenge of equity applies and the solutions there can apply here to proactively address each of the challenges identified. Engagement with community groups is essential in co-production of the solution

The Patient-Reported Outcome and Quality of Life Database (PROQOLID)

The PROQOLID project contains over 600 known PROMs curated by the Mapi Research Trust.
- The database provides the ability to find information, psychometric properties, and validity data on an extensive range of PROMs from generic measures to disease-specific PROMs, and PROMs focused on a particular population.
- Tables 16.5 and 16.6 provide information regarding several well-validated and commonly used PROMs.

Table 16.5 Examples of generic patient-reported outcome measures

EQ-5D™ (available at: ℜ https://euro qol.org, accessed 10 September 2023)	Simple, widely used, generic, and evidence-based, in which patients tick boxes and rate overall health on an analogue scale. Patients score on five domains of mobility, self-care, usual activities, pain and discomfort, and anxiety and depression	Available in over 200 languages for a wide range of conditions and populations.
WHOQOL tools (available at: ℜ https://www.who.int/tools/who qol, accessed 10 September 2023)	A range of free QoL assessment tools created by WHO in 15 international field centres to aim to develop cross-culturally relevant measures, initially for mental health and substance use, but subsequently validated in various diseases and populations	Available in multiple languages and measures QoL in six domains (physical capacity, psychological, level of independence, social relationships, environment, and spirituality), with an 'overall' impression

QoL, quality of life; WHO, World Health Organization.

Table 16.6 Examples of condition-specific patient-reported outcome measures

Depression Hospital Anxiety and Depression Scale (HADS)	Seven questions on anxiety and seven on depression interspersed
Heart failure Minnesota Living with Heart Failure Questionnaire (MLHFQ)	Self-administered 21-item disease-specific scoring on a 6-point Likert scale
Asthma Asthma Quality of Life Questionnaire (AQLQ)	32 items which aim to measure functional impairments in adults arising from asthma. Validated as the most valid PROM in asthma (Worth et al., 2014)
Multiple sclerosis Multiple Sclerosis Quality of Life Inventory (MSQLI)	Self-administered battery of 10 individual scales assessing pain, fatigue, bowel and bladder control, impact of visual impairment, mental health, perceived deficits, sexual satisfaction, overall health, and social supports

A question to be addressed is whether this makes a difference to clinical care and to outcomes. It is a correlation of improved outcomes if PROMs are measured, and an example is provided in Box 16.5.

An example of how PROM data has been used in England to inform hip replacement surgery outcomes for clinicians and patients is shown in Box 16.6.

The use of PROMs in cancer has been demonstrated to improve clinical outcomes. In a study on over 700 patients with metastatic cancer, randomized into an intervention PROM group and a non-PROM group, it was shown that integration of patient-reported outcomes (PROs) using a PROM into routine care was associated with increased survival, compared to usual care. After 7 years of follow-up and an overall mortality of 67%, there was a 5-month increase in life expectancy in the PROM group, which was statistically significant. This could be because those in the PROM group alerted clinicians to symptoms early and therefore had earlier remedial intervention.

Basch et al., 2017.

A comprehensive PROM programme has been implemented in NHS England since 2009. The programme has covered the following conditions:
* Elective surgery for hip replacement, knee replacement, groin hernia repair, and varicose vein surgery;
* Coronary revascularization;
* Long-term conditions;
* Survival in breast, colorectal, non-Hodgkin lymphoma, and prostate;
* Dementia.
Disease-specific and generic PROMs are used.

An illustrative example is unilateral hip replacement. Prior to operations, consent was obtained and the generic PROMs EQ-5D™ Index and EQ-VAS™, as well as the specific condition PROM Oxford Hip Score, were completed. These data have been used by providers to identify areas where patients think they perform well and areas where they can improve, and by commissioners to identify and share areas of good practice and encourage improvement. The same data have been used by service users to review where they may wish to choose for their procedure if this is available.

NHS Digital, 2023

Signposting

Mapi Research Trust. Available at: ℜ https://mapi-trust.org (accessed 10 September 2023).
PROMIS® Health Organization (n.d.). *What is PROMIS?* Available at: ℜ https://www.promishealth. org/57461-2/ (accessed 10 September 2023).

Further reading

Doward, L.C., Gnanasakthy, A., and Baker, M.G. (2010). Patient reported outcomes: looking beyond the label claim. *Health and Quality of Life Outcomes*, 8(1), p. 89. doi: 10.1186/1477-7525-8-89.
Nelson, E.C., Eftimovska, E., Lind, C., Hager, A., Wasson, J.H., and Lindblad, S. (2015). Patient reported outcome measures in practice. *BMJ*, 350, p. g7818. doi: 10.1136/bmj.g7818.

Williams, K., Sansoni, J., Morris, D., Grootemaat, P., and Thompson, C. (2016). Patient-reported outcome measures: literature review. *Australian Health Services Research Institute*. Available at: 🔗 https://ro.uow.edu.au/ahsri/818/ (accessed 10 September 2023).

Wilson, I.B. (1995). Linking clinical variables with health-related quality of life. *JAMA*, 273(1), p. 59. doi: 10.1001/jama.1995.03520250075037.

References

Basch, E., Deal, A.M., Dueck, A.C., Scher, H.I., Kris, M.G., Hudis, C. and Schrag, D. (2017). Overall Survival Results of a Trial Assessing Patient-Reported Outcomes for Symptom Monitoring During Routine Cancer Treatment. *JAMA*, 318(2), pp. 197–198. doi: 10.1001/jama.2017.7156

Calvert, M., Kyte, D., Price, G., Valderas, J.M., and Hjollund, N.H. (2019). Maximising the impact of patient reported outcome assessment for patients and society. *BMJ*, 364, p. k5267. doi: 10.1136/bmj.k5267.

Calvert, M., Thwaites, R., Kyte, D., and Devlin, N. (2015). Putting patient-reported outcomes on the 'Big Data Road Map'. *Journal of the Royal Society of Medicine*, 108(8), pp. 299–303. doi: 10.1177/0141076815579896.

Calvert, M.J., Cruz Rivera, S., Retzer, A., *et al.* (2022). Patient reported outcome assessment must be inclusive and equitable. *Nature Medicine*. 28(6), 1120–1124. doi: 10.1038/s41591-022-01781-8.

Hughes, S., Aiyegbusi, O.L, Lasserson, D., Collis, P., Glasby, J., and Calvert, M. (2021). Patient-reported outcome measurement: a bridge between health and social care? *Journal of the Royal Society of Medicine*, 114(8), pp. 381–8. doi: 10.1177/01410768211014048.

World Health Organization (2013). *Programme on mental health: WHOQOL user manual, 2012 revision*. Available at: 🔗 https://www.who.int/publications/i/item/WHO-HIS-HSI-Rev.2012-3 (accessed 10 September 2023).

NHS Digital (n.d.). *Patient-reported outcome measures (PROMs)*. Available at: 🔗 https://digital.nhs.uk/data-and-information/data-tools-and-services/data-services/patient-reported-outcome-measures-proms#top (accessed 10 September 2023).

Worth, A., Hammersley, V., Knibb, R., Flokstra-de-Blok, B., DunnGalvin, A., Walker, S., Dubois, A.E.J. and Sheikh, A. (2014). Patient-reported outcome measures for asthma: a systematic review. *npj Primary Care Respiratory Medicine*, [online] 24(1). doi.org/10.1038/npjpcrm.2014.20.

Patient-reported experience measures

Patient experience encompasses the range of interactions that patients have with the healthcare system at all levels, from consultation with a staff member to interaction with the organization overall through a given pathway of care, and may even include integration of pathways with each other.

PREMs capture 'what' happened during an episode of care, and 'how' it happened from the perspective of the patient.
- These may be functional (e.g. availability of services) or relational (e.g. relationship with staff).
- PREMs gather information on patients' perceptions of their experience while receiving care, and are an indicator of its quality rather than a direct measure.
- They have been in use since the early 2000s since the Picker Institute developed the National Inpatient Survey for use in the National Health Service (NHS) in England.

PREMs are questionnaire-based instruments and have been designed to obtain information about patient experience in a variety of conditions (e.g. cancer, hip surgery, bipolar disorder), settings (inpatient, outpatient, community services), and breadth quality (domain-specific vs multiple domains or overall).
- A systematic thematic review characterized how the PREMs in current use broadly matched the quality domains described by the Institute of Medicine (IOM), as well as being in keeping with NHS England and the National Institute for Health and Care Excellence (NICE) objectives in measuring patient experience (Figure 16.2) (Bull et al., 2018).

A PREM must include psychometric properties in that they measure what they intend to measure reliably.
- Bull et al. (2019) identified 88 PREMs across a variety of healthcare settings and assessed them against 10 validity and reliability criteria, as defined in the consensus-based standards for the selection of health status measurement instruments (Prinsen et al., 2018).

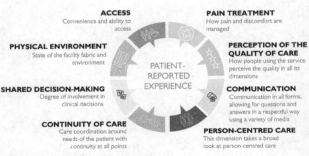

ACCESS
Convenience and ability to access

PAIN TREATMENT
How pain and discomfort are managed

PHYSICAL ENVIRONMENT
State of the facility fabric and environment

PERCEPTION OF THE QUALITY OF CARE
How people using the service perceive the quality in all its dimensions

SHARED DECISION-MAKING
Degree of involvement in clinical decisions

PATIENT-REPORTED EXPERIENCE

COMMUNICATION
Communication in all forms, allowing for questions and answers in a respectful way using a variety of media

CONTINUITY OF CARE
Care coordination around needs of the patient with continuity at all points

PERSON-CENTRED CARE
This dimension takes a broad look at person-centred care

Figure 16.2 Themes for PREMs in current use.
Adapted from Bull, Byrnes and Mulhern, 2018.

- They identified that >50% of these tools had not been rigorously assessed by using studies to explore internal consistency, structural validity, and content validity, and cautioned that careful consideration should be given when selecting suitable PREMs to measure change over time for meaningful healthcare evaluation.
- When choosing a PREM, the validity and reliability of the selected measure must be evaluated.

Several examples of PREMs used in clinical practice are given in Tables 16.7 and 16.8, and are selected from those which scored well in the systematic review.

- Some of these relate to mental health settings, which may be indicative of the longer-standing role of patient psychometric assessments in clinical practice in this field.
- In an improvement project, you may consider using one of these as a measure of improvement in the experience of patients.

Table 16.7 Selection of setting-focused patient-reported experience measures

Inpatient care	
HCAHPS 'Hospital Consumer Assessment of Healthcare Providers and Systems' (HCAHPS, 2019)	USA-focused, initiated in 2002, and reported publicly. Standardized national instrument of 29 questions about recent hospital stay (e.g. communication with nurses and doctors, responsiveness of staff, cleanliness and quietness of environment, discharge information, recommendation to others), as well as questions to adjust for case mix across hospitals. Administered to a random sample of adults across medical conditions between 48 hours and 6 weeks post-discharge. Available in multiple languages and available online
PIPEQ-OS (Psychiatric Inpatient Patient Experience Questionnaire—On Site) (Bjertnaes et al., 2015)	Initially developed as part of the Norwegian health programme to support institution-level quality improvement, hospital management, free patient choice, and public accountability; adapted for on-site use, consisting of 41 close-ended items, mostly scored on a 5-point response
Primary care	
EUROPEP (EQuiP, n.d.)	23-item standardized measure, developed between 1995 and 1998 as an international tool for patient evaluations of general practice care. Scored on a 5-point response. Available in multiple languages and well validated (Grol and Wensing, 2000)

Table 16.8 Selection of condition-focused patient-reported experience measures

Maternity	
ReproQ (Scheerhagen et al., 2019)	PREMs are based on the principles of the 'WHO responsiveness to care' model; designed to measure experiences of maternity care. Five sections asking about: • Current care process information (e.g. location and main Healthcare Professional (HCP) involved) • Clinical outcome for mother and child, as perceived by the mother in non-medical terms • Client experiences within the WHO responsiveness model domains • Information about previous pregnancies • Socio-demographic information

Substance dependence	
PEQ-ITSD (Patient Experience Questionnaire for Interdisciplinary Treatment for Substance Dependence) (Haugum et al., 2017)	Developed in Norway as part of the Norwegian Institute of Public Health PREMs (in conjunction with the PIPEQ community version) and describing three scales of experience: treatment and personnel; milieu of substance use treatment setting; and patient-perceived outcome

Individual children/adolescents	
ChASE (Child and adolescent service experience) (Day et al., 2011)	This questionnaire tool was co-produced with children who had been discharged from Child and Adolescent Mental Health Services (CAMHS) within the last 12 months. A 13-item tool measuring the domains of relationships, privacy, and session activity in service delivery was produced

Signposting

Picker (n.d.). *The highest quality person centred care for all, always.* Available at: ℬ https://picker.org/ (accessed 10 September 2023).

Further reading

De Vos, M.S., Hamming, J.F., and Marang-van de Mheen, P.J. (2018). The problem with using patient complaints for improvement. *BMJ Quality and Safety*, 27(9), pp. 758–62. doi: 10.1136/bmjqs-2017-007463.

Johnston, B.C., Patrick, D.L., Devji, T., et al. (2022). Patient-reported outcomes. In: Higgins, J.P.T, Thomas, J., Chandler, J, et al., eds. *Cochrane Handbook for Systematic Reviews of Interventions*, version 6.3 (updated February 2022). Available at: ℬ https://training.cochrane.org/handbook (accessed 10 September 2023).

Tzelepis, F., Sanson-Fisher, R., Zucca, A., and Fradgley, E. (2015). Measuring the quality of patient-centered care: why patient-reported measures are critical to reliable assessment. *Patient Preference and Adherence*, 9(1), pp. 831–5. doi: 10.2147/ppa.s81975.

References

Bjertnaes, O., Iversen, H.H., and Kjollesdal, J. (2015). PIPEQ-OS: an instrument for on-site measurements of the experiences of inpatients at psychiatric institutions. *BMC Psychiatry*, 15(1), pp. 234–42. doi: 10.1186/s12888-015-0621-8.

Bull, C., Byrnes, J., Hettiarachchi, R., and Downes, M. (2019). A systematic review of the validity and reliability of patient-reported experience measures. *Health Services Research*, 54(5), pp. 1023–35. doi: 10.1111/1475-6773.13187.

Bull, C., Byrnes, J., and Mulhern, B. (2018). We respect their autonomy and dignity, but how do we value patient-reported experiences? *MDM Policy and Practice*, 3(2), p. 238146831880745. doi: 10.1177/2381468318807458.

Day, C., Michelson, D., and Hassan, I. (2011). Child and adolescent service experience (ChASE): measuring service quality and therapeutic process. *British Journal of Clinical Psychology*, 50(4), pp. 452–64. doi: 10.1111/j.2044-8260.2011.02008.x.

EQuiP. Available at: https://www.qualityfamilymedicine.eu/page/europep (accessed 10 September 2023).

Grol, R. and Wensing, M. (2000). *Patients evaluate general/family practice: The EUROPEP instrument.* [online] *EQuiP*. Available at: https://www.qualityfamilymedicine.eu/page/europep (accessed 10 September 2023).

Haugum, M., Iversen, H.H., Bjertnaes, O., and Lindahl, A.K. (2017). Patient experiences questionnaire for interdisciplinary treatment for substance dependence (PEQ-ITSD): reliability and validity following a national survey in Norway. *BMC Psychiatry*, 17(1), pp. 73–83. doi: 10.1186/s12888-017-1242-1.

HCAHPS (2019). Available at: https://www.hcahponline.org (accessed 10 September 2023).

Prinsen, C.A.C., Mokkink, L.B., Bouter, L.M., et al. (2018). COSMIN guideline for systematic reviews of patient-reported outcome measures. *Quality of Life Research*, 27(5), pp. 1147–57. doi: 10.1007/s11136-018-1798-3.

Scheerhagen, M., van Stel, H.F., Franx, A., Birnie, E., and Bonsel, G.J. (2019). The discriminative power of the ReproQ: a client experience questionnaire in maternity care. *PeerJ*, 7, p. e7575. doi: 10.7717/peerj.7575.

Correlations of PREMs and PROMs

The challenge with collecting patient-reported outcomes and experience is to correlate the different measures—do they have any relationship (Box 16.7); for example, if the experience is good, does it mean the outcome is good as well, and if the experience is poor, can the outcome be good?

Box 16.7 Correlating PREMs and PROMs and outcomes

Case study 1

A systematic review of 55 studies on the association of PREMs and effectiveness and safety across diverse settings, from primary to secondary and tertiary care, was undertaken to assess whether a higher PREM was associated with better outcomes such as mortality, physical symptoms, length of stay, and adherence to treatment (Doyle et al., 2013). The review concluded that patient experience is consistently positively associated with patient safety and clinical effectiveness across a wide range of disease areas, as well as positive PROMs. Other health-related activities, such as preventative care, were also positively associated.

Case study 2

In a review of PREMs and PROMs in a study of elective surgical patients in England using the national PROM data set for patients undergoing hip replacement, knee replacements, and groin hernia repairs, the relationship between the experience scores and patients' characteristics experience with effectiveness and safety, and the influence that patient characteristics had on this relationship were studied (Black et al., 2014).

There was a significant positive association between a patient's overall PREM score and their PROM change score for all three procedures, with the strongest being on communication and trust. There was a significant negative association between patient experience and the reporting of post-operative complications. Patient experience cannot be used as a proxy for outcome. They concluded that patients distinguish between the three domains of quality when reporting their experience and outcome. The association is not necessarily causal, though if it is, it would have implications for improvement.

Doyle, Lennox and Bell, 2013; Black, Varaganum and Hutchings, 2014

References

Black, N., Varaganum, M., and Hutchings, A. (2014). Relationship between patient reported experience (PREMs) and patient reported outcomes (PROMs) in elective surgery. BMJ Quality and Safety, 23(7), pp. 534–42. doi: 10.1136/bmjqs-2013-002707.

Doyle, C., Lennox, L., and Bell, D. (2013). A systematic review of evidence on the links between patient experience and clinical safety and effectiveness. BMJ Open, 3(1). doi: 10.1136/bmjopen-2012-001570.

Using PROMs and PREMs in your project

Now that the potential for PROMs and PREMs has been discussed, the questions remains as to how we can be person-centred in our improvement projects and whether we can use measures such as PREMs and PROMs in our improvement management strategy and plan.

The following steps are recommended to help you decide how to proceed.

1. Involve patients at the start of the project, so that they can be part of the decision-making process.
2. Once the aim of the project has been determined, decide what the outcome for the patient group will be and whether it could be measured by a PROM and/or a PREM.
3. If the system already has a PREM and/or a PROM as part of routine quality data collection, try to use these measures.
4. If there are no patient-reported measures, then you can select one that is appropriate for the patient group, but answer the questions in Table 16.9.

The use of PREMs and PROMs can provide objective measures and can be part of a wider qualitative approach to developing a picture of what really matters to patients and improving their experience and outcomes.

Table 16.9 Questions to ask when considering using patient-reported measures

Leadership	What is the organizational and team culture?
	Do we have leadership support to provide resources?
Selection of measure	What do we want to measure—experience, outcomes, or both?
	Is there a measure which was developed with patients?
	What is the evidence base for the measure?
	Can we assess reliability, validity, and responsiveness of the measure?
	Will it provide the answer that we want—that is, will it enable us to tell us whether there is improvement?
Patients	How will we engage with the patient group?
	Can we ensure we have equitable application of the measures?
	How will we report back to the patients on the outcome of the project?
Clinicians	Are the clinicians on board, and how will we report data to them?
	Can it be part of routine work?
Infrastructure and resources	Do we have IT infrastructure to collect data?
	Can we integrate data collection into clinical processes?
	How will we analyse the data?
	Is it part of a national process?

Adapted from Øvretveit et al., 2017 and Gleeson et al., 2016.

Further reading

Bastemeijer, C.M., Boosman, H., van Ewijk, H., de Jong-Verweij, L.M., Voogt, L., and Hazelzet, J. (2019). Patient experiences: a systematic review of quality improvement interventions in a hospital setting. *Patient Related Outcome Measures*, 10, pp. 157–69. doi: 10.2147/prom.s201737.

International Journal for Quality in Health Care. Supplement on PROMs. Volume 34 (Supplement 1), 20 April 2022. Available at: ✂ https://academic.oup.com/intqhc/issue/34/Supplement_1 (accessed 10 September 2023).

Prodinger, B. and Taylor, P. (2018). Improving quality of care through patient-reported outcome measures (PROMs): expert interviews using the NHS PROMs Programme and the Swedish quality registers for knee and hip arthroplasty as examples. *BMC Health Services Research*, 18(1), pp. 87–99. doi: 10.1186/s12913-018-2898-z.

Weinfurt, K.P. and Reeve, B.B. (2022). Patient-reported outcome measures in clinical research. *JAMA*, 328(5), pp. 472-473. doi: 10.1001/jama.2022.11238.

References

Gleeson, H., Calderon, A., Swami, V., Deighton, J., Wolpert, M., and Edbrooke-Childs, J. (2016). Systematic review of approaches to using patient experience data for quality improvement in healthcare settings. *BMJ Open*, 6(8), p. e011907. doi: 10.1136/bmjopen-2016-011907.

Øvretveit, J., Zubkoff, L., Nelson, E.C., Frampton, S., Knudsen, J.L., and Zimlichman, E. (2017). Using patient-reported outcome measurement to improve patient care. *International Journal for Quality in Health Care*, 29(6), pp. 874–9. doi: 10.1093/intqhc/mzx108.

Top tips

- Ensure any PROM or PREM measures the intended outcome.
- Use international databases of PROMs and PREMs to identify the characteristics which are applicable to your clinical situation or project.
- Identify PROMs and PREMS to be used with patients and clinicians in a co-production process.
- Do not use tools which are resource- or time-heavy.
- Triangulate data from PROMs and PREMs with other data to provide a contextualized system of quality of care and areas for improvement.

Summary

As we move from Quality 1.0 to Quality 2.0, and finally to Quality 3.0, we are passing through a series of measurement approaches that are all required for quality improvement.

PROMs and PREMs provide a unique opportunity to improve care on what really matters to people receiving care.

There are challenges in using PROMs and PREMs, and as you enter the new world of measurement, you will see that if we have a valid standardized measurement system, then a new dimension will be added to it. Both our clinical practice and our improvement work, as we go from asking 'What is the matter?' to 'What matters to you?'.

Application of QI methods

Preparing your QI project

Key points

- Quality improvement is a complex set of interactions that requires careful planning to succeed.
- Application of the theories of improvement science and the Lenses of Profound Knowledge will provide a theoretical construct for your project.
- Before any improvement, one must identify a problem and the rationale.
- Studying a process and then analysing the variation within the process are the foundation of an improvement project.
- All those involved in the process should be listened to, and their support harnessed to deliver on the outcomes.
- Patients must be involved at all stages of the project, unless it is a process that is not relevant (e.g. in the laboratory).
- All projects should have a sponsor, an improvement team, and a patient member.

Introduction

> 'Quality is never an accident; it is always the result of high intention, sincere effort, intelligent direction and skillful execution; it represents the wise choice of many alternatives.'
>
> William A. Foster

In previous chapters, we have provided the theories that underpin quality improvement, as well as the rationale for improvement. In ⊃ Chapter 1, the domains of quality were discussed. As you now move on to applying these theories and methods, you need to decide:

- *What* you want to improve (i.e. identify a problem or challenge for staff or patients);
- *Why* you want to improve this problem—this is essential if you want others to change the way they think and the way they work;
- *How* you are going to improve.

In this and ⊃ Chapter 18, we will take the theory and methods discussed in previous chapters and apply them to solving quality challenges. You will learn how to apply the Lenses of Profound Knowledge (⊃ Chapter 3) to your problem and follow a project through by using improvement methodology:

- Assess the problem within the *system*;
- Find *unwarranted variation* in the processes of the system;
- Understand the beliefs and attitudes of the *people* in the system;
- Develop a *theory of change*.

There are five steps to take to prepare for your improvement project, each of which involves the theory discussed so far. The steps often take place simultaneously (Figure 17.1).

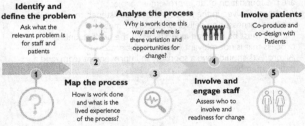

Figure 17.1 Steps to prepare for your quality improvement project.

How to start an improvement project

Define the problem/quality issue

'*What bugs you?*' is often the first question when getting started with an improvement project. This frustration with the status quo needs to be converted into a clear aim, but the problem needs to be identified and clearly articulated first, to build a case for change and engage others (Box 17.1).

- A starting point is to ask '*What matters*' to staff and '*What matters*' to patients and their families (see ➲ Chapters 8, 10, and 11).
- You may also want to think about what good-quality care looks like (see ➲ Chapter 1) and where care in your team, department, or institution could be better.
- To identify the problem or quality issue, you may look into registries, audits, safety events or incidents, global trigger tools, and clinical incident reports.
- It is often helpful to think about what works well in other places where you have worked or learn from presentations of improvement work at conferences and reports in the literature.

You may want to brainstorm your ideas with your team by using the Donabedian model for quality of care (see ➲ Chapters 3 and 12). In Table 17.1 questions that will help you define a problem are listed.

In Table 17.2, possible problems are listed against the quality domains.

Box 17.1 Identifying a problem

Clare noticed that she is called to review a lot of babies on the postnatal ward who are cold. This is frustrating because she knows it is avoidable, impacts their health, and diverts her away from sick babies on the neonatal intensive care unit (NICU). She discovered that an audit of hypothermic babies had been presented to the department, which had demonstrated some areas for improvement, but none of these had been put into place. The audit helped her to demonstrate this quality issue and build a case for change.

Table 17.1 Questions to ask to define a problem

Structures	What are the infrastructure issues that impact quality of care? For example, are staffing ratios a problem on the postnatal ward?	• How do we organize our work? • What are the tasks we need to do? • Do we have the right technologies? • Is the environment well planned (e.g. the drug room)? • How do we work together as a team?

Table 17.1 (*Contd.*)

Processes	Are our processes delivered reliably—activity which occurs for patients every time as per available evidence and agreed operating procedures?	• Is the operating procedure being followed? (e.g. all babies should have their temperature recorded on admission to the postnatal ward) • Does everyone follow the guidelines? (e.g. prescriptions written correctly for antibiotic prescribing)
Outcomes	Are our outcomes as good as they should be in comparison to other similar units?	• Are we above the average? (e.g. mortality from sepsis) • Who is the best that we need to emulate? (i.e. learning from others)

Table 17.2 Examples of quality improvement problems

Domain	Examples
Person-centred care	'Hello my name is' initiative Ask 'What matters to you?' (patients and staff) Increase integration of care Improve coordination of care Introduce shared decision-making
Safety (usually to prevent a complication)	Medication errors Hospital-acquired infections—central line infections, surgical site infections, and ventilator-acquired pneumonia Deterioration Falls Delirium Psychological safety Handovers
Efficiency	Lean approach to equipment Standardized blood-taking trolley Clinics starting and ending on time Operations starting on time Reducing duplication of blood tests
Effectiveness	Protocols are followed Care bundles are followed
Timely care	No delays in appointments Decreasing waiting time in emergency departments
Equitable care	Decreasing disparities in outcomes for LGBT+ Decreasing disparities for ethnic minorities Increasing diversity in the workplace Improving use of interpreting services
Sustainable care	Decreasing use of non-reusable plastics Decreasing use of water and electricity Decreasing carbon footprint of an operating theatre or clinic

Writing a powerful problem statement

A problem statement should communicate why you are doing this improvement work, what the problem is, and why it matters. Most importantly, it needs to demonstrate how the problem impacts the patient. A succinct statement using plain English and avoiding medical terminology is very effective in engaging both staff and patients in your improvement work, to start conversations.

A well-constructed statement should include:

- A description of the problem (factual observation) and its consequences;
- Quantitative data about the problem to connect with their minds (factual consequence);
- Qualitative data about the problem to connect with their emotions (emotional consequence);
- Approximately 25–30 words in short sentences, avoiding abbreviations and medical terminology.
- In Table 17.2 a case study on defining a problem is described.

Box 17.2 Defining a problem

Mohamed was frustrated with poor-quality weekend handovers. He wrote the following problem statement:

'*Weekend handover is inconsistent, unstructured, informal, and untraceable. Time is wasted, essential tasks are missed, patient safety is compromised, and healthcare professionals are left frustrated.*'

Pooja noticed that there were delays with administration of medication in her inpatient unit, causing patients to fall. Her problem statement was: '*Our patient's medications are time-critical. Delays are life-threatening. In the last month, at least three patients fell and in the last year, one patient died as a result.*'

Using 5Ps to improve clinical microsystems

- In Chapter 12, the concept of the clinical microsystem was introduced. In a complex adaptive system, these are the building blocks of a healthcare organization.
- It is likely that you will be improving your clinical microsystem (i.e. care provided by your team or department).
- The 5Ps framework can help examine the microsystem, to build an understanding across the teams and help select areas for improvement.

In Table 17.3, an example is provided as to how you can apply the 5Ps to your project (see Chapter 12).

Table 17.3 Application of the 5Ps method

Focus	Action	Example: cystic fibrosis outpatient clinics
Purpose	By writing a purpose statement, the team may discuss their shared goal and aim	To enable people with cystic fibrosis to live as normal a life as possible
Patients	Sharing knowledge of your patient population, the demographics, and their experience of care is important for all members of the microsystem team	A patient survey showed that the psychologist's and social worker's availability fall on different days of the week but could be combined to save extra trips to the hospital
Professionals	Every member of the microsystem team who contributes to the care of patients should be regarded as a professional, and learning more about the staff is important. Staff surveys are actually a good way to find out what would make the care better for patients	More flexible appointment times would improve working efficiency and reduce waiting times for patients
Processes	An opportunity for the team to review different processes of patient care by mapping, exploring interactions, and measuring how long the process steps take. The team rarely has time to review these and consider different views and perspectives	Understanding the process for admission from outpatient clinics, including the supporting microsystems such as physiotherapy, pharmacy, radiology, and microbiology
Patterns	There are patterns in every microsystem, but these are often unnoticed. It is helpful to look at outcome measures and trends over time, and the team should meet regularly to review these patterns to improve care	Weekly multidisciplinary team meetings to discuss patients attending clinics and explore social patterns within the microsystem, and team improvement meetings to discuss outcome measures such as number of days of home intravenous antibiotics a year

Stroke is the leading cause of long-term disability in developed countries and one of the top causes of mortality worldwide. With the introduction of thrombolysis and thrombectomy, the outcome has improved dramatically and early identification of people who would benefit from the treatment is essential so that they can be transferred to a stroke treatment centre and/or treatment can be initiated.

What is the theoretical basis?

In the case of acute stroke, every 9 minutes of delay will damage 1% of the brain and have an impact on long-term recovery. The aim is to have the door-to-decision time for thrombolysis or thrombectomy within 30 minutes of arrival in the emergency department.

Problem statement

Time is brain cells when a person has a stroke. Arrival in hospital to decision time for thrombolysis needs to be less than 30 minutes for the patient to avoid brain damage.

Microsystem assessment

In most hospitals, there were up to nine different microsystems which were required to come together to ensure all the steps were minimized. From the time of the stroke to the decision to treat, these microsystems need to interact with each other at the same time as they have to attend to all their other priorities: patient—ambulance—emergency department—computed tomography—stroke team.

Each of these was composed of smaller microsystems that were required to synchronize.

This QI project example is based on a Stroke Collaborative conducted in Ireland by the Royal College of Physicians (RCPI).

Signposting

Institute for Excellence in Health and Social Systems. (2023) Generic Microsystem Workbooks. Available at: https://clinicalmicrosystem.org/knowledge-center/workbooks (accessed 10 September 2023).

Sheffield Coaching Academy (2019) Microsystem one page books. Available at: https://www.sheffieldmca.org.uk/members/category/7 (accessed 10 September 2023)

How to study and analyse the process

It is important to understand how and why a problem has arisen before you start to tackle it.
- A common mistake is to jump to potential solutions, but you will risk tackling the symptoms of the problem, and not the root cause.
- It is useful for a range of staff and patients to help with this crucial step and that you take time to gather the right data.

Here are some tools which may be relevant to your problem.

Process mapping

In → Chapter 13, the methods for process mapping were introduced. It can help a team understand both individual steps and the process as a whole.
- The first step is to define the start and end points of the process to be mapped, so it is manageable.
- It is important for the team, including all stakeholders if possible, to identify the steps in the process, as one individual rarely understands all the steps.

QI project example: improving stroke care, part 2: Mapping the process

Key people in the different microsystems came together to map the process, first using Post-it notes, so that they could visualize what really happened (Figure 17.2).

Swim lane diagrams have the benefit of dividing the process into 'lanes', illustrating who is responsible for certain actions.

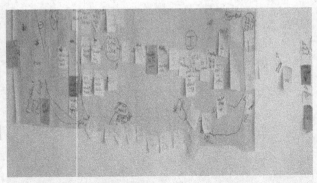

Figure 17.2 Mapping the process.

A swim lane map showed where the handoffs are and who has responsibility for each stage (Figure 17.3).

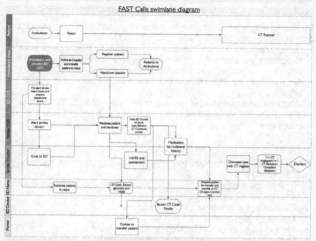

Figure 17.3 Process map for the stroke pathway.
Reproduced with permission from James Murphy © xcUH.

Patient journey mapping

One of the best ways for the team to really understand a problem from the patient's perspective is through mapping the patient journey.

- The patient is usually the only person who has experienced the whole process, so this can help a team understand, sometimes for the first time, how complicated the system can be for patients (such as number of waits, visits, and different people they meet).
- It can help plan effectively where to test ideas for improvement that are likely to have the greatest impact.
- Mapping is best done as a fun interactive event, with sufficient planning to engage senior leaders (or sponsors), change agents (respected staff who facilitate change and provide expertise), champions, and the patient group whose care would benefit most from redesign.
- An independent facilitator is useful to ask challenging questions without risking a breakdown in working relationships, and to create a safe environment to encourage honesty.
- By making the event practical, visual, and fun, it may generate lots of comments and ideas, but do not be tempted to solve problems until you have fully mapped and analysed the patient journey.

Top tips
- Take photos.
- Display the process map in offices/staff rooms for further comment.
- Make process mapping a frontline ownership event.

Waste walk tool

Eliminating waste while focusing on value for our patients is an important part of quality improvement (see ⊃ Chapter 14).
- For an activity to be considered as 'adding value', it should be of value to patients, transform the service in some way, and be correct the first time (e.g. diagnostic time or treatment intervention).
- Activities such as wait time and duplicate tests are 'non-value-added' activities.
- Waste consumes resources without adding value (Box 17.3), so if we eliminate waste, we will have more resources with which to work more effectively.

Box 17.3 Waste mnemonic: TRIMWOOD

TRIMWOOD is a mnemonic to remember the eight types of waste (see ⊃ Chapter 11):
1. **T**ransportation (e.g. patients moving to multiple appointments due to test results not being available);
2. **R**esource (e.g. equipment used infrequently);
3. **I**nventory (e.g. overstocked items);
4. **M**otion (e.g. equipment located far from the ward area);
5. **W**aiting (e.g. patients waiting for appointments);
6. **O**verproduction (e.g. unnecessary blood tests);
7. **O**verprocessing (e.g. chasing up appointments);
8. **D**efects (e.g. medication errors).

- The longer we work in a team or department, the easier it is to accept things and not see waste, but taking a 'waste walk' is a way to make waste visible again.
- The tool is a quick and easy way to identify areas for improvement; individuals or groups can complete a template to note down examples of the eight types of waste, as they walk around their department, asking questions such as '*Is the space underutilized?*' and '*Is equipment sitting idle in the corridor?*'.
- It is useful to include patients or someone from another department with a fresh pair of eyes.
- In Table 17.4 the elements of the Gemba waste walk are described.

Table 17.4 Gemba waste walk

Type of waste	Example	Possible cause	Action
Transportation	Multiple appointments for cardiology test results which are not yet available	Delay in test result reporting in cardiology due to physiologist vacancy	Prioritize test result sign-off by remaining physiologists to reduce the wait
Overproduction	Duplicate recording of information on admission to day-case unit	Information entered in the healthcare assistant's (HCA) notes, nursing records, and medical clerking	Streamline admission paperwork to avoid duplication
Inventory	Storing excessive medication on the ward, resulting in out-of-date medicines	Pharmacy supplies medication to the ward weekly without stock check-in	Monitor quantities of medication daily/weekly, and supply only those in short supply
Overprocessing	Chasing up appointments for referrals to dieticians	Referral pathway to dieticians is unclear, and inbox is not monitored, resulting in lost referrals	Improve referral pathway and acknowledge referrals with appointment date
Waiting	Patients waiting after scheduled arrival time for appointment	Clinic time slots are not appropriate or matched to clinical need	Improve clinic scheduling with clinician input
Motion	Nurses walk to the adjacent ward to locate ECG machine at least twice a day	Only one ECG machine available for all three wards	Locate ECG machine on the ward that uses it most frequently or at a central location (if no resource to purchase additional machines)
Defects	Wrong medications for asthma discharge	Unclear guideline for asthma discharges	Asthma medication discharge checklist led by asthma nurses
Underutilized skills	Poorly designed ambulatory unit with only one sink	No nursing or medical input into the design	Multidisciplinary team engagement for future plans of clinical areas

Waste identification

The focus was to decrease waiting between each step in the process.
- The stroke teams at each site looked carefully at the process and analysed how they could take out unnecessary waiting.
- They found that many of the processes could move from being sequential to being done at the same time; for example, during transport to hospital, the paramedical team could stabilize the patient, do the registrations, take baseline blood tests, and obtain consent for the computed tomography scan.

Value stream mapping

Value stream mapping visualizes every step or action required to complete a process from start to finish. By mapping the flow of information or materials, improvements can be identified to optimize flow by reducing waste or increasing speed.

The first step (the patient has a stroke and the ambulance is called) is represented by a rectangle and the total time the patient spends at this step (the cycle time) (Figure 17.4). Value added (VA) is when something happens (e.g. paramedics taking blood and stabilizing).

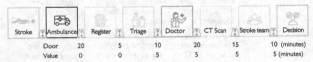

	Stroke	Ambulance	Register	Triage	Doctor	CT Scan	Stroke team	Decision
Door		20	5	10	20	15		10 (minutes)
Value		0	0	5	5	5		5 (minutes)

Figure 17.4 Value stream for the stroke pathway.

Non-value added is time waiting

At the hospital, each time waiting is broken down into VA where action is taken, and non-value added (NVA) where patients are waiting. The yellow triangles between each step show how much time the patient waits for the next process to take place. In a stroke project, the aim is to reduce NVA, so that the total time in the process from registration to decision is less than 30 minutes.

The VA time is calculated as how long it takes to complete each step. Decreasing to zero means that step could be eliminated and can be done simultaneously, for example:
- In the ambulance before the clock starts, the paramedics do the triage and preregistration and take blood samples;
- Triage and first assessment and consent are done together;
- The only fixed rate-limiting step is performing the computed tomography scan, which can be read as it is being performed, so a decision can be made.

Signposting

East London Foundation Trust QI Programme (2023). Understanding the problem. Available at: https://qi.elft.nhs.uk/collection/understanding-the-problem/ (accessed 10 September 2023)
NHS Institute for Innovation and Improvement (2005). Process mapping, analysis and redesign. Available at: https://www.england.nhs.uk/improvement-hub/wp-content/uploads/sites/44/2017/11/ILG-1.2-Process-Mapping-Analysis-and-Redesign.pdf (accessed 10 September 2023)
NHS England (2017) Bringing Lean to Life. Available at: https://www.england.nhs.uk/improvement-hub/wp-content/uploads/sites/44/2017/11/Bringing-Lean-to-Life.pdf (accessed 10 September 2023)

How to analyse the process

Analysis of the process requires the team to come together in a safe environment to study the process they have mapped and to assess why there is variation in the process. This requires the use of the techniques discussed in ⮕ Chapters 10 and 13.

Appreciative inquiry

(See ⮕ Chapter 10.)

Appreciative inquiry methods can be used to draw out what is working and what can work better if the team were to change the process.

- It is always a good idea to have a positive approach to solving problems.
- The aim is to draw on the strengths of the team and on what is working well.
- This will allow the team to discuss what could be better, what needs to be done to be better, and how to achieve better outcomes.
- This will develop a shared ownership of the problem and the solution.

QI project example: improving stroke care, part 6—appreciative inquiry

Twelve teams in each collaborative came together and used appreciative inquiry to develop solutions:

- *Discovery*: the teams explored where the best practice was happening in order to identify and appreciate '*what best is*'. For example, one team held simulated patient journeys on a regular basis.
- *Dream*: each team then discussed '*what might be*'—how the service could look after the interventions, with every person with a stroke assessed within 30 minutes of arrival.
- *Design*: the teams then designed the process based on their vision of '*what might be*', as well as on their assessment of '*what best is*', and with review of the value stream map and process map, a new process could be developed, which was appropriate for their own context.
- *Destiny*: the teams designed the new process—'*what can be*'—and also used co-production methods, so that all staff and patients were part of the solution rather than part of the problem.

Six Thinking Hats

(See ⮕ Chapter 11.)

As the process is analysed, the method of using thinking hats can be used to involve different members of your team to analyse, debate, and challenge the proposed solutions within a safe environment (Box 17.4).

Box 17.4 Example of Six Thinking Hats in use

The ambulatory unit is considering a new initiative of direct paramedic referral of patients in the community, rather than the existing pathway of referral via the emergency department (ED) after initial assessment and ED nurse triage. The team decided to meet to discuss, as there are different viewpoints and perspectives.

The Six Thinking Hats approach is chosen, so everyone thinks in parallel by using only one hat at a time:

1. *Blue hat*: the leader of the session manages the time, keeps the group focused, and actively contributes to the thinking associated with one hat at a time, then summarizes findings and what happens next;
2. *White hat*: what data do we have or need? (e.g. number of paramedic referrals to the ED and number of those that are safe to refer to the ambulatory unit (following triage), or time of day of referrals);
3. *Black hat*: what could go wrong? What are the disadvantages? (e.g. discussion of the risks of direct referral of patients to the ambulatory unit and governance of the new initiative);
4. *Yellow hat*: consideration of all the benefits (e.g. improving flow in the ED, improving patient experience);
5. *Green hat*: is there a different way of looking at this? How could the idea be further developed? (e.g. discussion of alternative approaches such as doctor telephone referral/advice, primary care or community nursing support);
6. *Red hat*: how do you feel about this? What is your gut feeling? For example, this is an innovative and exciting initiative, but we need to consider governance of the process carefully and the impact on other ambulatory unit activities and staffing.

- The Six Thinking Hats method encourages the group to try on other hats, so those with entrenched views may consider the idea from different perspectives.
- It is a very good way to generate ideas and build a common purpose for the project.

The 5 Whys

(See ⮕ Chapter 13.)

A method from the Lean methodology, the 5 Whys can be a quick and useful way to do a mini-root cause analysis of why the process is working or why it is not working (Box 17.5). The theory is that by asking a question five times (as a rule of thumb), one usually reaches the root cause of the problem or of the success.

Joanne is an anaesthetics trainee who is frustrated that she misses her lunchtime teaching every week because her morning operating list overruns:
- The theatre 1 operating list always overruns. *Why?*
- There is a long delay between patients on the list. *Why?*
- The porters do not collect the patients on time when called. *Why?*
- The porters cannot find a spare trolley. *Why?*
- Many of the theatre 1 trolley safety rails are broken. *Why?* (and so forth)

- It can be a very good learning tool for team members if used carefully. It was developed by Toyota as part of problem-solving training for their production system.
- However, problems are often more complex and require both depth and breadth analysis, so this approach may oversimplify the process of problem exploration. This risks a single root cause as a target for solutions.
- As noted in ⟳ Chapter 13, the tool must be used carefully, so that a simplistic analysis is avoided.
- Using an appreciative inquiry approach may be helpful to elicit the root cause.

QI project example: improving stroke care, part 7—the '5 Whys'

The team at one hospital wanted to find out how they could decrease the time waited by a patient to be assessed by the stroke team.
- The patient arrived without warning. *Why?*
- The paramedics called the hospital switchboard, but the message did not get through. *Why?*
- The switchboard paged only the middle-grade doctor on call. *Why?*
- The middle-grade doctor on call did not respond to the page. *Why?*
- Their bleep was not working. *Why?* (and so forth)

Cause-and-effect diagram/fishbone

In ⟳ Chapter 13 where variation was discussed, a 'cause-and-effect', or 'fishbone', diagram is designed to help teams identify all the possible causes of a problem, not just the obvious ones, and uncover the root causes (Box 17.6).
- It is a visual tool to help categorize the potential causes of a problem, with the problem/effect displayed at the head of the fish, a central spine, then several branches representing different categories like the skeleton of a fish.
- It is good to use the elements of the work system in the Systems Engineering Initiative for Patient Safety (SEIPS) model (see ⟳

Anna designed this fishbone diagram to look at the causes of a long waiting time for review in an outpatient clinic (Figure 17.5).

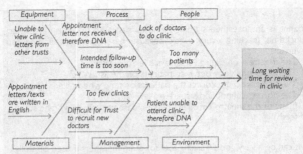

Figure 17.5 Example of a fishbone analysis.
Quality Improvement Clinic Ltd.

Chapters 12 and 14) as the main headings for each branch of the
diagram. This also incorporates the 5Ps and ensures a systems approach
is undertaken in assessing the process:

- Organization;
- Environment;
- Tools and technology;
- Tasks to be completed;
- People—the staff;
- People—the patients.

**QI project example: improving stroke care, part 8
Fishbone Analysis**

The stroke pathway can be analysed using a cause and effect or fishbone
diagram as shown in Figure 17.6. This will allow you to determine which
problems meed to be addressed.
(See Figure 17.6.)

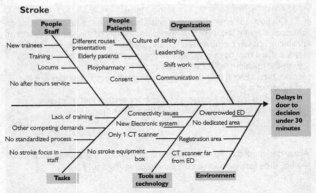

Figure 17.6 Fishbone analysis for the stroke pathway.

Pareto charts

(See ➔ Chapter 13.)

Once a process has been analysed, the problems identified as contributing to the outcome are organized into a Pareto chart, which is a bar chart, in descending order of frequency (see ➔ Chapter 13).

- The Pareto chart allows you to identify the most significant causes (the vital few) of the problem and where the improvement team can concentrate their change ideas (Box 17.7).
- It is similar to the way you would arrange the possible causes in a differential diagnosis, as common causes are first excluded, rather than starting with the rare ones.

Box 17.7 A Pareto chart example.

In this project the aim was to improve the time doctors were leaving at the end of the day so that they could keep to the agreed working hours. Hajera identified the causes that were responsible for her colleagues leaving work late using a Pareto chart as shown in Figure 17.7. She focused her change ideas on the most significant identified problem.

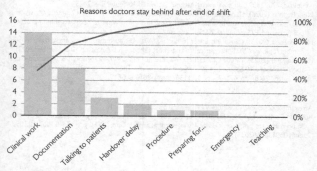

Figure 17.7 Example of a Pareto analysis.
Quality Improvement Clinic Ltd.

QI project example: improving stroke care, part 9

In the stroke project, the teams looked at where the most delays were occurring and used the Pareto chart to decide where to start (Figure 17.8).

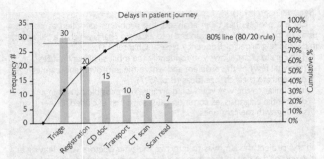

Figure 17.8 Pareto for the stroke pathway.

Signposting

NHS England (2023). Six Thinking Hats® Available at: https://www.england.nhs.uk/wp-content/uploads/2022/02/qsir-six-thinking-hats.pdf (accessed 10 September 2023).

NHS England (2023). Using five whys to review a simple problem. Available at: https://www.england.nhs.uk/wp-content/uploads/2022/02/qsir-using-five-whys-to-review-a-simple-problem.pdf (accessed 10 September 2023).

NHS England (2023). Cause and Effect (fishbone). Available at: https://www.england.nhs.uk/wp-content/uploads/2021/12/qsir-cause-and-effect-fishbone.pdf (accessed 10 September 2023).

NHS England (2023). Pareto Chart Tool. Available at: https://www.england.nhs.uk/pareto-chart-tool/ (accessed 10 September 2023).Card, A.J. (2016). The problem with '5 Whys'. *BMJ Quality and Safety*, 26(8), pp. 671–7. doi: 10.1136/bmjqs-2016-005849.

Further reading

An example of appreciative inquiry in a general practice:

Ruhe, M.C., Bobiak, S.N., Litaker, D., et al. (2011). Appreciative inquiry for quality improvement in primary care practices. *Quality Management in Health Care*, 20(1), pp. 37–48. doi: 10.1097/qmh.0b013e31820311be.

How to involve and engage staff

In ⟩ Chapters 10 and 11, the theories and methods that one can use to engage staff in an improvement project were discussed. This is a vital part of any improvement project and runs through the whole process. In essence, it is building the desire or *will* for change, so that people involved in the process are part of the solution, not the problem.

The key points are:

- Focus on *what really matters* to people—the *why* they come to work;
- Concentrate on the positives, rather than focusing only on what has to be changed;
- Create a vision for change, and create early wins;
- Always celebrate success;
- Build agency by using an appreciative inquiry approach;
- Tools such as Liberating Structures (https://www.liberatingstructures.com/) can assist (see ⟩ Chapter 11).

The following improvement tools can help you in the assessment of how people are going to respond to change.

Stakeholder mapping

Stakeholder mapping allows you to assess who has influence that may impact the success of the project. This will allow you to consider what actions are needed to ensure the project is successful.

- A 3 × 3 table may be used, as shown in Figure 17.9.
- Consider all people who may be involved or affected by the project, both staff and patients.
- Then make an assessment where they are in terms of influence and support. For example, a consultant may have high influence, but low support; a trainee may have less influence, but more support, etc.

The next step is to translate the influence map into an action plan, as indicated in QI project example, part 10.

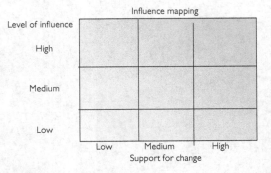

Figure 17.9 Influence or stakeholder map.

QI project example: improving stroke care, part 10

(See Figure 17.10).

This approach allows you to pre-empt problems, and by using the methods from ➲ Chapters 10 and 11, you engage effectively with the people involved in the process.

Stakeholder	Level of support	Level of influence	Key concern	Steps to get buy in
Nurses	Medium	medium	More work No time	Involve in service redesign
Trainee doctors	Low	Low to medium	Rotation does not allow involvement	Regular updates
Consultants	Medium	High	No evidence it wil work	Have a consultant champion Communication and data
Registration staff	Low	Low	No time	Ensure the workload issues are addressed, involve in planning

Figure 17.10 Stakeholder map.

Readiness assessment

A readiness assessment can also be undertaken by using the readiness tool, as discussed in ➲ Chapter 4. Readiness assessments aim to understand the factors that facilitate, or are barriers to, change so that implementation can be successful.

Diffusion of innovation

Diffusion of innovation postulates that there is a normal distribution of people who range from innovators to those who oppose change (Figure 17.11). The theory is that there are five groups of people and that one should assess the people in the team, so that your change approach can be adapted. This is reflected in the stakeholder analysis of the level of support.

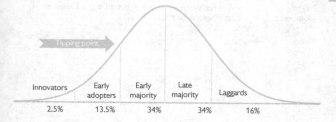

Figure 17.11 Rogers' diffusion of innovation.

- *Innovators* like change.
- *Early adopters* first want to see the change work, and then they will try it for themselves.
- The *early majority* will make a change when they see it works well and the implementation problems have been resolved. When this starts, it is called the *tipping point* and the innovation will soon become the way in which work is done.
- The *late majority* will adopt the change once it has been implemented by the early majority.
- Finally the *laggards* are the small number of people who only change when there is no other alternative.

It is useful to undertake this assessment at various stages during the project. People can move between different groups, depending on how much the innovation matters to them. In ⊃ Chapter 11, how to develop the clinical team was discussed. As you start your project, consider who the project members will be. In Table 17.5, the team members for the stroke project are shown.

Table 17.5 Quality team members in the stroke project

Clinical leadership	The stroke team requires a consultant responsible for stroke management
Technical expertise	Technical expertise is provided by members from different parts of the pathway: <ul><li>Paramedics</li><li>Registration</li><li>Triage and emergency department</li><li>Computed tomography radiographer and radiologist</li><li>Stroke nurse</li><li>Improvement lead</li></ul>
Day-to-day leadership	The lead for the project could be the stroke nurse and registrar who oversee the data collection and implementation of change on a daily basis. They work closely with the other team members to address issues at each step in the pathway
Patient	A person who has experienced the pathway is a valuable member of the team
Project sponsorship	The sponsor is the clinical director for the division or an executive director

Adapted from ᕫ www.ihi.org.

Signposting

NHS England (2023). Stakeholder analysis. Available at https://www.england.nhs.uk/wp-content/uploads/2022/02/qsir-stakeholder-analysis.pdf (accessed 10 September 2023)

Wanderman Center (2019) Readiness Thinking Tool (RTT). Available at: https://www.wandersmancenter.org/using-readiness.html (accessed 10 September 2023)

Health Foundation (2015) Communications in health care improvement - a toolkit. Available at: https://www.health.org.uk/publications/communications-in-health-care-improvement-a-toolkit (accessed 10 September 2023)

Liberating Structures. Available at: https://www.liberatingstructures.com/ (accessed 10 September 2023)

How to involve patients

The importance of co-production cannot be overemphasized and has been discussed in ⊃ Chapters 2, 8, 11, and 14. An improvement project should:

- Address what matters to the people who receive care, as well as what matters to the providers of care;
- Invite, if possible, a patient representative to be an equal and active member of the project team. They may ask questions that may not appear apparent to the service provider such as '*Why are you doing it this way?*' or '*Is this really person-centred?*';
- Ensure that you are inclusive and responsive to any suggestion made if you include patients;
- Make sure that you are improving *what really matters* to the patients and their families;
- Be realistic and not promote or promise something you cannot deliver;
- Not compromise on being truthful as to what can be improved and what can be achieved.

Ideally, co-production of solutions, as described in ⊃ Chapters 2, 11, and 14, will result in a person-centred solution to your project. This will involve working with user groups to redesign a service. The co-production ladder can help you decide how far you are on the co-production journey in your project (Figure 17.12).

Experience-based design, as described in ⊃ Chapter 14, is a specific methodology that builds improvement on the lived experience of users and providers of a service.

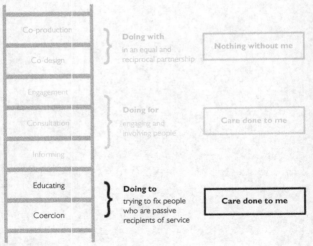

Figure 17.12 The co-production ladder.

Adapted with permission from ℐ℗ https://www.thinklocalactpersonal.org.uk/co-production-in-commissioning-tool/co-production/In-more-detail/what-makes-co-production-different/ (accessed 3 January 2023).

Top tips

Summary

Acknowledgements

Top tips

- Do not come with a preconceived solution to a problem, as this may not be the solution. Use the domains of quality to identify where you want to improve.
- Study the process where the problem has been identified.
- Involve staff and patients when you study the process, as this can build the desire to change.
- When studying the process, measure the baseline.
- Analyse the process with a fishbone/cause-and-effect diagram and then represent the causes on a Pareto chart.

Summary

Quality improvement is one part of quality management. As discussed in ⊃ Chapter 3, when approaching a quality improvement initiative, there are three steps, as part of the Juran Trilogy.

The first step is to plan:
- What is the problem?
- Why is it a problem—study the process?
- What do patients think?
- What do staff think?

The second step is to set controls:
- Do we have baseline data, and if not, how do we obtain the data?

The third step is to improve:
- Once we have identified and analysed the problem, we can move to the improvement process, which is discussed in ⊃ Chapter 17.

Acknowledgements

Thank you to London School of Paediatrics doctors in training Dr Anna Rzeskiewicz and Dr Hajera Sheikh for use of their quality improvement project examples, supported by © Quality Improvement Clinic Ltd. 2022. Reproduced with permission.

Application of QI methods

Key points

- Quality improvement projects must follow a rigorous methodology.
- The hypothesis for change—what needs to be done to achieve the outcome—is presented in a driver diagram.
- Methods commonly used are the Model for Improvement, Lean, and Six Sigma, all of which will have a Plan–Do–Study–Act (PDSA) learning cycle as part of the method.
- A test of change—PDSA—will always have a prediction to be tested.
- Measurement is essential to know that any change is an improvement.
- PDSA cycles can never be too small but can be too big.

Introduction

In ⊃ Chapter 17, the first five steps in the improvement process were described. Once you have identified the problem, studied the process, and looked for opportunities to improve, then one can move on to the improvement process.

In this chapter, we will discuss how to improve, based on the theories from ⊃ Chapter 17. The improvement theory and method are based on viewing the improvement process through the four *Lenses of Profound Knowledge* (see ⊃ Chapter 3):

- Understand the *system*;
- Identify and study *variation* within the system;
- Consider the *psychology*—how people behave;
- Have a theory of change—*knowledge*.

The lenses have been considered in previous chapters. In this chapter, we will consider the Lens of Knowledge (how to change) in the steps of the improvement process, as indicated in in Figure17.1 (part 1) and Figure 18.1 (part 2). The steps often take place concurrently.

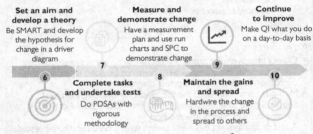

Figure 18.1 Steps to do a quality improvement project, part 2.

How to do your improvement project

How to do your improvement project

In any improvement project, once the problem has been identified and the potential opportunities for improvement recognized, the aim of the project must be formulated. The Model for Improvement is the method used widely (Figure 18.2), as discussed in ➲ Chapter 14.

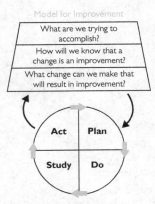

Figure 18.2 Model for Improvement.

Aim statement

'Aims Create Systems.'

W. Edwards Deming

The aim of the project will guide the project and should cover its scope. It is similar to the hypothesis of a research project. There are three steps to take, as shown in Table 18.1:

Table 18.1 Forming an aim statement

1. Decide on the purpose	Decide on the purpose of the project and which domain of quality is the focus
2. Frame the extent	Decide on the extent of the change—how much do you want to change?
3. Focus the aim	Write a SMART aim statement, including one or more of the following: • Safety: 'Decrease harm …' • Person-centredness: 'Improve experience …' • Effectiveness: 'Increase reliability …' • Equity: 'Improve provision …' • Timeliness: 'Reduce waiting …' • Efficiency: 'Reduce waste …' • Ecological: 'Improve sustainability …'

The components of a SMART aim statement are shown on Table 18.2. When you construct a SMART aim, the construct shown in Box 18.1 can be used.

Table 18.2 Components of an aim statement

Specific	States where it will happen and in which population group—a defined scope
Measurable	If you cannot measure it, then you cannot show there is an improvement
Actionable and Achievable	If you cannot implement the initiative, then it cannot be done—this is where tools such as the readiness test and stakeholder analysis are important
Relevant	Must address what really matters to patients and staff
Timely	Must have a specific time frame

Box 18.1 Construct of a SMART aim statement

We will increase/decrease: _____(outcome)
from: _____(baseline %, rate, #, etc.)
to: _____(future state %, rate, #, etc.)
by: _____(date, 3- to 6-month time frame)
in: _____(population impacted)
where: _____(place and context)

To decrease the door-to-decision time for thrombolysis or thrombectomy from 135 minutes to less than 30 minutes from arrival at the emergency department front door for all people with stroke by 1 December
2023 at hospital XYZ.

For the aim, keep it simple and do not include the intervention in the aim,
as that may change over time.
- Seek usefulness over perfection, as aims change.
- Formulate aims as a team, so that there is a shared purpose.
- Take the aim of testing with others to see if it makes sense.
- Have a definition for every term and measure.
- Ask whether you are aiming to optimize (first-order change) an existing
  system, or whether you should consider redesigning (second-order
  change) a new one.
- In Box 18.2 examples of Aim statements are provided.

Box 18.2 Example of an aim statement

Once you have a succinct problem statement, it can be converted easily
into an aim statement by using the construct shown in Box 18.1.

Melody's problem statement
'We cause distress (and blood loss) to babies who we are supposed to be
looking after by doing frequent blood tests that could be avoided.'

The problem statement leads to this aim statement
'To reduce the number of rejected group and save blood samples taken on
babies on the neonatal unit from 12 per week to less than 8 per week by 1st
February 2020.'

Quality Improvement Clinic Ltd.

Driver diagrams

Driver diagrams help an improvement team to visualize which 'drivers' are
required in order for the goal of their improvement aim to be realized (e.g.
'reducing deep vein thrombosis ...') (Figure 18.3; Box 18.3).
- The aim underpinning a driver diagram should be SMART.
- Drivers are considered within different levels:
  - *Primary drivers* are the overarching driving forces required for the aim
    to be achieved (e.g. prevention of deep vein thrombosis);
  - *Secondary drivers* feed into primary drivers; these are more specific
    and may relate to one or more primary drivers (e.g. education of
    healthcare professionals);
  - *Change ideas* are smaller-scale, practical, achievable changes that
    can be made into a process or system to facilitate the primary and
    secondary drivers (e.g. targeted e-learning course).

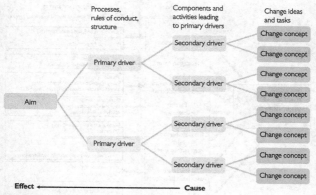

Figure 18.3 Format of a driver diagram.

Driver diagrams:

- Provide the hypothesis for change—your theory of what must be done to achieve the aim;
- Break a broad aim graphically into increasing levels of detailed actions that must or could be done to achieve the stated aim;
- Encourage the team to expand their thinking;
- Keep thinking linked with the overall aim;
- Allow participants and reviewers to see the logical links and completeness at every level of the plan;
- Support the development of measures to be embedded in the diagram;
- Encourage the development of measures at the early stages;
- Require operational definitions.

The driver diagram in Figure 18.4 is an example of a high-level hypothesis for what is required to achieve safety on a paediatric ward. Each primary driver will then become a subsequent driver diagram, with its own aim and hypothesis for change (Box 18.4).

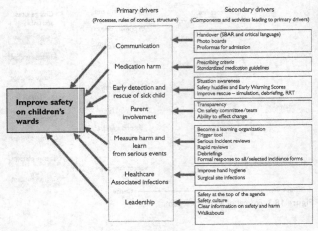

Primary drivers
(Processes, rules of conduct, structure)

Secondary drivers
(Components and activities leading to primary drivers)

Figure 18.4 Example of a global driver diagram.

Box 18.4 Example of a hypothesis for change

The driver diagram in the QI project example in Figure 18.5 shows how one can develop a hypothesis for a focused programme. In Figure 18.5, the problem was the high level of prescribing rates for sedative medications in this General Practice (GP). The aim was to reduce the total amount of sedative medications prescribed by 66% in all patients attending the GP centre by 1 July 2020. This outcome measure represents a reduction in the total number of milligrams of the six most commonly prescribed sedative medications (diazepam, alprazolam, temazepam, lormetazepam, zopiclone, and zolpidem). The theory of change was developed and presented in a driver diagram.

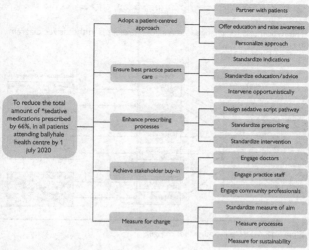

Figure 18.5 Example of a theory of change for a focused problem.

QI Project example: improving stroke care, part 12: How to do your improvement project

The hypothesis for change in the stroke project is in the driver diagram in Figure 18.6.

(See Figure 18.6.)

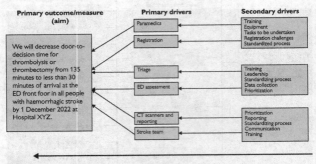

Figure 18.6 Stroke hypothesis for change.

Signposting

Bennett, B., Provost, L. (2015) What's your Theory? Available at https://www.apiweb.org/QP_whats-your-theory_201507.pdf (accessed 10 September 2023).

How to use data and interventions

How to use data and measurement

(See ⊃ Chapters 13 and 15.)

The second question in the Model for Improvement asks the question 'How will you know that the change you test has made a difference?'. Unless one measures the impact of the test or intervention over time, one cannot answer this question.

In ⊃ Chapter 13, the measurement of variation is discussed, and in ⊃ Chapter 15, the development of a measurement plan and how to measure are explained. Patient-focused measures are discussed in ⊃ Chapter 16. In Box 18.5 the different types of measures are described.

Box 18.5 Types of measures

1. *Outcome* measures are usually what happen to the patient or the system. These are in the SMART aim statement and in the driver diagram.
2. *Process* measures are measures of what you have to change in the system to achieve the desired outcome. In the driver diagram, they are usually measures of the primary, and sometimes secondary, drivers.
3. *PDSA* measures measure the impact of the test of change. These are iterative and may change as the PDSAs are tested.
4. *Balancing* measures include positive or negative unintended consequences of the intervention.
5. *Sustainable* measures indicate the impact the intervention has on the environment (⊃ Chapter 5).
6. *Equity* measures ensure all is improving (⊃ Chapter 6).
7. *Economic and/or financial* measures indicate the cost-effectiveness or cost benefit of the intervention (⊃ Chapter 7).
8. *Patient-reported* measures measure experience (PREM) and outcome (PROM) (⊃ Chapter 8).

Choosing measures

For your improvement project:
- Study the process and measure baseline data before you start.
- The aim statement will have the outcome measure.
- The outcome measure may be a process measure as well (if you are improving a process), but remember that the purpose of improvement is to improve outcomes for the people in the system.
- Ask which measures are required, so that you develop a series of measures—usually one outcome measure, 4–5 process measures, and 1–2 balancing measures.
- When designing the project measurement plan, ask whether there is any chance that there may be a disproportionate impact on a group of patients. If this is a possibility, for example, the intervention may not benefit a person from a different ethnic background or from the LGBT+ community as much as a person from the dominant population group, you need to segment the data, as discussed in ⊃ Chapter 6.

Displaying measures

In ⊃ Chapters 13 and 15, the ways in which you can display measures were discussed.
- In most cases, either annotated run charts or a safety cross will tell the story of your improvement project (Box 18.6).

- Sometimes an annotated statistical process control (SPC) chart will be a better option.
- Always include people's stories as a part of the measure display.

Box 18.6 Measures and a run chart example

It is important to define the measure carefully, so it can be replicated by others, and document the Plan–Do–Study–Act (PDSA) cycles, as demonstrated in this example (Figure 18.7).

Quality Improvement Clinic Ltd.

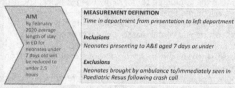

AIM
By February 2020 average length of stay in ED for neonates under 7 days old will be reduced to under 2.5 hours

MEASUREMENT DEFINITION
Time in department from presentation to left department

Inclusions
Neonates presenting to A&E aged 7 days or under

Exclusions
Neonates brought by ambulance to/immediately seen in Paediatric Resus following crash call

PDSA Test #	PLAN	DO	STUDY	ACT
1a	**Information sharing:** Highlighting problem to departmental lead & neonatal registrars	Face-to-face meeting & presentation	Support given, change ideas offered escalated importance of issue in department	Share information with ED team, update change ideas
1b	**Information sharing:** with ED team	Presentation and WhatsApp message	Some reduction in variability in waiting times, idea for clear escalation plan	Build escalation plan with MDT team & prep dissemination
1c	**Idea sharing:** with cross trust peers	Small group presentation & discussion	Increased confidence in presenting issue, confirmation on process taken	Present updated progress to ED/Neonatal team
1d	**Update feedback** to collective MDT at local quality & safety meeting	Presentation with bulletin follow-up	Reduced waiting times following further highlighting of issue, further call for clear escalation plan	Formulate escalation plan
2a	Formulate **escalation plan**	Written escalation plan formulated agreed with all consultants involved	Consensus consultant support gained	Distribute escalation plan to ED & neonatal teams
2b	**Disseminate escalation plan**	Escalation plan presented &placed on shared drive	Escalation plan accepted well and used, some further reduction in length of stay	Keep and reassess
3a	MDT business plan to purchase **Transcutaneous bilirubin machine**	Meet with Consultants ED/Neonates to build business plan for Transcutaneous bilirubinometer	Spare transcutaneous bilirubinometer located and unused in linked department	Implement training for ED nursing staff to implement use
3b	Dissemination of **Transcutaneous bilirubin** for used at ED triage	Demonstration given to ED nurses, user guide sheet written	Transcutaneous bilirubin readings undertaken at triage, communicated to Registrar →reduced length of stay	ED nurses to continue to teach other nurses. Reassess

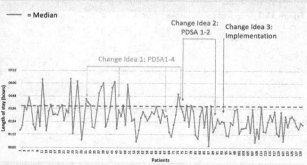

—— = Median

Change Idea 2: PDSA 1-2

Change Idea 3: Implementation

Change Idea 1: PDSA1-4

y-axis: Length of stay (hours) — 07:12, 06:00, 04:48, 03:36, 02:24, 01:12, 00:00

x-axis: Patients

Figure 18.7 Measures and run chart.

- *Outcome*:
  - Percentage of patients seen within 30 minutes of arrival in the emergency department (ED);
  - Experience of the patients and families with a patient-reported experience measure (PREM)
  - Outcome of the intervention in patients with a patient-reported outcome measure (PROM)
- *Process*: each step of the pathway is measured; the rate-limiting step is the time in the computed tomography (CT) scanner. The process measures will be the time it takes in each step—the cycle time.
- *Balancing*: waiting times of other patients in the ED.
- *Financial*: cost benefit of decreased long-term impact versus investment in the new service?
- *Equity*: assessment of the impact on different patients, based on ethnicity and socio-economic status.
- *Sustainable*: measurement of the carbon footprint of each step, in terms of consumables and use of CT.
- In Figure 18.8 the SPC chart for the stroke project is shown, demonstrating the improvement made.

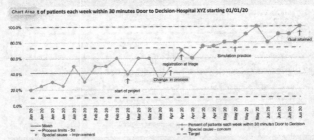

Figure 18.8 SPC chart for the stroke project.

How to test change ideas

In all the methods used in quality improvement and in implementation science, the process of testing changes is fundamental.

There are two types of changes:
- *First-order* changes are incremental changes restoring the equilibrium (e.g. making the system more efficient to produce the same outcomes);
- *Second-order* changes are transformational and change the process and eventual outcome.

The ideas for change will be tested in a Plan–Do–Study–Act (PDSA) cycle. In Box 18.7 a few tips to help you test changes are given.

Box 18.7 Tasks and tests

Top tip

Before you commence on testing, you will need to decide what tasks need to be completed in order to do the test. To be a test, there must be a prediction. It is important to distinguish between the *tasks* that have to be done to prepare for the test and a *test* (PDSA) itself.

For example, if you want to have a new referral form for your clinic, the task will be preparing the form. The test will be the PDSA, where there is a prediction as to whether the form will be used or not, and whether it does what it is intended to do.

Therefore, one needs to prepare before one starts a PDSA cycle.

The PDSA cycle is shown in Figure 18.9

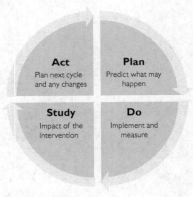

| **Act**
Plan next cycle
and any changes | **Plan**
Predict what may
happen |
| **Study**
Impact of the
intervention | **Do**
Implement and
measure |

Figure 18.9 PDSA cycle.

There are several rules for a PDSA:
- A PDSA can never be too small; hence they are called small tests of change. However, a PDSA can be too large.

- A PDSA must have a prediction; otherwise there is no test.
- A PDSA is about learning and each cycle must add to your understanding of whether the intervention is going to work or not.
- Multiple cycles of PDSAs can be done at the same time.
- In Table 18.3 the different parts of the PDSA cycle are shown.
- Just like a scientific experiment, PDSAs must have a well-defined methodology, be described each time, and carried out in a rigorous fashion.
- In a report on an improvement project, the PDSA must be described to show how the project was conducted.
- PDSA recording is important, so that learning can be documented.

Table 18.3 PDSA

Plan and Predict	*Plan:*
	What tasks need to be undertaken to prepare for the test?
	What is to be tested?
	Who will do the test?
	Where will it be done?
	How will it be measured?
	Predict:
	What will happen?
	Will the test be done?
	Will it work?
Do	The test is implemented.
	Collect the data.
	Ask how it worked.
	Gather information from those doing the test and from others impacted.
Study	Study what happened and assess if it worked or not.
Act	Learn and make changes for the next cycle.

In Box 18.8 an example of how we perform PDSA cycles within clinical practice is described.

Box 18.8 Clinical example of a PDSA

We use PDSAs in clinical practice every time we try an intervention on a patient. For example, if a child presents with petit mal epilepsy, we follow each stage of the cycle.

- *Plan:* prescribe medication; inform the parents of side effects; co-decide on how to measure seizures and how to record them in a seizure diary.
- *Predict:* will the parents give the medication or not? Will there be side effects? Is the dose sufficient to decrease or eliminate the seizures?
- *Do:* the parents give the medication and record seizure activity and any side effects.
- *Study:* the data are reviewed at the follow-up clinic.
- *Act:* the dose is increased or decreased, or the medication changed, depending on the outcome of reviewing what happened.

QI project example: improving stroke care, part 14—testing ideas

Depending on the analysis of the problem, the outcome of the appreciative inquiry, and the co-design of the service, several change ideas could be tested with PDSAs:

- *Ensuring as many steps in the process can be done simultaneously;*
- *Paramedics can take the blood tests prior to arrival;*
- *Paramedics can obtain initial consent;*
- *Registration can be performed simultaneously with the first assessment;*
- *Triage can be eliminated;*
- *Consent for investigation and treatment can be confirmed with the family at the time of the CT.*

Further reading

Reed, J.E. and Card, A.J. (2016). The problem with Plan–Do–Study–Act cycles. *BMJ Quality and Safety*, 25(3), pp. 147–52. doi: 10.1136/bmjqs-2015-005076.

How to maintain the gains made and spread your project to others

Quality improvement initiatives are often difficult to sustain once the initial project has been completed. It is important to include sustainability in the initial planning phase, so that it has a better chance of being hardwired into the system. This means that the new process becomes the way things are done and it is not easy to revert to the old way of doing things.

In ➲ Chapter 4, the theories of implementation science were discussed and they can provide you with methods to facilitate a sustained project.

Sustainability or maintaining the gains has been defined as the extent to which 'an evidence-based intervention can deliver its intended benefits over an extended period of time', either after the improvement process has ended or after external support from the donor agency has been terminated (Rabin et al., 2008).

An intervention may drift (i.e. the outcome is not that which was ideally intended in the testing phase) or there may be a drop of voltage (i.e. the impact lessons over time) (Chambers et al., 2013). It is for this reason that the theories and methods discussed in ➲ Chapter 4 are of relevance.

The sustainability (maintaining gains) model presented in ➲ Chapter 11 provides the factors that are important:

1. The new process needs to fit in with the culture of the organization or team.
2. Support of the organization and clinical leadership are essential.
3. The infrastructure needs to support the intervention.
4. Capability to do the intervention may require training.
5. The new process must have a relative advantage over the old process and be adaptable to the local context.
6. There must be credibility to the benefit of the improvement.
7. The new process should be easier to do—both simple to apply and easy to test.
8. There need to be intrinsic benefits for the people in the process, as well as extrinsic benefits for the patients.
9. The benefits should be easily seen.
10. Measurement of the outcomes are important to demonstrate success.

These factors are also important when you aim to spread the intervention and change to another context.

When one spreads other units, one can also use the diffusion of innovation model that was discussed earlier. Another way to look at it is the classic version of the diffusion bell curve shown in Figure 18.10.

Just as you have individuals who are innovators, as you spread, you will have clinical teams who are early adopters, etc.

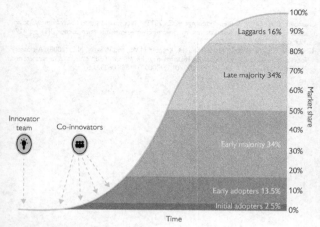

Figure 18.10 Diffusion of innovation.
With permission of Health Foundation.

QI project example: improving stroke care, part 15—spread of ideas

It is important to spread ideas as part of the planning of an improvement project. In the stroke collaborative, there was a gradual development of the spread strategy over the 2 years of the programme.

* *The first teams developed the ideas for the intervention.*
* *Innovator teams were recruited to join the first wave, and they tested and shared ideas.*
* *In subsequent sessions, ideas were cascaded from the innovator teams, so that in time, the lessons from what worked and what did not were spread rapidly.*
* *Concept cafes were held as part of the programme, to facilitate the spread of ideas.*

Signposting

Healthcare Improvement Scotland (2013) Guide on spread and sustainability. Available at: https://www.healthcareimprovementscotland.org/about_us/what_we_do/knowledge_management/knowledge_management_resources/spread_and_sustainability.aspx (accessed 10 September 2023).

NHS Institute for Innovation and Improvement (2010) Sustainability Model. Available at: https://www.england.nhs.uk/wp-content/uploads/2021/03/qsir-sustainability-model.pdf (accessed 10 September 2023).

Further reading

Horton, T. and Illingworth, J. (2018). *The spread challenge.* Available at: https://www.health.org.uk/publications/the-spread-challenge (accessed 10 September 2023).

References

Chambers, D.A., Glasgow, R.E., and Stange, K.C. (2013). The dynamic sustainability framework: addressing the paradox of sustainment amid ongoing change. *Implementation Science*, 8(1), pp. 117–127. doi: 10.1186/1748-5908-8-117.

Rabin, B.A., Brownson, R.C., Haire-Joshu, D., Kreuter, M.W., and Weaver, N.L. (2008). A glossary for dissemination and implementation research in health. *Journal of Public Health Management and Practice*, 14(2), pp. 117–23. doi: 10.1097/01.phh.0000311888.06252.bb.

Continuous Improvement

Continuous improvement

'In healthcare everyone has two jobs: to do your work and to improve it.'

Paul Batalden

In this chapter, we have synthesized the theories and methods discussed in previous chapters into a plan of action. The aim is for you to be a constant continual improver by asking the five questions contained in the Quintuple Aim discussed in ⮕ Chapter 1, with the addition of sustainable quality improvement (Box 18.9).

Box 18.9 The aims of quality improvement

- How can we make the processes of care better to improve the outcomes of care?
- How can we improve the experience of people receiving care?
- How can we improve the experience of the people delivering care?
- How can we ensure that the care we deliver is equitable?
- How can we achieve this at a lower cost?
- How can we improve the impact of healthcare on the environment?

To achieve these objectives in our quest for continual improvement, we need a theory, a method, and measurement of what we do.

1. Identify the problem to improve, what is important, and why.
2. Engage the people involved—staff and patients.
3. Use methods such as Systems Engineering Initiative for Patient Safety (SEIPS) and the microsystem to assess the system.
4. Map the current process, and plan the future one.
5. Analyse the process with the 5 Whys, fishbone, and Pareto to identify areas for improvement.
6. Develop a SMART aim and hypothesis for change—the driver diagram.
7. Use the Model for Improvement, or 5S or Define, Measure, Analyse, Improve, and Control (DMAIC), to test change ideas with PDSAs.
8. Measure the process and outcomes, and illustrate with a run chart, an SPC chart, or a safety cross.
9. Build in sustainability from the start.
10. Learn and adapt as you learn.

Top tips

Many improvement projects suffer from a lack of preparation and poor methodology. For your project to be successful:
- Engage staff and patients, and harvest ideas;
- Study the process for the problem;
- Develop a SMART aim with the team;
- Develop a hypothesis for change—the theory of what has to be done to achieve improvement;
- Separate tasks from tests;
- Start small with one patient, one healthcare worker, and one intervention;
- Be rigorous in the measurement of PDSAs;
- Have a good family of measures.

Summary

- Quality improvement is dependent on having a strong theoretical background and a rigorous methodology. Without these, the spread of a successful intervention will not be possible, as the theory of change will not have been tested and there will be no fidelity.
- Careful planning and then deciding on which method to follow are essential.
- Measurement is important, and must be feasible and relevant.
- Implementation is dependent on the context, readiness for change, and the people involved.
- Patients and families should always be part of the improvement process.

Acknowledgements

Thank you to London School of Paediatrics doctors in training Dr Melody Bacon and Dr Segn Nedd for use of their quality improvement project examples, supported by © Quality Improvement Clinic Ltd. 2022. Reproduced with permission.

Quality improvement, research, ethics, and publishing

Key points
- Quality improvement (QI) and research have many features in common.
- It is important to identify whether your project is research or not.
- If the project is considered as research, then it must comply with the requirements of your local ethics committee.
- If it is a QI project, then ethical considerations must be made even if it does not require formal ethics committee approval.
- Research on QI is essential to demonstrate it works.
- Data protection guidance and law must be adhered to, regardless of whether a project is considered QI or research.
- Publication of QI projects and programmes is important to build the evidence base for QI.
- The SQUIRE 2.0 guidelines provide the framework for publication.

Research and quality improvement

Deciding whether project is quality improvement or research

It is important to determine whether your quality improvement (QI) project is research or not, as this will determine whether you require approval from an ethics committee. This is essential for the governance of your project, and to protect you as well as the patients or staff involved in the project. In Table 19.1, research and QI are compared.

Table 19.1 Comparison between research and quality improvement

	Research	Quality improvement
Definition	Research is designed and conducted to generate new generalizable or transferable knowledge (Health Research Board, Ireland)	QI uses existing knowledge to improve health outcomes Lynn et al. (2007) defined QI as 'systematic, data-guided activities designed to bring about immediate improvements in health care delivery in particular settings'
What it is not	Service evaluation Clinical audit Review of existing evidence	Determining new interventions Invasive procedures Testing new treatments
Types of studies	It includes both quantitative and qualitative studies that aim to generate new hypotheses, as well as studies that aim to test existing or new hypotheses Working with human tissue	Implementation of patient safety interventions that have been proven to work Use of PDSA cycles within MFI, Lean, Six Sigma, and co-production methods
Design	Hypothesis set and then study design decided and does not change	Hypothesis set and expected to change iteratively as ideas are tested and implemented
Knowledge management	Seeking to establish new knowledge above that of routine care, based on current knowledge	Learning about implementation in different contexts is the foundation of QI
Subjects	Depending on research-defined subjects; in an RCT, two controlled groups	Subjects could be everyone who fit the criteria for the intervention without exclusion
Management of risk	Research has inherent risk that is managed with consent	Patients should not be placed at risk
Hypothesis	To be proven or not	Constantly testing
Data	p-values, confidence intervals	Run charts and SPC charts
Scope	To answer a research question	To improve care

Table 19.1 (Contd.)

	Research	Quality improvement
Ethics approval	Always required	May be required

MFI, Model for Improvement; PDSA, Plan–Do–Study–Act; QI, quality improvement; RCT, randomized controlled trial; SPC, statistical process control.

Based on links listed under ➔ Signposting, p. 436.

Criteria for a project being a research project

Casarett et al. (2000) proposed the following criteria that will make any project research rather than QI:

- Your project aims to ascertain fundamental new knowledge on something not previously studied.
- There is randomization, with one group receiving the intervention and one group not.
- You have a fixed hypothesis to be tested with a fixed protocol.
- Caregivers are blinded to the intervention.
- You are evaluating a new drug or clinical device.
- The intervention is an untested clinical intervention.
- Any additional intervention to a patient that they would not have received otherwise (e.g. venepuncture, radiology, etc.).
- The project has external funding from a research body.
- You are interviewing people and their well-being, and identity or anonymity needs to be protected.

Difference between quality improvement and evaluation of quality improvement

It may be useful to separate the quality intervention from the research evaluation of the intervention's processes and enablers. Much of what is published in the quality and patient safety literature are research evaluations of QI programmes or the processes of QI, such as development of measures or social engagement strategies (Figure 19.1).

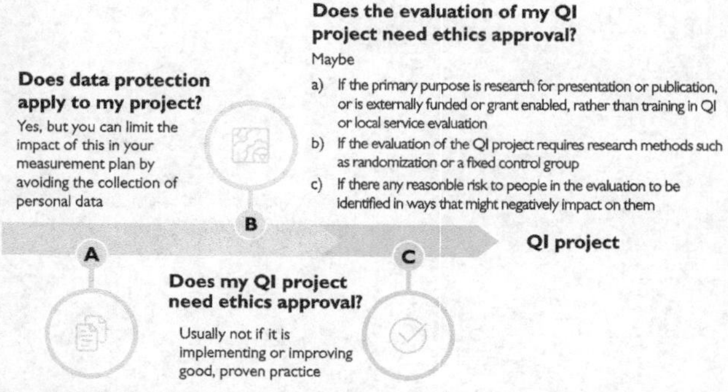

Does the evaluation of my QI project need ethics approval?

Maybe

a) If the primary purpose is research for presentation or publication, or is externally funded or grant enabled, rather than training in QI or local service evaluation

b) If the evaluation of the QI project requires research methods such as randomization or a fixed control group

c) If there any reasonable risk to people in the evaluation to be identified in ways that might negatively impact on them

Does data protection apply to my project?

Yes, but you can limit the impact of this in your measurement plan by avoiding the collection of personal data

Does my QI project need ethics approval?

Usually not if it is implementing or improving good, proven practice

QI project

Figure 19.1 Considerations for data protection, ethics, and research classification when doing quality improvement.

In these research settings, it is usually healthcare staff or systems that are being examined, rather than patients, as they deliver clinically validated interventions.

Signposting

UK Medical Research Council. (2023) Decision Tree tool – Is my study research? Available at http://www.hra-decisiontools.org.uk/research/index.html (accessed 10 September 2023).

Further reading

Al-Surimi, K. (2018). Research versus quality improvement in healthcare. *Global Journal on Quality and Safety in Healthcare*, 1, pp. 25–7.

Backhouse, A. and Ogunlayi, F. (2020). Quality improvement into practice. *BMJ*, 368(1), p. m865. doi: 10.1136/bmj.m865.

Kline, J.N. and Payne, A.S. (2020). Improvement science is a partner in basic and clinical research. *Journal of Investigative Medicine*, 68(3), pp. 724–7. doi: 10.1136/jim-2019-001260.

Mormer, E. and Stevans, J. (2019). Clinical quality improvement and quality improvement research. *Perspectives of the ASHA Special Interest Groups*, 4(1), pp. 27–37. doi: 10.1044/2018_pers-st-2018-0003.

References

Casarett, D., Karlawish, J.H.T., and Sugarman, J. (2000). Determining when quality improvement initiatives should be considered research. *JAMA*, 283(17), p. 2275. doi: 10.1001/jama.283.17.2275.

Ireland Health Research Board. (2023) Is my project research evaluation or audit? Available at https://www.hrb.ie/funding/gdpr-guidance-for-researchers/gdpr-and-health-research/what-is-research/ (accessed 10 September 2023).

Lynn, J. (2004). When does quality improvement count as research? Human subject protection and theories of knowledge. *Quality and Safety in Health Care*, 13(1), pp. 67–70. doi: 10.1136/qshc.2002.002436.

Data protection and quality improvement

Data protection and quality improvement

Regardless of whether you are conducting research or QI, or whatever your intentions for publication may be, you must comply with local data protection law and guidance (such as the European Union (EU) or UK General Data Protection Regulation (GDPR)).

This applies to personal data gathered on any individual, including patients, families, and staff. There are several principles which help to reduce issues with data protection for QI:

- Avoid collecting personal data, unless it is essential. Most data for improvement are focused on process or outcome measures which do not require personal information on individuals.
- Anonymize qualitative data at the time of collection or when sharing, so that there are no personal features (name, age, location) that would make the person identifiable. Pseudonymization involves the use of a substitute identifier such as a number or an alternative name. If data exist which may be able to 'unblind' these actions, then it is subject to data protection rules.
- Aggregate data in such a way as to ensure individuals cannot be identified. For example, if presenting falls data, this may involve combining features such as age into ranges (75–80 years) or locations ('hospital' or 'nursing home').

If appropriate, appoint a gatekeeper who will be the only person who has access to personal identifiable data. In some jurisdictions (e.g. the EU), the designation of data roles and responsibilities (processor, controller) are mandated by law (e.g. GDPR).

Signposting

Information Commissioner's Office (2022). *Guide to the General Data Protection Regulation (GDPR)*. Available at: ℘ https://ico.org.uk/for-organisations/guide-to-data-protection/guide-to-the-general-data-protection-regulation-gdpr/ (accessed 10 September 2023).

Intersoft Consulting (2013). *General Data Protection Regulation (GDPR)*. Available at: ℘ https://gdpr-info.eu (accessed 10 September 2023).

Ethics of quality improvement

Ethics of quality improvement

Defining ethics

There are four principles of medical ethics to consider when undertaking an assessment (Varkey, 2021) (Table 19.2).

Table 19.2 Principles in ethics

Principle	Definition
Beneficence	In healthcare, we are obliged to act in the best interests of patients, including preventing harm and supporting those who have special needs or disabilities and those who are at risk of any untoward event.
Non-maleficence	This principle is the obligation not to cause harm from the proposed intervention, with the need to consider the risks and benefits of the treatment and to advise on the one that causes the least harm and the most benefit.
Autonomy	This principle assumes that patients as people have the freedom to make their own decisions within the limits of accepted medical practice. This can be overridden if there is an urgent clinical need or if the person is not capable of making a decision. The principle is in keeping with principles of person-centred care, although clinical indication and patient choice need to be balanced.
Justice	Justice is about equity in healthcare and everyone having an equal opportunity for the best-quality care possible. This is managing resources, conflicts of interests, beliefs, and attitudes. In quality improvement, the domain of equity focuses on this principle. In addition, it should ensure that people are treated fairly and the burden of experimentation is not only on the disadvantaged, but also on all.

These principles are applied to our day-to-day clinical work, research, and QI. They are sometimes at odds with each other, and it is good practice to constantly ask whether care provided is ethical, and for a QI project, it could be:

- Benefit for all;
- Causing no harm;
- Equitable impact; and
- Co-produced with people.

What are the ethical issues in quality improvement?

The ethical challenges of QI have not been explored in detail in the past. Questions of ethics were usually based on deciding whether or not the planned project constituted research or not, as discussed above. However,

QI has its own ethical considerations and these need to be considered in your project. Hunt et al. (2021) summarized the key issues to be addressed, as follows:

- Have patients and families been engaged and informed? Are the aims of the project clear to them and is there a need for informed consent?
- If there are qualitative data to be collected, has this been in a way that protects the participants?
- Have staff been engaged, and will they have time, training, and support for the project?
- Is there any potential for physical or psychological harm?

Mitchell et al. (2021) have raised the ethics of routinely measuring without ensuring that there will be improvement following the measurement. They question whether routine collection of data is ethically justified if there is no improvement.

Why is ethics in quality improvement important?

Essential to QI is an understanding of what quality means from the viewpoint of all people in the process (i.e. the *lived human experience*) (see ⊙ Chapter 8). The perspectives will allow you to assess the trade-offs made when deciding on what to improve.

- QI is about changing important features such as care or human (patient and staff) lived experience or treatment outcomes. This means that decisions regarding quality interventions are serious and need to be respected.
- Resources for QI efforts that could be used to directly change experience or provide care must be justified and accountable by results.
- There must be a tolerance of learning when people and organizations engage in QI. The safe acceptance of failure is a key feature of QI learning. Appropriate mentoring and coaching support must be provided to ensure successful learning, as well as implementation.
- This 'seriousness and respect' could be addressed through good engagement (co-creation) with staff and patients under an ethical framework.

Fiscella et al. (2015) argued the distinction between *QI* and *QI research* is not distinct, especially if one considers the internal validity of the outcome (i.e. if the findings are invalid or the intervention did not succeed and resources were wasted). Generalizability is present in both. A challenge is that the traditional ethics committees do not understand the QI methodology and often assess the projects on the basis of biomedical research with a fixed hypothesis and protocol.

Cribbs et al. (2020) argued that even if QI is different from research, it still has ethical considerations that we need to consider. QI is a complex endeavour, which mainly involves changing the way in which people interact within a complex system.

Ethical issues to be considered are summarized in Table 19.3.

Table 19.3 Ethical issues

Criteria	Issues to be addressed
Priority	• Deciding which programme to undertake; for example, should one prioritize a programme that brings greater efficiency over a programme that brings greater safety?
	• Determining how to allocate resources
	• If one knows whether an intervention works (e.g. a safety bundle assessing whether one is obliged to implement it above other interventions)
Effectiveness	• Ethical considerations on staff who do not implement the programme that one knows will work
Risk	• If there is any risk involved, should one undertake the intervention?
Human centredness	• Deciding how to define effectiveness and person-centred care
	• Asking whether patients always have to be co-producers of the QI project
	• Consideration of the ethical aspects in reporting the outcomes
	• Acknowledgement of the difficulty to measure patient experience
	• Balancing what matters to people with what can be provided

How do you manage the ethical issues?

As you start your project, you can follow the three steps in Figure 19.2, which will help you decide whether you need to seek ethics approval and to be prepared for submission.

- When you start a QI project, use the guidance given to assess whether it is research or QI.
- If the project is research, then submit the protocol to the local ethics committee for approval.
- If it is QI, continue to assess the ethical aspects of the project and how you will deal with them.
- If you are planning to publish, then consider the requirements of the chosen journal, as some will request ethics approval or a statement of how you assessed the ethical issues.
- Ask the local ethics committees to learn about QI and deepen their understanding of what their role is in enabling good QI work and research.

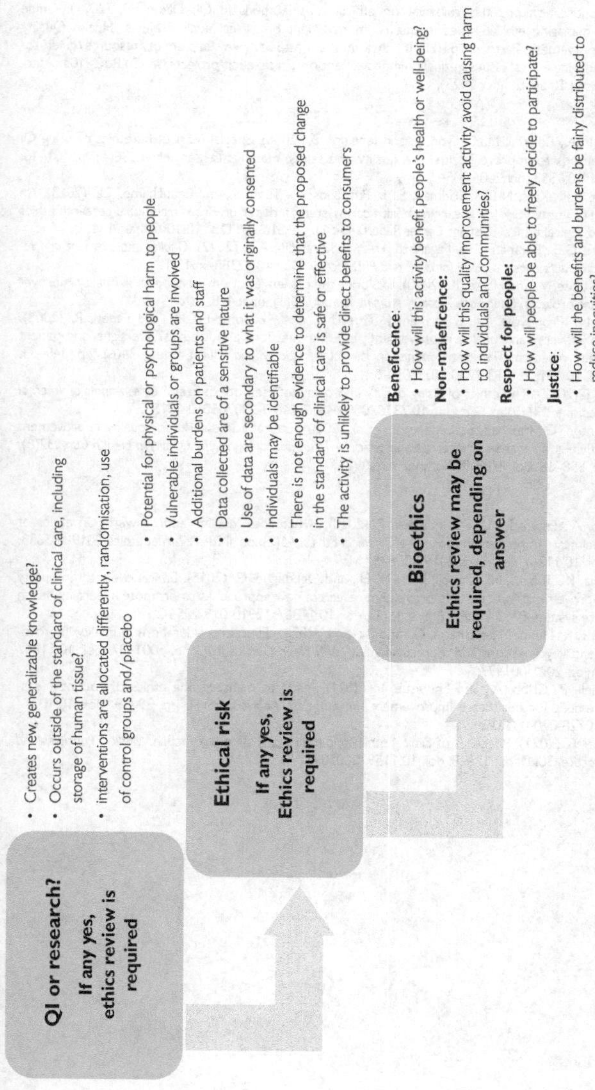

QI or research?
If any yes,
ethics review is
required

- Creates new, generalizable knowledge?
- Occurs outside of the standard of clinical care, including storage of human tissue?
- interventions are allocated differently, randomisation, use of control groups and/placebo

Ethical risk
If any yes,
Ethics review is
required

- Potential for physical or psychological harm to people
- Vulnerable individuals or groups are involved
- Additional burdens on patients and staff
- Data collected are of a sensitive nature
- Use of data are secondary to what it was originally consented
- Individuals may be identifiable
- There is not enough evidence to determine that the proposed change in the standard of clinical care is safe or effective
- The activity is unlikely to provide direct benefits to consumers

Bioethics
Ethics review may be
required, depending on
answer

Beneficence:
- How will this activity benefit people's health or well-being?

Non-maleficence:
- How will this quality improvement activity avoid causing harm to individuals and communities?

Respect for people:
- How will people be able to freely decide to participate?

Justice:
- How will the benefits and burdens be fairly distributed to reduce inequities?

Figure 19.2 Steps to decide whether you need ethics approval.

Signposting

This publication provides guidance on ethical considerations in QI: Dixon, N. (2021). Guide to managing ethical issues in quality improvement or clinical audit projects. Health Quality Improvement Partnership (HQIP) Available at: https://www.hqip.org.uk/resource/guide-to-managing-ethical-issues-in-quality-improvement-or-clinical-audit-projects/#.Y3YRdC-l10s (accessed 10 September 2023).

Further reading

Baily, M.A., Bottrell, M.M., Lynn, J., and Jennings, B. (2006). Special report: the ethics of using QI methods to improve health care quality and safety. *Hastings Center Report*, 36(4), pp. S1–40. doi: 10.1353/hcr.2006.0054.

Faden, R.R., Kass, N.E., Goodman, S.N., Pronovost, P., Tunis, S., and Beauchamp, T.L. (2013). An ethics framework for a learning health care system: a departure from traditional research ethics and clinical ethics. *Hastings Center Report*, 43(S1), pp. S16–27. Doi: 10.1002/hast.134.

Gilbert, G.E., Bauman, E.B., Paganotti, L.A., and Franklin, A.E. (2022). *Quality improvement and research differences: a guide for DNP and PhD faculty*. Doi: 10.32388/xp13f1.

Hall, S., Lee, V., and Haase, K. (2020). Exploring the challenges of ethical conduct in quality improvement projects. *Canadian Oncology Nursing Journal*, 30(1), pp. 64–8.

Kass, N., Pronovost, P.J., Sugarman, J., Goeschel, C.A., Lubomski, L.H., and Faden, R. (2008). Controversy and quality improvement: lingering questions about ethics, oversight, and patient safety research. *The Joint Commission Journal on Quality and Patient Safety*, 34(6), pp. 349–53. doi: 10.1016/s1553-7250(08)34044-6.

Lynn, J. (2007). The ethics of using quality improvement methods in health care. *Annals of Internal Medicine*, 146(9), p. 666. doi: 10.7326/0003-4819-146-9-200705010-00155.

Naughton, C., Meehan, E., Lehane, E., et al. (2020). Ethical frameworks for quality improvement activities: an analysis of international practice. *International Journal for Quality in Health Care*, 32(8), pp. 558–66. doi: 10.1093/intqhc/mzaa092.

References

Cribb, A., Entwistle, V., and Mitchell, P. (2020). What does 'quality' add? Towards an ethics of healthcare improvement. *Journal of Medical Ethics*, 46(2), pp. 118–122. medethics-2019-105635. doi: 10.1136/medethics-2019-105635.

Fiscella, K., Tobin, J.N., Carroll, J.K., He, H., and Ogedegbe, G. (2015). Ethical oversight in quality improvement and quality improvement research: new approaches to promote a learning health care system. *BMC Medical Ethics*, 16(1). doi: 10.1186/s12910-015-0056-2.

Hunt, D.F., Dunn, M., Harrison, G., and Bailey, J. (2021). Ethical considerations in quality improvement: key questions and a practical guide. *BMJ Open Quality*, 10(3), p. e001497. doi: 10.1136/bmjoq-2021-001497.

Mitchell, P., Cribb, A., and Entwistle, V. (2021). Made to measure: the ethics of routine measurement for healthcare improvement. *Health Care Analysis*, 29(1), pp. 39–58. doi: 10.1007/s10728-020-00421-x.

Varkey, B. (2021). Principles of clinical ethics and their application to practice. *Medical Principles and Practice*, 30(1), pp. 17–28. doi: 10.1159/000509119.

Publishing quality improvement

Publishing quality improvement

Why should we publish quality improvement?

As noted in → Chapter 1, one of the main issues facing QI is the lack of published evidence showing that QI actually works. While there has been an increase in the volume of QI publications, there remains an issue with the quality of published papers. Knudsen et al. (2019) reviewed the quality of the published work and concluded that 'even though a majority of the QI projects reported improvements, the widespread challenges with low adherence to key methodological features in the individual projects pose a challenge for the legitimacy of PDSA-based QI. This review indicates that there is a continued need for improvement in quality improvement methodology.'

It is often difficulty to attribute the outcome of the intervention to the improvement initiative and therefore it can be difficulty to apply to other settings. Dixon-Woods (2019) has called for more research on QI, stating: 'without sound evaluation, patients may be deprived of benefit, resources and energy may be wasted on ineffective QI interventions or on interventions that distribute risks unfairly, and organisations are left unable to make good decisions about trade-offs given their many competing priorities.'

A major problem has been the lack of robustness in the application of the PDSA methodology. Either this is not reported or it is reported inconsistently, so that papers cannot be compared, nor the fidelity of the intervention assured (McNicholas et al., 2019). Therefore, it is important to publish QI, and this will require the same type of rigour as you would have in publishing a research paper. We encourage you to include publication as part of your QI journey and to plan to publish from the outset.

Principles to apply when publishing

Several principles should be considered:
- It is important that you consider the impact of the context on the project and describe the context in detail.
- If readers want to implement a similar programme, discussion on the context will aid them to see what is required for successful implementation.
- A clear theory of change is essential.
- A coherent implementation strategy must be described.
- The PDSA methodology must be rigorous and well explained.
- Measurement should include processes and outcomes, and measurement over time (annotated run charts and statistical process control (SPC) charts) should be used.
- Data with a story will be more powerful than data alone.

Format for publishing

QI publications should be structured using the SQUIRE 2.0 guidelines, which mirror a project charter. The guidelines have been developed to ensure that QI reports follow a defined format, and they are summarized in Table 19.4.

Table 19.4 Summary of publication requirements

	Question	Details
Introduction	Overview	Provide the context for the project, as this will provide the reader with a wider understanding of the project
Rationale	Why did you undertake the project?	• What is the problem? • Why is it a problem? • What is known about solutions? • Baseline data to demonstrate the problem • Assessment and analysis of the process • Aim statement for the project • Hypothesis for change in a driver diagram • Proposed intervention and evidence
Method	How did you do the project?	• Who is involved? • Measurement strategy? • Tasks undertaken • Tests of change • Analysis • Plans for sustaining the gains
Results	Results: what did you achieve?	• Report on what happened • Explain tests of change (PDSA) to ensure rigour and fidelity (often a weakness in QI reports) • Report on what happened and the story of the improvement • Measures in run charts or SPC charts for outcome, process, balancing, cost effectiveness and benefit, equity, and sustainable QI—both quantitative and, if appropriate, qualitative
Learning	What did you learn?	• Limitations of the project • Reflections on your learning • Lessons for others • Transferable learning • Conclusions

Signposting

SQUIRE 2.0. (2016) SQUIRE Guideline. Available at: https://www.squire-statement.org/ (accessed 10 September 2023).

Further reading

Budrionis, A. and Bellika, J.G. (2016). The learning healthcare system: where are we now? A systematic review. *Journal of Biomedical Informatics*, 64, pp. 87–92. doi: 10.1016/j.jbi.2016.09.018.

Franklin, B.D. and Thomas, E.J. (2022). Replicating and publishing research in different countries and different settings: advice for authors. *BMJ Quality and Safety*, 31(9), pp. 627–30. bmjqs-2021-014431. doi: https://doi.org/10.1136/bmjqs-2021-014431.

Kaplan, H.C., Brady, P.W., Dritz, M.C., et al. (2010). The influence of context on quality improvement success in health care: a systematic review of the literature. *Milbank Quarterly*, 88(4), pp. 500–59. doi: 10.1111/j.1468-0009.2010.00611.x.

Ogrinc, G. (2021). Measuring and publishing quality improvement. *Regional Anesthesia and Pain Medicine*, 46(8), pp. 643–9. rapm-2020-102201. doi: 10.1136/rapm-2020-102201.

Ogrinc, G., Davies, L., Goodman, D., Batalden, P., Davidoff, F., and Stevens, D. (2016). SQUIRE 2.0 (Standards for QUality Improvement Reporting Excellence): revised publication guidelines from a detailed consensus process. *BMJ Quality & Safety*, 25(12), pp. 986–92. https://doi.org/10.1136/bmjqs-2015-004411

Pearlman, S.A. and Swanson, J.R. (2021). A practical guide to publishing a quality improvement paper. *Journal of Perinatology*. 41(6), pp. 1454–8 doi: 10.1038/s41372-020-00902-w.

Reed, J.E. and Card, A.J. (2016). The problem with Plan–Do–Study–Act cycles. *BMJ Quality and Safety*, 25(3), pp. 147–52. doi: 10.1136/bmjqs-2015-005076.

Schondelmeyer, A.C., Brower, L.H., Statile, A.M., White, C.M., and Brady, P.W. (2017). Quality improvement feature series article 3: writing and reviewing quality improvement manuscripts. *Journal of the Pediatric Infectious Diseases Society*, 7(3), pp. 188–90. doi: 10.1093/jpids/pix078.

Wong, B.M. and Sullivan, G.M. (2016). How to write up your quality improvement initiatives for publication. *Journal of Graduate Medical Education*, 8(2), pp. 128–33. doi: 10.4300/jgme-d-16-00086.1.

References

Dixon-Woods, M. (2019). How to improve healthcare improvement—an essay by Mary Dixon-Woods. *BMJ*, 367, pp. l5514–17. doi: 10.1136/bmj.l5514.

Knudsen, S.V., Laursen, H.V.B., Johnsen, S.P., Bartels, P.D., Ehlers, L.H., and Mainz, J. (2019). Can quality improvement improve the quality of care? A systematic review of reported effects and methodological rigor in plan-do-study-act projects. *BMC Health Services Research*, 19(1), pp. 683–95. doi: 10.1186/s12913-019-4482-6.

McNicholas, C., Lennox, L., Woodcock, T., Bell, D., and Reed, J.E. (2019). Evolving quality improvement support strategies to improve Plan–Do–Study–Act cycle fidelity: a retrospective mixed-methods study. *BMJ Quality and Safety*, 28(5), pp. 356–65. doi: 10.1136/bmjqs-2017-007605.

Journals for publishing quality improvement

There are several options for publication. The choice of journal depends on the purpose for the publication.
- Decide who the target audience is. If you want to influence colleagues in your clinical specialty, it may be the journal of that subspecialty, or you may wish to publish in a specific QI or patient safety journal.
- Once the audience has been decided, then target your message to that audience and context.

The selected journals shown in Table 19.5 are mainly the ones that focus on QI and patient safety. General journals, such as *BMJ*, *New England Journal of Medicine*, and *JAMA*, publish papers on QI and patient safety, as do most specialty journals. Many of the journals have a specific QI section and an editorial process.

Table 19.5 Selected journals to consider

Journal*	Focus
BMC Health Services Research https://bmchealthservres.biomedcentral.com	BMC Health Services Research is an open-access, peer-reviewed journal that considers articles on all aspects of health services research. The journal has a special focus on digital health, governance, health policy, health system quality and safety, healthcare delivery and access to healthcare, healthcare financing and economics, implementing reform, and the health workforce.
BMJ Open Quality http://quality.bmj.com/	BMJ Open Quality is an online workspace that supports individuals and teams to work through quality improvement ideas, make an intervention, and publish their results while developing their knowledge and skills.
BMJ Quality and Safety https://qualitysafety.bmj.com/	BMJ Quality and Safety (previously Quality and Safety in Health Care) is an international peer-reviewed publication providing research, opinions, debates, and reviews for academics, clinicians, and healthcare managers, focused on the quality and safety of healthcare and the science of improvement.
Implementation Science https://implementationscience.biomedcentral.com/	Implementation Science is an open-access, peer-reviewed online journal that aims to publish research relevant to the scientific study of methods to promote the uptake of research findings into routine healthcare in clinical, organizational, or policy contexts.

Table 19.5 (Contd.)

Journal*	Focus
Implementation Science Communications https://implementationsciencecomms.biomedcentral.com/	*Implementation Science Communications*, an official companion journal to *Implementation Science*, is a forum to publish research relevant to the systematic study of approaches to foster uptake of evidence-based practices and policies that affect healthcare delivery and health outcomes in clinical, organizational, or policy contexts.
International Journal for Quality in Health Care https://academic.oup.com/intqhc	The *International Journal for Quality in Health Care* (*IJQHC*) is a leading international peer-reviewed scholarly journal addressing research, policy, and implementation related to the quality of healthcare and health outcomes to populations and patients worldwide.
IJQHC Communications https://academic.oup.com/ijcoms	*IJQHC Communications* publishes papers in all disciplines related to the quality and safety of healthcare, including health services research, healthcare evaluation, technology assessment, health economics, utilization review, cost containment, and nursing care research, as well as protocols and clinical research related to the quality of care.
The Joint Commission Journal on Quality and Patient Safety https://www.jointcommissionjournal.com/	*The Joint Commission Journal on Quality and Patient Safety* is a peer-reviewed publication dedicated to providing health professionals with new ideas and information to improve the quality and safety of healthcare. The journal invites manuscripts on development, adaptation, and implementation of innovative concepts, strategies, methodologies, and practices in quality and patient safety.
Journal for Healthcare Quality (JHQ) https://journals.lww.com/jhqonline/pages/default.aspx	The *Journal for Healthcare Quality* (*JHQ*), a peer-reviewed journal, is an official publication of the National Association for Healthcare Quality. *JHQ* is a professional forum that continuously advances healthcare quality practice in diverse and changing environments and is the first choice for creative and scientific solutions in the pursuit of healthcare quality.

(Continued)

Table 19.5 (*Contd.*)

Journal*	Focus
Journal of Patient Safety https://journals.lww.com/journalpatientsafety/pages/default.aspx	The *Journal of Patient Safety* is dedicated to presenting research advances and field applications in every area of patient safety. While the journal has a research emphasis, it also publishes articles describing near-miss opportunities, system modifications that are barriers to error, and the impact of regulatory changes on healthcare delivery.
Journal of Patient Safety and Risk Management https://journals.sagepub.com/home/cri	The *Journal of Patient Safety and Risk Management* considers patient safety and risk at all levels of the healthcare system, from patients to practitioners, managers, organizations, and policymakers. It publishes peer-reviewed research papers, reviews, and commentaries on patient safety and medico-legal issues.
NEJM Catalyst https://catalyst.nejm.org/	*NEJM Catalyst* brings healthcare executives, clinical leaders, and clinicians together to share innovative ideas and practical applications for enhancing the value of healthcare delivery. From a network of top thought leaders, experts, and advisors, the digital, peer-reviewed journal, live-streamed events, and qualified Insights Council provide real-life examples and actionable solutions to help organizations address urgent challenges affecting healthcare.

* All websites accessed on 10 September 2023.

Summary

Top tips

- Make an assessment of whether your project is research or not.
- Undertake an evaluation of the ethical issues to be considered in your project.
- If it is research, consult the ethics committee.
- Plan the publication of your project as part of your project charter.
- Use the SQUIRE 2.0 guidelines as the template for your charter.

Summary

As QI and patient safety initiatives have spread and developed over the past 20 years, the ethical considerations have become more apparent.

While most projects will not require ethical approval, it is important to assess the ethical issues that may arise.

Publication is important and should be part of the planning process from the start. Publications can be in specialty journals, general journals, or journals focusing on QI and patient safety.

Resource Hyperlinks

BMJ QI series

The series provides papers from leading thinkers and researchers on quality improvement.
BMJ Series on Quality Improvement https://www.bmj.com/quality-improvement

AURUM Institute

This guide is an easy-to-use version of the *Improvement Guide*.
Guide to Quality Improvement (free) https://online.fliphtml5.com/hgjjt/nchh/#p=1
The following health service improvement departments have many useful resources.

NHS England resources

NHS England Impact https://www.england.nhs.uk/nhsimpact/
East London NHS Trust QI https://qi.elft.nhs.uk/
NHS Improvement Hub https://www.england.nhs.uk/improvement-hub/

NHS Scotland resources

Healthcare Improvement Scotland http://www.healthcareimprovementscotland.org/
Knowledge Network Scotland Human Factors https://www.knowledge.scot.nhs.uk/hfe.aspx

Ireland Health Service Executive (HSE) resources

The toolkit provides easy-to-use references on quality improvement.
https:// www.hse.ie/eng/about/who/nqpsd/qps-education/qualityimprovem enttool kit. html

World Health Organisation

Quality Toolkit 2022
https://qualityhealthservices.who.int/quality-toolkit/qt-home
WHO Global Learning Laboratory
https://www.who.int/initiatives/who-global-learning-laboratory-for-quality-uhc

Microsystems theory

In ◉ Chapter 12, the microsystem theory was introduced. There are several good websites to explore this methodology.

Dartmouth Institute for Excellence in Health and Social Systems https://
clinicalmicrosystem.org
Sheffield Microsystems Coaching Academy https://www.sheffieldmca.
org.uk/

Learning Health Systems

This resource is about bringing systems together for improvement.
Free Systems Convening Book https://www.wenger-trayner.com/
systems-convening-book/
This reference is about how to develop a learning health system which
aims to continually learn and improve.
Learning Health Systems https://learninghealthcareproject.org.

Person-centred care

Several websites provide information on the philosophy, theory, and
practice of person-centred care.
Beryl Institute https://www.theberylinstitute.org/
Institute for Patient and Family Centred Care https://www.ipfcc.org/
International Consortium for Healthcare Outcome Measures https://
www.ichom.org/
International Alliance of Patients' Organizations: (IAPO) https://www.
iapo.org.uk/
Picker Institute https://www.picker.org/
Planetree International https://www.planetree.org/
Point of Care Foundation https://www.pointofcarefoundation.org.uk
World Patient Alliance https://www.worldpatientsalliance.org/

Quality improvement organizations

IFIC- Integrated Care Foundation https://integratedcarefoundation.org
International Society for Quality in Healthcare https://www.isqua.org/

Clinical Excellence Commission NSW https://www.cec.health.nsw.gov.
   au/CEC-Academy/quality-improvement-tools

Healthcare Excellence Canada https://www.healthcareexcellence.ca/

Health Foundation https://www.health.org.uk/
Kings Fund https://www.kingsfund.org.uk/
Q Community https://q.health.org.uk/

Agency for Healthcare Research & Quality https://www.ahrq.gov/pati
   ent-safety/index.html
Institute for Healthcare Improvement www.ihi.org

Glossary of terms

Term	Explanation
Agency	Agency is the ability to choose to act with purpose
Appreciative inquiry	A positive approach that looks for strengths and opportunities in teams and systems to build the opportunity for improvement
Belonging	A concept where a team member has a sense of being an accepted part of a team or organization
Carbon emissions	Often used synonymously with greenhouse gas emissions. The amount of carbon dioxide that is released as a result of an activity
Carbon footprint	The total volume of carbon emission (or greenhouse gas emissions) associated with a group of activities (e.g. over a person's lifetime or during a manufacturing process)
Carbon literate	An awareness of the carbon dioxide costs and impacts of everyday activities and the ability and motivation to reduce emissions
CFIR	Consolidated Framework for Implementation Research: an implementation science framework
Climate resilience	The ability to plan for, respond to, and recover from climate risks
Co-production QI	Working and utilizing the skills of all the healthcare team/professionals to deliver quality improvement
Co-production clinical	Co-production recognizes that optimizing available therapies and techniques with the patient's own goals for their treatment can provide measurable improvement in their care
CT scan	Computed tomography scan: a type of scan that combines X-rays and computers to produce detailed internal images of the body
Cultural competence	An appreciation and understanding of people from diverse cultures and backgrounds and respect for values, beliefs, attitudes, behaviours, and needs that may differ from one's own
Diffusion of innovation	A theory of how change is spread through a system
DMAIC	An improvement method with five steps: Define, Measure, Analyse, Improve, and Control

Term	Explanation
Driver diagram	Provides the hypothesis for change, as well as a schematic overview of the theory of what must be done to achieve the aim of a project
ED	Emergency department, also known as accident and emergency department and as emergency room
EHR	Electronic health record, which is a comprehensive digital tool to integrate the case notes of a patient, including electronic prescribing, computerized order sets for laboratory test ordering, and telehealth capability
EMR	Electronic medical record, which is a digital version of the paper patient medical notes
ERIC	Expert Recommendations for Implementing Change: an implementation science framework
Five (5) Ps	Five characteristics of a microsystem: Purpose, Patients, Professionals, Processes, Patterns
Five (5) Whys	An assessment tool which identifies the root causes of a problem
GDPR	General Data Protection Regulation, defining how data must be protected
Greenhouse gas (GHG)	A gas which traps heat in the atmosphere. Includes gases such as carbon dioxide, methane, water vapour, and nitrous oxide
Greenhouse gas (GHG) emission factor	A coefficient which allows the conversion of an activity into GHG emissions
Haemodialysis	A procedure where a dialysis machine and a special filter are used to clean blood
Health disparities	Preventable differences in health and healthcare experienced by socially disadvantaged groups
Health equity	Every person is given the opportunity to be as healthy as possible by mitigating obstacles that result in health disparities
HFE	Human factors and ergonomics: a unique academic, transdisciplinary subject that brings together knowledge from multiple disciplines, such as psychology, anatomy, and physiology, and organization management in order to design a safe system, taking into account human capabilities and characteristics
Hierarchy of needs	A theory by Maslow that postulates that humans have five levels of needs, ranging from survival and security to love and integration, and from self-esteem to self-actualization
House officer	A term used to describe a doctor in their first year of postgraduate medical training

Term	Explanation
Implicit bias	Subconscious and unintentional biases that influence decision-making, behaviours, and interactions
Integrated care	Partnerships or relationships between organizations/patients/services that come together to plan and deliver joined-up health services, to improve the lives of those who live and work in the area
Ishikawa diagram	'Fishbone' diagram suggesting possible explanations or hypotheses that could explain or contribute to the problem under review
Juran Trilogy	Three interacting components of quality management: planning, control, and improvement
Lean 5S	An improvement method with five steps: Sort, Set in Order, Shine, Standardize, and Sustain
LHS	Learning healthcare systems: defined by the Institute of Medicine (2011) as systems where 'Science, informatics, incentives, and culture are aligned for continuous improvement and innovation, with best practices seamlessly embedded in the delivery process and new knowledge captured as an integral by-product of the delivery experience'
Macrosystem	A higher strategic organization, including all parts of the organization
Mesosystem	A part of the organization that consists of a number of microsystems serving a defined population (e.g. a division in a hospital)
Microsystems	Smaller parts of an organization delivering care or a service (e.g. a clinical team)
NHS	National Health Service: the health delivery service in the United Kingdom
Pareto chart	Organized data in ascending or descending order on a bar chart identifying the top factors relating to a problem, to demonstrate the 80–20 rule—80% of outcomes result from 20% of all causes for a problem
PARIHS	Promoting Action on Research Implementation in Health Services Framework: an implementation science framework
Patient safety	Refers to the prevention of errors and adverse effects to patients associated with healthcare
PDSA cycle	A method to test changes in four steps: Plan–Do–Study–Act
Person-centred care	A model of care that puts the patient at the centre

Term	Explanation
Pollution	The introduction of harmful materials into the environment which can modify natural characteristics, including soil, water, and air pollution
PREM	Patient-reported experience measure: a method to measure patient experience
Pressurized metered-dose inhalers	Inhalers which deliver a measured amount of medication in a burst created by the pressurized propellant in an aerosol chamber
PRO	Patient-reported outcome from the patient's perspective
Process map	Visual representation of individual processes and outcomes making up a system
Profound Knowledge	Developed by Deming to understand improvement (i.e. the four lenses of systems, variation, psychology, and theory of knowledge)
PROM	Patient-reported outcome measure: a measure to report outcomes from the patient's perspective
Psychological safety	The belief that one will not be punished or humiliated for speaking up with ideas, questions, concerns, or mistakes
QI	Quality improvement: a process to improve the quality of care within the domains of quality
Quintuple Aim	Five aims of improving the experience of care, improving the health of populations, improving healthcare workers' experience, ensuring equity of care, and reducing per capita costs of healthcare
RE-AIM	Reach, Efficacy, Adoption, Implementation, and Maintenance: an implementation science framework
Readiness assessment	Assessment of whether a team is ready to undertake an improvement project
Run chart	Graphically represents data trends over time
Safety cross	A graphic demonstration of an event each day
Scale-up of a project	Better for complicated problems; is usually top–down, takes place more rapidly, and needs leadership from the top to ensure take-up
Scripts	A shorthand for 'prescriptions'
SEIPS	Systems Engineering Initiative for Patient Safety: a human factors method to assess systems and processes that produce outcomes
Self-actualization	The realization or fulfilment of one's talents and potentialities

Term	Explanation
SMAC	Sequential multi-channel analysis: Blood test taken for a panel of multiple components, including kidney function, glucose, and cholesterol
SMART	Specific, Measurable, Achievable, Relevant, Time-bound: a method to describe the aim of an improvement project
SPC chart	Statistical process control chart: tracks and analyses variation over time with statistical control limits
SPO	The theory proposed by Donabedian that outcomes are determined by the structure of a system and the processes within the system
Spread of a project	Generally built bottom–up at grassroots or frontline level. It will develop over time and usually requires customization to the local context
SQUIRE 2.0	Standards for QUality Improvement Reporting Excellence 2.0: provides a method for writing up quality improvement reports
Stakeholder map	A table that assesses the engagement and influence of key people in a project
Sustainability	The ability to meet the needs of the present without compromising the ability of future generations to meet their own needs
Sustainability of a project	The extent to which an intervention or improvement is sustained over time once funding or the project has ended
Telemedicine	The remote delivery of healthcare using telecommunications technology (e.g. web conferencing)
Triple Aim	Three aims of improving the experience of care, improving the health of populations, and reducing per capita costs of healthcare
Unwarranted variation	Unwarranted clinical variation is variation that cannot be justified by the condition of the person receiving care
Value stream mapping	Visualizes every step or action required to complete a process from start to finish
Virtuous cycle	A series of events in which a positive outcome or experience results in another positive outcome, which, in turn, promotes the next one or enhances the initiating one

Economic terms (in ⮕ Chapter 7)

Partial health economic evaluation	Measures cost and/or health outcomes, but does not have a comparator and does not relate costs to outcomes
Full health economic evaluation	Compares the costs, resource use, and effects of an intervention in comparison to an alternative, and relates the costs to the effects in a summary metric
Unit cost	The cost of one unit of resource use
Opportunity cost	The potential benefit of a foregone alternative
Cost savings	The quantity of resource use and costs (i.e. the value of resource use) saved
Costs avoided	Cost of an event that is avoided
Cost-effectiveness analysis	Analyses the costs of two or more similar initiatives in comparison to their effects by using a context-specific measure
Cost utility analysis	Analyses the costs of two or more initiatives in comparison to their effects, where the measure of effectiveness is in quality-adjusted life years. Identifies 'value for money' across initiatives with different target outcomes
Quality-adjusted life year (QALY)	A composite measure of health-related quality of life and mortality. One QALY denotes a full year with perfect health. Fractions of a QALY denote a year with imperfect health
Incremental cost-effectiveness ratio (ICER)	Estimates the ratio of additional costs to additional outcomes associated with a new intervention in comparison to current practice
Cost-effectiveness (CE) threshold	Refers to the maximum amount a decision-maker is prepared to pay for an additional unit of health effect. Typically defined as a monetary amount per QALY
Net costs	The accumulation of all costs and savings related to an activity, that is, the sum of costs related to the intervention, future cost savings, and avoided costs
Net health effects	The accumulation of all health effects related to an activity, that is, the sum of health effects over time

Acronyms

Acronyms	In full
5Ps	Purpose, Patients, Professionals, Processes, and Patterns
5S	Sort, Set in order, Shine, Standardize, and Sustain
CE	Cost-effectiveness
CEA	Cost-effectiveness analysis
CFIR	Consolidated Framework for Implementation Research
CUA	Cost utility analysis
DMAIC	Define, Measure, Analyse, Improve, and Control
ED	Emergency department
EHR	Electronic health record
EMR	Electronic medical record
ERIC	Expert Recommendations for Implementing Change
GDPR	General Data Protection Regulation
HFE	Human factors and ergonomics
ICER	Incremental cost-effectiveness ratio
LHS	Learning healthcare systems
NHS	National Health Service
PDSA	Plan–Do–Study–Act
PREM	Patient-reported experience measure
PRO	Patient-reported outcome
PROM	Patient-reported outcome measure
QALY	Quality-adjusted life year
QI	Quality improvement
RE-AIM	Reach, Efficacy, Adoption, Implementation, and Maintenance
SEIPS	Systems Engineering Initiative for Patient Safety
SMAC	Sequential Multiple Analyzer Chemistry panel of blood tests
SMART	Specific, Measurable, Achievable, Relevant, Time-bound
SPC	Statistical process control
SPO	Structure–process–outcome
SQUIRE 2.0	Standards for QUality Improvement Reporting Excellence 2.0

Index

For the benefit of digital users, indexed terms that span two pages (e.g., 52–53) may, on occasion, appear on only one of those pages.

Tables, figures, and boxes are indicated by t, f, and b following the page number